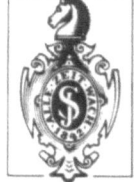

H. W. Sutherland · J. M. Stowers
D. W. M. Pearson (Eds.)

Carbohydrate Metabolism in Pregnancy and the Newborn · IV

With 60 Figures

Springer-Verlag
London Berlin Heidelberg New York
Paris Tokyo

H. W. Sutherland, MBChB, FRCOG
Clinical Reader in Obstetrics and Gynaecology, Aberdeen Maternity Hospital,
Foresterhill, Cornhill Road, Aberdeen, AB9 2ZA, UK

J. M. Stowers, MA, MBChB, MD, FRCP, FRCOG
Emeritus Professor of Dietetics and Endocrinology, University of Aberdeen,
13 Westerton Road, Cults, Aberdeen, AB1 9MR, UK

D. W. M. Pearson, MBChB, MRCP
Consultant Physician, Diabetic Clinic, Woolman Hill, Aberdeen Royal Infirmary,
Aberdeen AB9 2ZB, UK

ISBN-13: 978-1-4471-1682-0   e-ISBN-13: 978-1-4471-1680-6
DOI: 10.1007/978-1-4471-1680-6

British Library Cataloguing in Publication Data
Carbohydrate metabolism in pregnancy and the newborn IV
1. Newborn babies & pregnant women. Carbohydrates. Metabolism   I. Sutherland,
Hamish W. (Hamish Watson), 1933– II. Stower, John M. (John Marcus), 1919–
III. Pearson, D.W.M. (Donald W.M.), 1950–   612′.396

Library of Congress Cataloging-in-Publication Data
Carbohydrate metabolism in pregnancy and the newborn IV/H.W. Sutherland, J.M.
Stowers, D.W.M. Pearson (editors). p. cm.
Based on the Fourth International Colloquium on Carbohydrate Metabolism in
Pregnancy and the Newborn held at the University of Aberdeen, Scotland in 1988.
Includes bibliographies and index.
1. Diabetes in pregnancy—Congresses.   2. Infants (Newborn)—Health and
hygiene—Congresses.   3. Carbohydrates—Metabolism—Disorders—
Congresses.   I. Sutherland, Hamish W.   II. Stowers, John M.   III. Pearson, D.
W. M. (Donald W. M.), 1950–   IV. International Colloquium on
Carbohydrate Metabolism in Pregnancy and the Newborn (4th: 1988: University of
Aberdeen [DNLM: 1. Abnormalities—etiology—congresses.   2. Carbohydrates—
metabolism—congresses.   3. Pregnancy in Diabetes—complications—
congresses.   4. Pregnancy in Diabetes—metabolism—congresses.   WQ 248 C2643
1988] RG580.D5C36 1989 618.3—dc19 DNLM/DLC for Library of
Congress 89-4291 CIP

Softcover reprint of the hardcover 1st edition 1989

Filmset by Wilmaset, Birkenhead, Wirral

2128/3916–543210   Printed on acid-free paper

Foreword

Traditions are dangerous; doubly so in science. Traditions are unchanging; science is about change. This was the 4th International Colloquium on Carbohydrate Metabolism in Pregnancy and the Newborn to be held in Aberdeen, and by now the form is set. How much its content has changed is a matter of nice judgement and not under the control of the organizers. It is not within their power to bring news of revolution, if there has been no revolution. Certainly many of the speakers had kent faces from previous Aberdeen meetings, but so they would be at any meeting on diabetes anywhere in the world.

The written proceedings of scientific conferences have purposes other than to record changes: sometimes they need to state a consensus. The 3rd Colloquium came to an agreement about the importance of prepregnancy recognition and control of abnormalities of carbohydrate metabolism. The 4th set out to examine what results it had achieved. Much of this book is taken up with follow-up studies of the applications of similar regimes in different parts of the world.

Since the first Aberdeen meeting in 1973, progress in the management of diabetic pregnancy has been slow and steady, but the change in the city and the society where the meetings took place has been fast. The foreword to the record of the 2nd Colloquium spoke of the lovely crown tower of the University that has brooded over the six centuries of academic comings and goings. The 3rd had no such tranquillity. It spoke instead of the economic blight that had wilted conferences but stated confidently that the University had survived many crises in its long history and would emerge from this one a bit battered and a good deal slimmer. In the short term, that confidence has been justified. This book proves that we met again, on schedule, 5 years later. If our masters in London mean what they say, the next one is in doubt.

It takes a lot of people to organize a conference and edit a book. It is invidious to select one person and say: "He did it". There may not be another opportunity to record one salient fact about all four of the Aberdeen Colloquia on Carbohydrate Metabolism in Pregnancy and the Newborn. Hamish Sutherland did it.

Aberdeen   Arnold Klopper
November 1988

Preface

This book is based on the concepts discussed, clinical practice described and ideas developed by the experts assembled at the Fourth Quinquennial International Colloquium on Carbohydrate Metabolism in Pregnancy and the Newborn held in the University of Aberdeen, Scotland, in 1988. The programme for the colloquium was planned to cover all aspects of clinical care for women with established diabetes and gestational diabetes mellitus. The aim of providing an up-to-date, comprehensive manual for use in clinical practice prompted the editors to include an additional chapter on obstetric aspects of diabetic pregnancy. We trust that the expertise of all authors will be appreciated by a wide clinical and scientific readership in addition to those physicians, obstetricians and paediatricians directly involved in metabolic and perinatal medicine. The over-riding theme is the importance of integrated care in the management of women with diabetes mellitus and this theme is paralleled by the interdisciplinary research approach. The editors are most grateful to the zeal and scholarship of the contributors and the expedition with which they produced their manuscripts.

Grateful acknowledgement is made to Novo Industries and Nordisk for sponsoring our Scandinavian colleagues and to Eli Lilly for sponsoring our American colleagues. The following companies were also generous to our travel fund: Boehringer, Bayer, Upjohn, Hypoguard, Syntex Pharmaceuticals Limited, Becton Dickinson, Boots & Company PLC, Clydesdale Bank, Rocket of London, Scientific Medical Systems Limited, Picker, R. L. Dolby & Co., Schering, Amex and Vickers Medical. Lipha Pharmaceuticals contributed generously to the preparation of the colour illustrations.

Regrettably, the stimulating discussion following the papers and posters at the colloquium is not included in this volume as we and the publishers were anxious to achieve an early date for publication.

We wish to record our thanks to Michael Jackson of Springer-Verlag for his help and understanding in bringing this to fruition. Lastly, we owe a great debt to the careful work of Mrs. Elaine Stirton and Mrs. Sheila Mearns in the University Department of Obstetrics and Gynaecology who have been tireless in their efforts to translate our concept to the Fourth Colloquium and now to this publication respectively and to Professor Templeton, Regius Professor of Obstetrics and Gynaecology for his enthusiastic support.

Aberdeen   Hamish W. Sutherland
November 1988   John M. Stowers
                                                   Donald W. M. Pearson

Contents

1. The Development of Diabetes and its Relation to Pregnancy: The Long-Term and Short-Term Historical Viewpoint

D. R. Hadden

An important historical discovery was made in 1987. Until then the base reference to diabetes in pregnancy was the review published by Matthews Duncan (1882), which is a compilation of 22 pregnancies in 15 women published up to that date, reviewed at a meeting of the Obstetrical Society of London: the fetus died in at least 13 out of 19 recorded pregnancies in 15 diabetic mothers and the mother herself died of diabetes within a year in nine of these cases. Duncan refers to the earliest case, that of Bennewitz, only in a brief summary translated into English in the *Edinburgh Medical Journal* of 1828.

At the meeting in Berlin in 1987 of the Diabetes Pregnancy Study Group of the European Association for the Study of Diabetes, I referred to this earliest report from Berlin and was very grateful when Dr. Barbara Hillebrand, who was in the audience, was able to obtain (from the library in Munich) a copy of Dr. Bennewitz's original thesis for the degree of doctor of medicine dated 1824. The thesis was in Latin, and has now been translated into English by Dr. A. B. Scott of the Department of Latin, The Queen's University of Belfast.

Heinrich Gottleib Bennewitz publicly defended his thesis at the University of Berlin on 24 June 1824. It is a simple case report and review of the literature on the causes and treatments of diabetes known at that time. It would not be inappropriate to imagine ourselves in Dr. Bennewitz's shoes at this moment and see how well we might defend our own theses on carbohydrate metabolism in pregnancy and the newborn!

He wrote with charm and simplicity and one can warm to him for his honest comments on the lack of understanding of what was happening to his patient, and the Herculean task he had set himself to review all the opinions on diabetes at that time. His Greek derivation of the word *diabetes* and his one-line definition of the symptoms are unchanged today – "urine differing in quality and quantity from the normal . . . accompanied by unquenchable thirst and eventual wasting".

He referred briefly to the thoughts of the ancient Greek physicians: Hippocrates who supposed that there might be ducts between the stomach and the urinary bladder to explain the excessive production of urine. Aretaeus the

DE
DIABETE MELLITO,
GRAVIDITATIS SYMPTOMATE.

DISSERTATIO

INAUGURALIS MEDICA
QUAM
GRATIOSI MEDICORUM ORDINIS
CONSENSU ATQUE AUCTORITATE
IN
UNIVERSITATE LITTERARIA BEROLINENSI
PRO SUMMIS
IN MEDICINA ET CHIRURGIA HONORIBUS
RITE OBTINENDIS
DIE XXIV. M. IUNII A. MDCCCXXIV
H. L. Q. S.
PALAM DEFENDET
AUCTOR
HENR. GOTTL. BENNEWITZ
BEROLINENSIS.

OPPONENTIBUS:
W. DE MOELLER, MED. ET CHIR. DDR.
A. TIETZEL, MED. ET CHIR. DDR.
O. ZIMMERMANN, MED. ET CHIR. DDR.

BEROLINI,
TYPIS IOANNIS FRIDERICI STARCKII.

DIABETES MELLITUS: A SYMPTOM OF PREGNANCY

An inaugural dissertation in medicine in which
its author
Heinrich Gottleib Bennewitz
of Berlin
will defend publicly with the consent and on the authority of the distinguished order of doctors in the University of Letters of Berlin to obtain in due order the highest honours in medicine and surgery, on the 24th day of the month of June in the year 1824.

HLQS.

The opponents being
W. de Moeller, Doctor of Medicine and Surgery
A. Tietzel, Doctor of Medicine and Surgery
O. Zimmermann, Doctor of Medicine and Surgery

Berlin, at the press of Johann Friederich Starck

Fig. 1.1. Frontispiece of Dr. Bennewitz's thesis with translation into English.

Cappadocian, who produced the still classical and perceptive description of diabetes as a "liquifying of the skin and body members into urine . . . this illness is persistent . . . of long incubation, but once matured man does not last long . . .". Galen preferred to consider it a primary disease of the kidneys. Given the imperfect knowledge of anatomy at that time, I suspect that if our present knowledge was derived only from autopsies of patients who had died from untreated ketoacidosis we might well reach similar conclusions.

Fifteen hundred years later, Thomas Willis, the English physician, is credited as being the first to discover sugar in the diabetic's urine, and to suspect that this was present to some extent even in the healthy state. Bennewitz summarized the current theories in 1824, and discarded the older concepts of climate, snake-bite, invisible ducts from stomach to bladder or primary renal or spermatic disease. He concentrated on possible causes of excess sugar production, whether from the stomach (Dr. John Rollo of London had written his monograph on dietary treatment 20 years previously), the reproductive system (which might be relevant in pregnancy) or elsewhere. He favoured the honest, if pragmatic, view that this excess production of sugar must be only "one aspect of a wider kind of disease not yet adequately researched".

One further warms to Bennewitz, in spite of his study of logic and metaphysics under Hegel in Berlin, for his simple scientific approach: "do not write a dissertation to adorn and praise the works of the learned:– rather to confirm and support your diagnosis. I have attempted to set forth a shapely and clear account of a remarkable illness . . .". Before giving the case history, he summarized his belief that the diabetic condition was in some way a symptom of the pregnancy, or due to the pregnancy. He noted that "other disorders . . . began to break out as the pregnancy matured . . . the little fires which had hidden beneath the smouldering deceiving ashes broke forth and devoured again the woman's condition in the most wretched manner". He was convinced that "the disease appeared along with pregnancy, and at the very same time . . . ; when pregnancy appeared, it appeared; while pregnancy lasted, it lasted; it terminated soon after the pregnancy". Finally, he showed a degree of humility when he remarked that his patient must be something of a rare bird!

The case history commences on 13 November 1823, when Frederica Pape, aged 22, was admitted at 7 months in her fifth pregnancy to the Berlin Infirmary. The first three pregnancies appear to have been unremarkable, but in the fourth in 1822 she had an onset of thirst and polyuria which had resolved spontaneously after delivery. These symptoms returned at an unspecified time in her fifth pregnancy. She had "a really unquenchable thirst – she consumed more than six Berlin measures of beer or spring water, although the quantity of urine greatly exceeded the amount of liquid consumed, and the urine itself smelt like stale beer. Her voice was weak, skin dry, face cold and she complained of a dragging pain in her back".

Treatment was more a matter of belief than of understanding, but apart from having withdrawn 360 ml of venous blood all at once (the equivalent of 36 10-ml routine blood tests today) and taking a high protein diet probably deficient in vitamins, she must have benefited from the rest and care. The measurement of 2 oz of sugar in 16 lb (224 oz) of urine which is equivalent to about 1% glycosuria was his only biochemical evidence of diabetes mellitus.

From about 32 to 36 weeks she had a recurrent sore throat and increased abdominal distension such that twins were suspected. When examined on 28 December 1823 the cervix was dilating and the fetal head already partially descended. On 29 December she had an obstructed labour, and the child died intrapartum, probably due to delay in the second stage. Bennewitz remarks that the baby was of "such robust and healthy character whom you would have thought Hercules had begotten". He weighed 12 lb, which fact was witnessed carefully.

Postpartum, in spite of continued dieting, sweating and purging, and the application of eight leeches, her strength improved daily, and sugar disappeared from her urine. "With nature to preserve and treat her, we dismissed our patient cured." Unfortunately there is no record of her subsequent health, perhaps because Dr. Bennewitz presented his thesis within 6 months and having been successful in obtaining his doctorate, dropped out of academic medicine.

If Dr. Bennewitz was a straightforward clinician, the simple observations which he made 165 years ago remain the challenge that brings us back to Aberdeen for this Fourth International Colloquium. The development of diabetes and its relationship to pregnancy, even if the pregnant diabetic woman is still something of a rare bird in general terms, continue to fascinate a broad group of investigators. The obstetrician still observes the problems of antenatal care and of delivery. The paediatrician is still concerned with the immediate perinatal problems of the large-for-dates infant. The diabetologist has much more effective treatment at his disposal but may still not achieve the goal of total normoglycae-mia throughout the pregnancy. Epidemiology, a discipline requiring careful record-keeping and long-term studies across generations, is concerned with the long-term outcome of both mother and child: how instructive it would be if we could follow up the family of Frederica Pape (from 1824 there would be at least six generations) to see if there was any special influence of pregnancy on the inheritance of diabetes in the offspring.

The most recent concepts on the possible interrelationships between diabetes and pregnancy have come from the geneticists, the molecular biologists and the immunologists. These disciplines come with a complex terminology, at times confusing to the clinician, but the recent development of gene probes and monoclonal antibodies has made it possible to ask much more searching questions. Finally, the biochemists are still essential: their techniques have improved since Bennewitz boiled off the 16 lb of urine to leave the 2 oz of sugar crystals, but by whatever method the excess sugar is identified, and whether in the fasting state, after a normal meal or after a bowlful of 75 g of pure glucose, the scientific assessment of the severity of the diabetic condition will ultimately depend on chemical measurement.

Dr. Bennewitz dismissed his patient cured, leaving nature to preserve and treat her. Although his concept of cure was merely to survive the hazard of the pregnancy, the disastrous results recorded by Matthews Duncan 60 years later show the major risks that existed to both mother and child from uncontrolled diabetes. The main aim of studying carbohydrate metabolism in pregnancy and in the newborn is to abolish those risks, but if at the same time we can throw further light on the actual cause of the diabetic condition, and if we can devise a treatment or technique to prevent it occurring at all, we will have done something to satisfy Bennewitz's enquring mind.

Insulin-Dependent Diabetes

If we accept for convenience the concept of two major forms of diabetes mellitus, and call them insulin-dependent and non-insulin-dependent diabetes, it is possible to make some observations on how pregnancy would interact either to precipitate or exacerbate each condition. In passing, it is interesting that there is no suggestion that the pregnant state alleviates diabetes, although this is recognized in many autoimmune disorders such as rheumatoid arthritis and systemic lupus erythematosus.

A logical (Hegelian) synthesis of current knowledge would have to admit two strands of thought on the aetiology of both types of diabetes – the genetic and immunological evidence, and the environmental evidence. Immunity can be studied both at humoral level (circulating in the blood) and at cellular level. The main body of work in this field is on circulating humoral immunoglobulins or antibodies, which are produced by the B cells, or plasma cells, in the bone marrow. Immunoglobulins active against the beta cells of the pancreatic islets, and against insulin itself, have been identified and may well be the most important marker for the active autoimmune state which precedes the clinical recognition of insulin-dependent diabetes. However, it is precisely that type of immunological reaction which might be expected to be ameliorated, not exacerbated, in pregnancy.

More recently, with the development of specific monoclonal antibodies, it has been possible to identify certain clones or groups of T cells, derived from the thymus gland (perhaps under the influence of the hormone thymulin). These cells may be helper or suppressor to the B cells or plasma cells in forming the immunoglobulins. A recent concept of the course of events would be that at some stage in development one or more of the beta cells of the pancreatic islets becomes immunogenic (in immunological language, it expresses a class 2 (DR) antigen on its cell membrane). This may be a genetically inherited tendency, but is probably also acquired due to interferon production following a virus infection or some other stimulus. Once the cell membrane becomes immunogenic the T cells in the thymus become activated. The T-helper cells then activate the B cells or plasma cells to make specific immunoglobulins (complement-fixing anti-islet-cell antibodies), which in turn cause the gradual destruction of the pancreatic beta cells and the eventual clinical presentation of insulin-dependent diabetes (Doniach et al. 1985). It is possible that the pregnant state might facilitate the activation of the T cells and thus pregnancy in some way might be truly diabetogenic.

We have addressed this problem by studying T cell regulation in a group of 15 women known to have developed islet cell antibodies during a recent pregnancy in which they had hyperglycaemia (diagnosed by 75-g oral glucose tolerance test (OGTT) and requiring either dietary management or insulin treatment during the pregnancy to maintain normal blood glucose levels) (Rodgers et al. 1988). Using flow cytometry we found no difference in the number of helper or suppressor T cells (Leu 2, Leu 3, Leu 8) in these subjects compared to 11 postgestational controls. But some of the women who had developed islet cell antibodies did show an increase in the number of lymphocytes expressing the T cell activation marker 1L2R when compared to controls. We conclude that even if there is no consistent alteration in T cell numbers to suggest active cellular immune processes in women who had hyperglycaemia during pregnancy, there may be some patients where the immune process has become activated following, or even during, the pregnancy.

An environmental interaction of the effect of pregnancy on the causation of insulin-dependent diabetes is even less well established. The curious group of insulin-dependent diabetic boys who were born in Iceland 9 months after their mothers had apparently consumed large quantities of nitrosamine containing partially smoked mutton (Helgason and Jonasson 1981) has prompted further investigation using an animal model in Aberdeen, and it is possible that a chemical substance could be in part responsible for activating the immune cascade or even for direct damage to the pancreatic beta cell. The remarkable difference between the prevalence of insulin-dependent diabetes between countries and even between the same racial groups in different countries, suggests that environmental causes still await discovery.

Non-Insulin-Dependent Diabetes

Current thought on the pathophysiology of non-insulin-dependent diabetes has a dualistic outlook on the result of defective insulin production and of increased resistance to the action of insulin. Both these factors affect the basal, or fasting, plasma glucose, and this appears to set the pattern for the post-food levels of plasma glucose.

There have been many studies of insulin production (usually in response to some form of glucose challenge) and of insulin resistance which can be assessed by glucose clamping techniques or by mathematical modelling concepts (Rudenski et al. 1988). In conjunction with long-term observation of the natural history of the diabetic condition in these patients (Hadden et al. 1986) it is possible to construct a scheme which will allow an explanation of the findings at the time of diagnosis of non-insulin-dependent diabetes, and during the long-term management of the disease (at least on diet only). The effect of pregnancy on this scenario can then be superimposed. At the time of diagnosis there will have been a relatively rapid rise in fasting plasma glucose, giving rise to recent symptoms of thirst and polyuria. At this time there is a relative deficiency in insulin production by the beta cell, and a relatively greater degree of insulin resistance. After establishing an appropriate long-term steady state, usually by eating less food, the fasting plasma glucose is considerably lower (though not necessarily normal) and symptoms have disappeared. From that point, provided excess food is avoided, there appears to be a slow but inexorable rise in fasting plasma glucose (about 0.2 mmol/l per year), which is consequent upon an equally slow, progressive fall in insulin production by the pancreatic beta cell, at about 1.5% per year. This fall in beta cell function might have started as early as age 20, although the rise in fasting plasma glucose might not become apparent above the upper end of the normal range until much later, perhaps at age 40.

The effect of a pregnancy during this protracted time span is probably dependent more on an increase in insulin resistance (due to the hormonal milieu of normal pregnancy) resulting in a rise in fasting plasma glucose in later pregnancy: there is no change in insulin production, and even some evidence of a fall in basal or fasting plasma glucose in early pregnancy, which may also be hormonally mediated. There is thus a change in carbohydrate metabolism in normal pregnancy and this change can be superimposed on the slowly evolving pathogenetic changes of non-insulin-dependent diabetes, but it is not necessary to suggest that pregnancy is truly diabetogenic in the long term. On the other hand, the hyperglycaemic maternal environment in these cases might well have a permanent effect on the fetal islet cell, which would have to respond with increased insulin production at an early stage in development. Whether this concept of fetal islet cell "sensitization" has any bearing on the prevalence of non-insulin-dependent diabetes in subsequent generations has not been adequately assessed in the human.

Gestational Diabetes, or the Onset of Hyperglycaemia in Pregnancy

Ever since the clear statement by Bennewitz that he dismissed his patient "cured" after her pregnancy there has been a belief in the concept of temporary gestational diabetes. Perhaps he should take some of the blame for not following up his patient, for in all likelihood her diabetes was not cured. The number of young diabetic mothers who died in diabetic ketoacidotic coma soon after pregnancy was shown by Matthews Duncan. It might even be that there was a worsening of autoimmune damage to the remaining beta cells shortly after delivery, by analogy with postpartum autoimmune thyroiditis. Taking the long-term epidemiological view, it is clear that there must be two processes at work, either of which may become temporarily involved in the duration of a pregnancy. The spontaneous onset of insulin-dependent diabetes in young adult women may occur with an annual incidence of about one in 1000: if pregnancy causes temporarily increased insulin resistance and this is superimposed on pre-existing but progressing beta cell autoimmune damage, the diagnosis of temporary, or gestational, insulin-dependent diabetes will be made: the mother will need insulin during the pregnancy but will probably be able to stop it temporarily postpartum. Whether the intervention of the pregnancy accelerates or ameliorates the progress of islet cell damage is uncertain: it may well have no permanent independent effect at all. From the severity of her symptoms, and her youth, it is most probable that Frederica Pape really had insulin-dependent diabetes, which just happened to be coincidental with her pregnancy.

In the past 20 years the increasing interest in the concept and the relative ease of carrying out glucose tolerance tests in pregnancy have produced an enormous literature on the subject. In most cases this represents the detection of glucose intolerance using an oral glucose load, often in late pregnancy when insulin resistance is greater. The O'Sullivan study in Boston has shown, and continues to show, the strength of this concept for diagnosing future non-insulin-dependent diabetic women. The World Health Organization tried to simplify the diagnostic criteria by applying the same cut-off levels after a 75-g glucose load in the non-pregnant and pregnant state. After several local and international studies of random normal pregnancies it is clear that a 2-h level of venous plasma glucose of 8.0 mmol/l will considerably overdiagnose the condition: a 2-h level of 9.0 mmol/l in the second or third trimester will still produce 5% of unselected pregnancies as "abnormal" (DPSG study 1988).

The largest prospective study was carried out on 917 unselected mothers in Aberdeen (Farmer et al. 1988), using the now unique 25-g intravenous glucose load. These authors confirmed a weak relationship between maternal glucose disposal and fetal weight and congenital malformations, but doubted the value of screening all pregnancies in this fashion.

It has now become clear that the non-pregnant female, and even the male, may have a prevalence of impaired glucose tolerance not greatly different from the results seen in the third trimester of pregnancy (Harris et al. 1987). This does not mean that knowledge of maternal blood glucose is not important – clearly the risk to the fetus of significant hyperglycaemia still remains in the short term. But it may result in still further upgrading of the level of acceptable plasma glucose in normal pregnancy.

Perhaps one of the problems has been too rigid adherence to the concept of glucose intolerance, which by definition needs a glucose load to identify. The risk is that of sustained hyperglycaemia and this is better defined by the fasting plasma glucose. There is surprisingly poor correlation between the results of a 75-g oral glucose tolerance test (OGTT) and those of a simple before and after meal profile of plasma glucose.

In conclusion, if Dr. Bennewitz was to attend this Fourth Aberdeen Colloquium, I have no doubt that he would take pleasure in having reported his "rare bird", a case of real diabetes mellitus: he would certainly be interested in the continued investigations into the cause of diabetes mellitus, and the discussion as to whether pregnancy has anything to do with it. But I feel that his logical mind would be surprised to find just quite so many cases of "gestational impaired glucose tolerance", and with his philosophy of letting nature take her course, I suspect that he would have been a non-interventionist in any case.

References

Bennewitz HG (1828) Symptomatic diabetes mellitus (abstracted from Osann's 12ter Jahresbericht des Poliklinischen Institutes zu Berlin, p 23). Edin Med J 30:217–218

Diabetes Pregnancy Study Group (1988) A multicentre study of the responses to the 75 g oral glucose tolerance test during pregnancy (in preparation).

Doniach D, Spencer KM, Bottazzo GF (1985) Immunology of insulin-dependent diabetes. In: Rose NR, Mackay IR (eds) The autoimmune diseases. Academic Press, New York, pp 227–242

Farmer G, Russell G, Hamilton-Nicol DR et al. (1988) The influence of maternal glucose metabolism on fetal growth, development and morbidity in 917 singleton pregnancies in non-diabetic women. Diabetologia 31:134–141

Hadden DR, Blair ALT, Wilson EA et al. (1986) Natural history of diabetes presenting age 40–69 years: a prospective study of the influence of intensive dietary therapy. Q J Med 230:579–598

Harris MI, Hadden WC, Knowler WC, Bennett PH (1987) Prevalence of diabetes and impaired glucose tolerance and plasma glucose levels in the US population aged 20–74 years. Diabetes 36:523–534

Helgason T, Jonasson MR (1981) Evidence for a food additive as a cause of ketosis-prone diabetes. Lancet II: 716–720

Matthews Duncan J (1882) On puerperal diabetes. Trans Obstet Soc Lond 24:256–285

Rodgers L, O'Brien CJ, Crockard A et al. (1988) A quantitative assessment of T-cell immunity in women subjects at high risk of developing insulin dependent mellitus. Poster presentation to the 4th Aberdeen International Colloquium on Carbohydrate Metabolism in Pregnancy and the Newborn, 12–14 April 1988

Rudenski AS, Hadden DR, Atkinson AB et al. (1988) Natural history of pancreatic islet B-cell function in type 2 diabetes mellitus studied over six years by homeostasis model assessment. Diab Med 5:36–41

2. Polyendocrinopathy

R. L. Himsworth

The occurrence of more than one endocrine disease in the same patient has intrigued first physicians and then endocrinologists, immunologists and geneticists. To paraphrase Oscar Wilde, to have one disease is permissible, to have two looks like immunological unruliness. As polyendocrinopathy is immunological in origin, the varieties of multiple endocrine adenomatosis will not be considered here. The overlap of organ-specific autoimmune diseases has been recognized for many years and eponyms such as Schmidt's syndrome have been applied to particular combinations. The target glands affected include pancreatic islets, thyroid, adrenals and gonads and also importantly the parietal cells of the stomach. The particular association of thyroid, gastric, adrenal and pancreatic autoimmune phenomena with either overt disease or the presence of antibodies is common and has been designated type II autoimmune polyglandular syndrome (Winter and Maclaren 1987); it has a strong association with HLA DR3 or DR4. The form of diabetes is insulin dependent, type I, and indeed has been termed type IB (Bottazzo et al. 1974), the form with a female preponderance, later onset and persistence of islet cell antibodies.

In considering autoimmune endocrine disease in relation to pregnancy we have to discuss the prevalence of each individual disease, both treated and untreated, the prevalence of the prodromal situation, the effects of these various different conditions on the outcome of pregnancy and the effects of the pregnancy on the development of the autoimmune disorder. We might also address other more nebulous questions: the effects, if any, of the genetic predisposition on pregnancy; and the effects, if any, of the fundamental immunological disorder on the pregnancy. We must also consider the effects of any hormonal imbalance on the development of the fetus, and importantly the impact on fetal development, and especially the development of the fetal endocrine system, of maternal immunoglobulins moving across the placenta. Finally, another layer of complexity is superimposed by the "polyendocrinopathy" and the implication of some form of synergism between co-existing organ-specific autoimmune diseases. This is a formidable agenda. Information on many of these matters, however, is either wholly lacking or imprecise. Moreover although the autoimmune endocrinopathies may incorporate all endocrine glands, most of the conditions are individually uncommon and still more rare in combination. The focus therefore will be on disorders of the thyroid gland in conjunction with diabetes.

Let us start by considering the genesis and evolution of an immunological endocrine disorder. First there is genetic predisposition. The evidence for this from epidemiological studies is overwhelming but this alone is not sufficient for the disease to occur because the concordance rates of monozygotic twins for type I diabetes and for thyroid disease do not exceed 50%. Attention has focused on the contribution of the class II antigens, especially DR3 and DR4, to this genetic susceptibility for both conditions. These antigens were originally defined serologically and are now known to be encoded by genes on chromosome 6 which are polymorphic. Recent evidence from the study of restriction fragment length polymorphisms (Hitman et al. 1986) has allowed the definition of still closer associations. Nevertheless it has been calculated (Rotter et al. 1986) that genes carried on chromosome 6 can only account for two-thirds of the genetic susceptibility to diabetes.

Against this genetic background an initiating event has been postulated. This is something which, given the protracted development of an autoimmune endocrine disorder, is very difficult to identify in retrospect. (Such an event should be clearly differentiated from an occurrence which precipitates overt endocrine failure, for instance an infection immediately preceding the onset of clinical diabetes.) There follows a prodromal period when organ-specific auto-antibodies are present. These may be indicators of immunological events rather than agents of cell destruction. In the latter part of this period the maximum secretory capacity of the gland is diminishing. The decline of secretory capacity may not however be steady, but may be interrupted by improvement shown either by recovery in maximal hormone output or by reduced antibody titres. Finally, hormonal secretion by the gland falls below a critical level and disease becomes manifest. Even after this, however, there may be residual function by the gland but with time this generally ceases.

Conception may occur at any stage in this progression. Towards the end there may be unrecognized endocrine failure in which case fertility is reduced, certainly in diabetes, hypothyroidism and Addison's disease and the pregnancy is unlikely to be carried to a successful conclusion. Equally, in the common exception to endocrine failure as a sequel to an autoimmune process, hyperthyroid Graves's disease, fertility is reduced and fetal loss is high in untreated patients. In every untreated endocrine autoimmune disease the hormonal and metabolic disorder is such that we need look no further for an explanation of the poor outlook.

But what if the disease has been treated or is in its prodromal phase? Will fertility or the outcome of pregnancy be affected? And, if there is a complex of organ-specific autoimmune disorders, does this combination make the outcome worse?

I shall not discuss here the effects of diabetes on conception, pregnancy, fetal malformation and neonatal morbidity. But there is one question to which there seems to be as yet no satisfactory answer. Is there any effect on pregnancy or the fetus of the prodromal phase of type IB diabetes? It would seem important to determine whether the reproductive performance of women who develop specifically type IB diabetes years after pregnancy is abnormal, and if so whether the effect relates to the proximity of pregnancy to the onset of clinical diabetes. This matter is important if we are to distinguish between the effects of a metabolic or endocrine derangement on the one hand and an immunological phenomenon on the other. A recent paper (Mills et al. 1988) has shown that malformation rates in infants of diabetic mothers may be unrelated to glycaemic control during organogenesis and serves to emphasize this point. There are plenty of examples, however, in which a treated immunological disease in the mother can affect the fetus by the transfer of maternal immunoglobulins across the placenta. In organ-specific disease fetal and neonatal hyperthyroidism due to maternal thyroid-stimulating antibodies, and neonatal hypothyroidism due to thyroid-stimulating hormone (TSH) receptor-blocking antibodies are classic examples. Myasthenia gravis, idiopathic thrombocytopenic purpura and congenital heart block are other examples. Furthermore there is evidence that less targeted autoimmune disorders in the mother adversely affect pregnancy, thus fetal loss is unduly high in systemic lupus erythematosus (reviewed by Mor-Yosef et al. 1984) and in rheumatoid arthritis (Kaplan 1986).

The question therefore arises as to whether these effects are due to the immunological disorder which lies behind the disease. In addressing this question one can look at two common situations. First, the progress and outcome of pregnancy in patients with auto-antibodies but either no disease or fully treated disease – here thyroid disease may provide a model. Second, the same parameters in the type I diabetic, with and without a second immunological disorder.

First, how common is autoimmune thyroid disease in its prodromal phase? Goitre and auto-antibodies are common in women in their reproductive years. A large-scale survey at Wickham in North-East England (Tunbridge et al. 1977) found goitres in 11%–15% of women between the ages of 18 and 44 years. In the same patients the prevalence of both cytopathic thyroid microsomal antibodies was 4.4%–6.3% and of an elevated TSH (>6 mU/l) was 4.0%–5.7%. Both of these findings indicate a significant prevalence of autoimmune disease without failure of hormone production. In South Wales Professor Hall and his colleagues (Fung et al. 1988) found 117 out of 901 women (13%) had thyroid auto-antibodies when booking at an antenatal clinic and the condition of transient postpartum thyroid dysfunction developed in an estimated 16.7% of the whole series of patients. These postpartum events show that the presence of auto-antibodies is no mere immunological phenomenon and indicate an immediate potential for disordered thyroid function. In this latter series, however, the outcome of pregnancy was no different amongst those with and without thyroid antibodies.

Hyperthyroid Graves's disease is common in the reproductive phase of life. In this disorder poor endocrine control is not only deleterious to the outcome of pregnancy but may also be a cause of fetal malformation (Momotani et al. 1984). Further, in this condition the fetal thyroid may be influenced by the transfer of maternal TSH receptor antibodies across the placenta. Fetal or neonatal hyperthyroidism is rare; still more uncommon is neonatal hypothyroidism due to TSH receptor-blocking antibodies which may be present in mothers with Hashimoto's thyroiditis (Matsuura et al. 1980). Thyroid microsomal antibodies are now known to be directed against the enzyme thyroid peroxidase which is essential for thyroid hormone synthesis. These antibodies could affect the fetal thyroid in either of two ways: they may be cytotoxic or they may block the active site on the enzyme.

After this protracted digression let me return to my main theme: polyendocrinopathy. As thyroid auto-antibodies are common in the general population it would be expected by chance alone that they would occur frequently in type I diabetic women, but as these two diseases are linked in polyendocrinopathy it comes as no surprise to find a higher prevalence of thyrogastric auto-antibodies in people with type I diabetes than in the general population. For example, Maclaren and Riley (1985) found such antibodies to be present in over 25% of diabetic girls below 10 years of age and this figure rose to over 50% in diabetic women aged between 31 and 40 years. Not only does the prevalence of these antibodies increase with age but it is highest in presumed type IB diabetics.

The opportunity therefore exists to look at reproductive performance of women with type I diabetes with and without a predisposition for another organ-specific autoimmune disease. There is evidence, assembled by Beral and her colleagues (1984), that the reproductive outcome in type I diabetic women is worse if they subsequently develop thyroid disease. They found a significantly increased risk of fetal or neonatal death which was independent of the severity of diabetes in such women. Moreover the risk of an unfavourable outcome increased with successive pregnancies. This last observation could be due to an evolving immunological disorder predisposing to rejection or an ill-effect on the fetus, or to developing thyroid gland failure. Scott and his colleagues from Leeds (Saad et al. 1984) disputed these findings but their figures included many patients with non-organ-specific autoimmune diseases.

In conclusion, autoimmune diseases in general have an adverse effect on the outcome of pregnancy. Untreated or inadequately treated autoimmune diseases of endocrine glands carry an avoidable penalty. Nevertheless the outcome may be worse than normal in treated patients. There is some evidence that in the prodromal phase the outcome may be adverse when organ-specific auto-antibodies are present but endocrine function is otherwise normal in insulin-dependent diabetics. It is not yet known whether pregnancy and fetal development are normal in patients with islet cell antibodies, whether or not they subsequently develop diabetes.

References

Beral V, Roman E, Colwell L (1984) Poor reproductive outcome in insulin dependent diabetic women associated with later development of other endocrine disorders in the mothers. Lancet I: 4–7

Bottazzo GF, Florin-Christensen A, Doniach D (1974) Islet-cell antibodies in diabetes mellitus with autoimmune polyendocrine deficiencies. Lancet II:1279–1283

Fung HYM, Kologlu M, Collison K et al. (1988) Postpartum thyroid dysfunction in Mid Glamorgan. Br Med J 296:241–244

Hitman GA, Sachs J, Cassell P et al. (1986) A DR-3-related DX alpha gene polymorphism strongly associated with insulin dependent diabetes. Immunogenetics 23: 47–51

Kaplan D (1986) Fetal wastage in patients with rheumatoid arthritis. J Rheumatol 13:875–877

Maclaren NK, Riley MD (1985) Thyroid, gastric, and adrenal autoimmunities associated with insulin-dependent diabetes mellitus. Diabetes Care [Suppl 8] 1:34–38

Matsuura N, Yamada Y, Hohara Y et al. (1980) Familial neonatal transient hypothyroidism due to maternal TSH-binding inhibitor immunoglobulins. New Engl J Med 303:738–741

Mills JL, Knopp RH, Simpson JL et al. (1988) Lack of relation of increased malformation rates in infants of diabetic mothers to glycemic control during organogenesis. N Eng J Med 318:671–676

Momotani N, Ho K, Hamada NN et al. (1984) Maternal hyperthyroidism and congenital malformation in the offspring. Clin Endocrinol 20:695–700

Mor-Yosef S, Navot D, Rabinowitz R, Schenker JG (1984) Collagen diseases in pregnancy. Obstet Gynecol Surv 39:67–83

Rotter JI, Vanheim CM, Raffel LJ et al. (1986) Genetic aetiologies of diabetes. Pediatr Adolesc Endocrinol 15:1–11

Saad E, Wales JK, Scott JS (1984) Pregnancy outcome in women with diabetes and other autoimmune disease. Lancet II:1283–1284

Tunbridge WMG, Evered D, Hall R et al. (1977) The spectrum of thyroid disease in a community: the Wickham Survey. Clin Endocrinol 7:481–493

Winter WE, Maclaren NK (1987) To what extent is 'polyendocrine' serology related to the clinical expression of disease? Clin Immunol Allergy 1:109–123

3. Obesity and Fat Distribution

M. E. J. Lean, H. W. Sutherland and P. Garthwaite

Introduction

Obesity has long been recognized as a risk factor for the development of diabetes mellitus, particularly in later life, and in young women it is widely thought to predispose towards impaired glucose tolerance and diabetes in pregnancy. This review tackles related questions but does not address obstetric issues or the management of the overweight during pregnancy. These were well reviewed by Campbell (1983) with the conclusion that weight loss should not be attempted during pregnancy. Several elements need to be considered: the presence of obesity before pregnancy, weight gain during the pregnancy (possibly at different stages of pregnancy) and the distribution of body fat. There may also be important aetiological factors common to the development of obesity and impaired carbohydrate tolerance, both genetic and environmental factors including diet.

Pregnancy is itself an interesting model for obesity, and many workers now feel that little or no increase in energy intake is necessary for the weight gain. The increase in body fat may however have been overestimated, and there may be superimposed alterations in fat distribution (Whitehead et al. 1981; Anderson and Lean 1986; Durnin 1987).

Metabolic Aspects of Obesity

Genetics

Obesity runs in families, but this does not necessarily mean that it is inherited genetically, rather than the result of social and environmental influences which are perpetuated through the generations. Extensive population surveys and large studies of twins and of adopted siblings have established that there is indeed a powerful genetic basis for obesity, with an inheritance of about 0.7–0.9. This compares with an inheritance of 1.0 for a totally genetic phenotypic variant such as eye colour, and about 0.6 for the inheritance of ischaemic heart disease which most clinicians would agree has a very significant genetic basis (Stunkard et al. 1986a,b; Bouchard 1987). Overfeeding studies by Bouchard and colleagues have also indicated interactive factors in weight gain such that there are genetically controlled differential responses to an environmental influence, overfeeding: about 90% of the variance in body fat changes is accounted for by genetic factors (Poehlman et al. 1986; Bouchard 1987). The inheritance is polygenic, i.e. more than one gene may be responsible, but specific chromosomal loci have not yet been identified for simple obesity. There are clues from population studies that the x chromosome may be involved with a "sex-linked recessive lethal gene" such that females are over-represented in the progeny of obese parents (Mayer 1968). A defect on chromosome 15 is probably responsible for the obesity in Prader-Willi syndrome (Butler et al. 1986).

The importance of establishing a genetic basis for obesity is that it can only become manifest, expressed in the phenotype, through specific metabolic mechanisms. In that sense, obesity must be considered a disease.

Metabolic Factors Causing Obesity

It is clearly insufficient just to demonstrate that purely genetic factors are involved in obesity. These determine susceptibility, but weight gain can only occur through a net imbalance in the energy balance equation (Fig. 3.1). For this to happen, either the appetite must be increased to provoke an energy intake greater than that required for weight maintenance (primary hyperphagia), or energy expenditure is reduced (Fig. 3.1). In fact, a combination of both these effects is probably necessary in most cases, to avoid compensatory adjustments.

The food intake of the obese has been the subject of repeated study. Almost all published results have failed to indicate that they overeat compared with thin

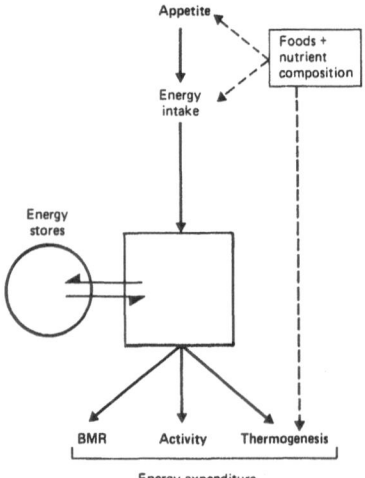

Fig. 3.1. The energy balance equation in schematic form.

controls. Such findings have often led to a variety of completely erroneous interpretations for the complex aetiology of obesity. The explanation lies in the major methodological problems in all approaches to the measurement of habitual food intake, most tending to underestimate. The apparent energy intake of the overweight is systematically under-recorded by about 20% by comparison with their energy requirement for weight maintenance from independent measurement of energy expenditure.

There is no clear evidence that the overweight expend less energy on physical exertion, on the contrary they may expend more because of the extra work required to move their bulk, and their basal metabolic rate is increased compared to thin people. Over 24 h as measured by whole-body calorimetry, or over several weeks as estimated by the doubly labelled water technique, the energy expenditure of the overweight is increased in proportion to their increased mass, or more accurately their increased (metabolically active) fat-free mass (James 1983; Jequier 1984; Prentice et al. 1986).

The clue to the still apparently mysterious mechanism of weight gain may lie in the rate of weight gain. One stone (7 kg) gain in a year would be considered a rapid rate, but if the energy content of adipose tissue is 7000 kcal/kg, then this rate of increase is 49 000 kcal/year which is only 6% of the energy balance of an average female subject (2100 kcal/d). Even with the highly sophisticated apparatus now available it is extremely difficult to measure energy balance with this degree of accuracy in human subjects, and smaller differences will continue to be missed. It is only possible to carry out relatively short-term experiments, so these must be conducted in the most rigorously controlled way in order to detect very small differences.

An area of recent interest emerging from studies in congenitally obese animal models has been in the role of "diet-induced thermogenesis" (DIT). Feeding leads to an increase in metabolic rate and a proportion of this, probably under sympathetic control, may have a regulatory role in determining energy balance and the stability of body weight. Several studies have indicated that subjects prone to obesity (those who have lost weight to become thin again, and thus suitable for comparison with non-obese controls) have reduced DIT following carbohydrate ingestion. We have recently studied the metabolic effects of isocaloric energy-balance diets with high fat/low carbohydrate content or vice versa and an overfed diet, using 24-h whole-body calorimetry, in groups of obese, post-obese and thin control subjects. Energy expenditure was found to be determined by the carbohydrate intake, not fat intake. There was a significant interaction between the subject group and DIT: the post-obese had reduced energy expenditure on a diet with 40% fat, 45% carbohydrate, i.e. a normal UK diet, but were able to generate DIT satisfactorily on a high carbohydrate/low fat diet (Lean and James 1988; Fig. 3.2).

Biochemical Effects of Obesity on Carbohydrate Tolerance

Many studies have examined endocrine and biochemical abnormalities in obesity, although many of these will be secondary to the obesity itself rather than aetiological factors. One of the most striking is the elevation of insulin secretion, which reflects resistance to the effects of insulin on glucose clearance in target tissues. The majority of non-insulin-dependent diabetics are obese, and impair-

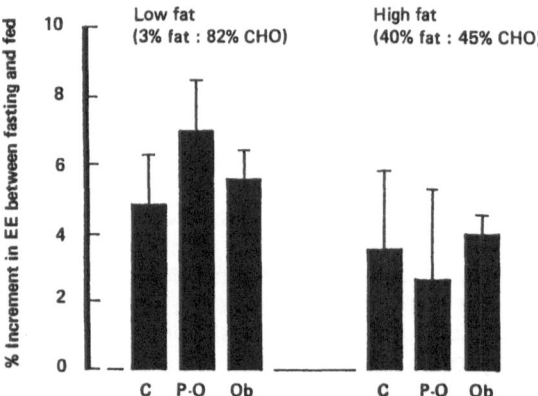

Fig. 3.2. Thermic effect (DIT) over 24 h from diets equal in energy content, and achieving precise energy balance (± 2%), but with either high-fat/low-carbohydrate or low-fat/high-carbohydrate content. Data from Lean and James (1988) in groups of control, obese and postobese (after slimming) women.

ment of glucose tolerance is predicted by obesity in population surveys such that its prevalence is approximately doubled when body mass index (BMI) is increased to 30. There seems to be a common aetiological link between obesity and diabetes since weight changes over a 10-year period do not appear to alter the frequency of diabetes in subjects who were previously overweight (Modan et al. 1986).

Both basal (Bogardus et al. 1985) and carbohydrate-stimulated (Prager et al. 1986) insulin secretion are increased in obesity and this is reversible with weight loss (Bagdade et al. 1967) but perhaps not to normal levels (Modan et al. 1986). The mechanism is unclear. Some animal evidence would suggest that hypersecretion of insulin is the primary event, under hypothalamic control. The mainly obese women with histories of gestational diabetes studied by Ward et al. (1985) appeared to have impaired insulin sensitivity compared to well-matched controls, and higher basal insulin but reduced glucose-stimulated insulin secretion. Alternatively, there may be an alteration in the action of internalized, receptor-bound insulin on the intracellular glucose transporters, leading to greater demand for insulin in order to normalize blood glucose. Hyperglycaemia and hyperinsulinism can also both result from feeding a high fat diet, which, as discussed above, may be a factor in causing obesity (Himsworth 1935; Clark et al. 1983). In obese subjects with impaired glucose tolerance or diabetes, plasma insulin concentration may become reduced compared with the non-diabetic obese, although it may often exceed that of normal non-obese subjects.

A second biochemical alteration of possible relevance to carbohydrate metabolism in pregnancy is the increased activity of aromatase in the enlarged adipose tissue mass of (non-pregnant) obese women, together with diminished serum sex hormone binding globulin (SHBG) activity. The end result is increased circulating free testosterone, and this is thought to contribute to the hirsutism and menstrual irregularities, with inadequate luteal phase, which are frequent in obesity. It is also a factor in determining the distribution of body fat, which relates to insulin sensitivity and carbohydrate tolerance (see below, Kissebah et al. 1985). The low SHBG is correctable with weight loss (O'Dea et al. 1979).

Effect of Pregnancy on Obesity and Body Fat Content

Many women date the onset of obesity to pregnancy. In the UK, only 13% of female teenagers aged 16–19 are obese (BMI>25), while 44% of women are obese by the age of 50–54. However, the figures at the same ages for men (who cannot blame pregnancy directly!) are 11% and 50%, so this may simply be an effect of age. Analysis is complicated by socioeconomic factors, and by confusion between the effects of pregnancy and childrearing (see the questionnaire in Knight 1984), but women of 50–54 who have had four or more children do have a slightly higher BMI (27.1 non-manual, 26.5 manual) than women who have had only one or two (24.6 non-manual, 25.4 manual) (Knight 1984).

Until recently it was generally accepted that during a normal pregnancy there is a significant increase in total body fat. A wide range is obviously compatible with successful outcome but the estimates of Hytten have often been accepted as the norm, with an average total weight gain of 12.5 kg, including a 3.5-kg increase in stored fat equivalent to over 30 000 kcal., and requiring an overall increase in energy intake to meet the energy costs of pregnancy of 300 kcal/d in the second and third trimesters (Hytten 1980). From evidence gathered in the Third World and in the UK it became clear that food intake during pregnancy is in fact almost identical with that when not pregnant (Durnin et al. 1985; Anderson and Lean 1986; Durnin 1987). This implies that there must be savings in energy expenditure during pregnancy, but while Western women may rest more in pregnancy, this is not the case in the Third World. It is possible that the body somehow becomes more efficient during normal activities or sleep (though strange if inefficiency were selected for the non-pregnant state) or that there is some specific metabolic adaptation during pregnancy. Either way, any energy saving, spread over 9 months, is a tiny proportion of total metabolism and usually undetectable by current methods of measurement. The data collected by Durnin in Scotland (Durnin et al. 1985; Durnin 1987), Lawrence et al. in Gambia (1984) and by Forsum et al. in Sweden (1985) appear to suggest that there is indeed a small reduction in basal metabolic rate (BMR) per unit body weight in the first few weeks of pregnancy, i.e. there is a lag in the increase in BMR after weight has begun to rise. Some of this will relate to alteration in body water content but the possibility of a metabolic factor remains. This effect is missed if measurements begin after pregnancy is established.

Metabolic Association of Body Fat Distribution

Recent interest in the importance to metabolism of fat distribution stems from the work of Vague (1954) which has gone on to demonstrate that women with an "android" type of fat distribution, predominantly in central, truncal, sites have a greater frequency of diabetes than those with a more peripheral "gynoid" fat distribution. Indeed, a central fat distribution in young women has been shown to predict the development of diabetes and hyperinsulinaemia up to 30 years later (Vague et al. 1986), and it carries similar risks in men (Krotkiewski et al. 1983; Ohlson et al. 1985).

The simplest measurement of fat distribution is a circumferential waist/hip ratio (WHR), made with a tape measure at the levels of the umbilicus and the superior anterior iliac crests (or alternatively the widest point over the hips). This ratio correlates with the proportion of abdominal adipose tissue which is internal as opposed to subcutaneous, and may thus reflect inversely the metabolic activity of the internal adipose tissue. High WHR and increased internal fat deposition are of course characteristic of Cushing's syndrome and polycystic ovarian disease as well as type II diabetes (Ashwell et al. 1985; Lean et al. 1987a,b).

Most studies have found WHR itself to be correlated modestly with obesity or BMI, but these combine as independent predictors of diabetes (Ohlson et al. 1985; Haffner et al. 1987; Lean et al. 1987a,b). High WHR is also associated with hypertension, increased serum triglyceride, reduced high-density lipoprotein (HDL) cholesterol, elevated serum testosterone and reduced SHBG (Kissebah et al. 1985; Haffner et al. 1987).

Effect of Obesity and Fat Distribution on Carbohydrate Tolerance in Pregnancy and Effects on the Newborn

Gestational diabetes is associated with neonatal problems, particularly macrosomia and hypoglycaemia, and also with the development of diabetes in the mother in later life (O'Sullivan 1975). The role of overweight in causing impaired glucose tolerance during pregnancy has been disputed and Treharne et al. (1979) related impaired intravenous glucose tolerance in pregnancy to an "android" fat distribution. We have recently carried out a study to examine the relationships of BMI and WHR, as indices of fatness and fat distribution, with glucose tolerance during pregnancy in an unselected sample of young women.

One hundred and one women attending the routine antenatal clinics and living within 10 miles of Aberdeen were recruited. Fourteen smoked during their pregnancy and a further five resumed smoking following delivery. Glucose tolerance was tested at 26–28 weeks gestation by a standard 75-g oral glucose tolerance test (OGTT) (WHO 1985). Prepregnant body weight was calculated from the first recorded value at the antenatal clinic using published data on weight gain in the same population (Altman and Cole 1980). Postpartum WHR and weight and infant's growth rate expressed as weight for age centile (Tanner and Whitehouse 1973) were measured and other details collected by a single observer on a visit to the subject's home 30±5 weeks postpartum. Waist was measured at the umbilicus and hips at the level of the anterior superior iliac spine using an inextensible tape with the subject vertical.

Fasting capillary plasma glucose was normal (<6 mmol/l; <108 mg/dl) in all cases. The 120-min sample from the OGTT was again normal in all cases according to the WHO criteria (1985) corrected for capillary plasma samples, i.e. <8.9 mmol/l (<160 mg/dl). The mean plasma glucose (±2 SD) at each time point during the OGTT is shown in Fig. 3.3. Figure 3.4 shows the distributions of BMI and WHR in the postpartum women, and in Fig. 3.5 the glucose tolerance is shown for women who were above or below the medians for BMI and WHR. Mean follow-up and prepregnant weights were almost identical for the whole study and the return towards prepregnant weight showed no bias on the basis

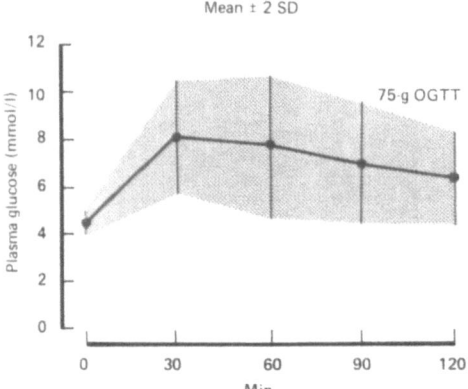

Fig. 3.3. Mean (±2 SD) plasma glucose during a standard OGTT in 101 unselected women at 26–27 weeks gestation.

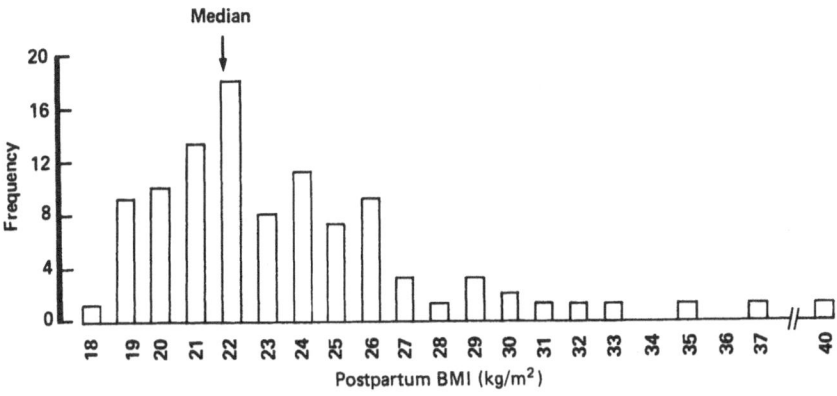

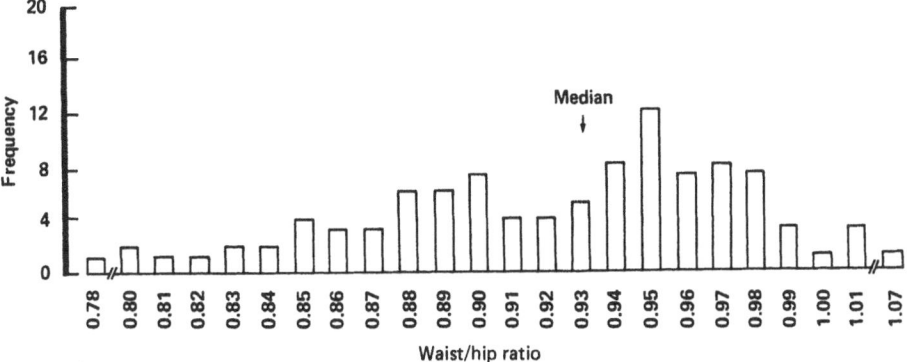

Fig. 3.4. Frequency histograms for postpartum waist/hip ratio and BMI in 101 women.

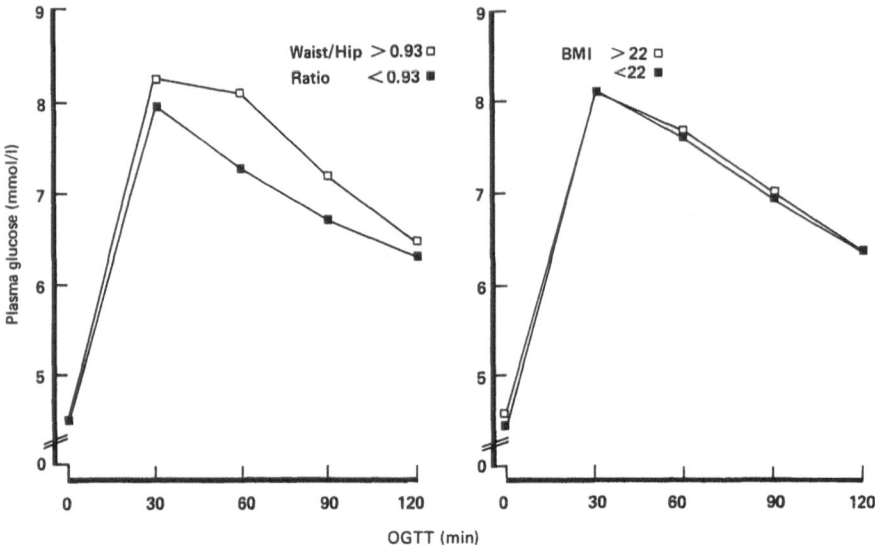

Fig. 3.5. Glucose tolerance of 101 pregnant women, divided as means of groups above or below the medians for postpartum BMI (22 kg/m^2) and waist/hip ratio (0.93).

of existing obesity. Forty-seven women were receiving the oral contraceptive pill at the time of follow-up: no significant differences were found between them and non-pill-users in terms of BMI or WHR. There was a significantly lower BMI ($P<0.05$) but no difference in WHR in women who had breast-fed for at least 1 week ($n=72$; BMI=22.9±3.5, WHR=92±5.4) compared with non-breast-feeders ($n=28$; BMI=25.0±4.7, WHR=93±5.5). Data for the 14 smokers were also analysed separately: birthweight centile was lower (mean 41.2, compared with 45.5 in non-smokers) but this difference was not significant and no other differences emerged.

As in other studies, there was a weak positive interrelation between BMI and WHR, though stepwise multiple regression analysis indicated a relationship between fasting plasma glucose and BMI, but *not* fasting glucose and WHR. On the other hand, while there was no indication of an effect of BMI on any aspect of glucose tolerance following a 75-g oral load, WHR correlated significantly ($P<0.05$) with plasma glucose at 60 min and 90 min, and with the fall in plasma glucose between 30 min and 60 min.

There was also an unexpected positive correlation between gestation at delivery and WHR ($P=0.002$). The only factor which showed a consistent relation to birthweight and birthweight centile was the plasma glucose 120 min after a standard test meal (see Sutherland et al. 1989, Chap. 24). This effect remained after controlling for BMI, WHR and fasting plasma glucose, as well as for maternal height which correlated negatively. Body mass index related to plasma glucose responses to this more physiological meal challenge.

As with obesity, the development of type II diabetes has a strong genetic element, but dietary and other environmental factors also operate. The development of diabetes in the genetically prone is enhanced by obesity. Since fatness (BMI) is positively correlated with intra-abdominal adipose deposition (Ashwell et al. 1985) and, as the present study confirms, with WHR, it seems that a common final mechanism may operate.

Measuring WHR is a very simple screening test to predict conditions related to fat distribution, and this study has shown it to be sensitive enough to detect variations in glucose responses and in birthweight within a normal pregnant population. It might be valuable to use such a measurement, either prepregnant or in early pregnancy, to predict problems. in individual pregnancies. The correlations are probably only strong enough to be able to indicate a subpopulation in whom testing for carbohydrate intolerance would be reasonable.

Conclusions

Obesity and weight gain have been for too long attributed to the deadly sins of greed and sloth. Environmental factors are of course necessary, but equally a genetically derived metabolic basis is necessary. Pregnancy is probably not an important cause of obesity in women, but may involve some subtle energy-saving mechanisms. The relationships between obesity, fat distribution and carbohydrate tolerance are still incompletely understood in the non-pregnant, and are explored here for the first time in relation to pregnancy. For future epidemiology, measurement of the WHR would be a useful addition to routine screening, with the possibility that it may be predictive of carbohydrate intolerance in pregnancy.

References

Altman DG, Cole EC (1980) Assessing weight for dates on a continuous scale. Ann Hum Biol 7:35–44

Anderson AS, Lean MEJ (1986) Dietary intake in pregnancy. Hum Nutr Appl Nutr 40A:40–48

Ashwell M, Cole TJ, Dixon AK (1985) Obesity: new insights into anthropometric classification of fat distribution shown by computed tomography. Br Med J 290:1692–1694

Bagdade JD, Bierman EL, Porte D (1967) The significance of basal insulin levels in the evaluation of the insulin response to glucose in diabetic and non-diabetic subjects. J Clin Invest 46:1549–1557

Bogardus C, Lillioja S, Howard BV, Reaven G, Mott D (1985) Relationships between insulin secretion, insulin action and plasma fasting glucose concentration in nondiabetic and noninsulin dependent subjects. J Clin Invest 74:1238–1246

Bouchard C (1987) Genetics of body fat, energy expenditure and adipose tissue metabolism. In: Berry EM, Blondheim SH, Eliahou HE, Shafrir E (eds) Recent advances in obesity research, V. J. Libbey, London, pp 16–25

Butler MG, Meaney J, Palmer CG (1986) Clinical and cytogenetic survey of 39 individuals with Prader–Labhart–Willi syndrome. Am J Med Genet 23:793–809

Campbell DM (1983) Dietary restriction in obesity and its effect on neonatal outcome. In: Campbell DM, Gillmer MG (eds) Nutrition in pregnancy. Royal College of Obstetrics and Gynaecology, London, pp 243–267

Clark MG, Rattigan S, Clark DG (1983) Obesity with insulin resistance: experimental insights. Lancet II: 1236–1240

Durnin JVGA (1987) Energy requirements of pregnancy: an integration of the longitudinal data from the five-country study. Lancet II: 1131–1133

Durnin JVGA, Grant S, McKillop FM, Fitzgerald G (1985) Is nutritional status endangered by virtually no extra intake during pregnancy? Lancet II: 823–825

Forsum E, Sadurskis A, Wager J (1985) Energy maintenance cost during pregnancy in healthy Swedish women. Lancet I: 107–108

Haffner SM, Stern MP, Hazuda HP, Pugh J, Patterson JK (1987) Do upper body and centralized adiposity measure different aspects of regional body-fat distribution? Relationship to non-insulin-dependent diabetes mellitus, lipids and lipoproteins. Diabetes 36:43–51

Himsworth HP (1935) The syndrome of diabetes mellitus and its causes. Lancet I:465–473

Hytten FE (1980) Weight gain in pregnancy. In: Hytten FE, Chamberlain G (eds) Clinical physiology in obstetrics. Oxford, Blackwell Scientific Publications, pp 193–233

James WPT (1983) Energy requirements and obesity. Lancet II: 386–389

Jequier E (1984) Energy expenditure in obesity. Clin Endocrinol Metab 13:563–580

Kissebah AH, Evans DJ, Peiris A, Wilson CR (1985) Endocrine characteristics in regional obesities: role of sex steroids. In: Vague J, Bjorntorp P, Guy-Grand B, Rebuffe-Scrive M, Vague P (eds) Metabolic complications of human obesities. Elsevier, Amsterdam, pp 115–130

Knight I (1984) The heights and weights of adults in Britain. OPCS, HMSO, London

Krotkiewski M, Bjorntorp P, Sjostrom L, Smith U (1983) Impact of obesity on metabolism in men and women. J Clin Invest 72:1150–1162

Lawrence M, Lamb WH, Lawrence F, Whitehead RG (1984) Maintenance cost of pregnancy in rural Gambian women and influence of dietary status. Lancet II: 363–365

Lean MEJ, James WPT (1988) Metabolic effects of isoenergetic nutrient exchange over 24 hours in relation to obesity in women. Int J Obes 12:15–28

Lean MEJ, Murgatroyd PR, Trayhurn P, Dixon AK (1987a) The case for brown adipose tissue function in humans: biochemistry, physiology and computed tomography. In: Berry EM, Blondheim SH, Eliahou HE, Shafrir E (eds) Recent advances in obesity research, V. J. Libbey, London, pp 109–116

Lean MEJ, Sutherland F, Sutherland HW (1987b) Fatness and fat distribution in relation to glucose tolerance in pregnancy. Proc Nutr Soc 46:151A

Mayer J (1968) Overweight. Causes, cost and control. Prentice-Hall, London, pp 45–57

Modan M, Karasik A, Fuchs Z, Lusky A, Shitrit A, Modan B (1986) Effect of past and concurrent body mass index on prevalence of glucose intolerance and Type 2 (non-insulin-dependent) diabetes and on insulin response. Diabetologia 29:82–89

O'Dea JP, Wieland RG, Hallberg MC, Llerena LA, Zorn EM, Genuth SM (1979) Effect of dietary weight loss on sex steroid binding, sex steroids and gonadotrophins in obese postmenopausal women. J Lab Clin Med 93:1004–1008

Ohlson LO, Larsson B, Svardsudd K et al. (1985) The influence of body fat distribution on the incidence of diabetes mellitus. Diabetes 34:1055–1058

O'Sullivan JB (1975) Prospective studies of gestational diabetes and its treatment. In: Sutherland HW, Stowers JM (eds) Carbohydrate metabolism in pregnancy and the newborn. Churchill Livingstone, Edinburgh, pp 195–204

Poehlman ET, Tremblay A, Despres J-P et al. (1986) Genotype-controlled changes in body composition and fat morphology following overfeeding in twins. Am J Clin Nutr 43:723–731

Prager R, Wallace P, Olefsky JM (1986) In-vivo kinetics of insulin action on peripheral glucose disposal and hepatic glucose output in normal and obese subjects. J Clin Invest 78:472–481

Prentice AM, Black AE, Coward WA et al. (1986) High levels of energy expenditure in obesity. Br Med J 292:983–987

Stunkard AJ, Foch TT, Hrubec Z (1986a) A twin study of human obesity. J Am Med Assoc 256:51–54

Stunkard AJ, Sorensen TIA, Hanis C et al. (1986b) An adoption study of human obesity. N Engl J Med 314:193–198

Tanner JM, Whitehouse RH (1973) Height and weight charts from birth to five years allowing for length of gestation. Arch Dis Child 48:786–804

Treharne IAL, Sutherland HW, Stowers JM, Samphier M (1979) Reproduction in obese women. In: Sutherland HW, Stowers JM (eds) Carbohydrate metabolism in pregnancy and the newborn, 1978. Springer-Verlag, Berlin, pp 479–499

Vague J (1954) La différenciation sexuelle humaine; ses incidences en pathologie. Masson, Paris

Vague Ph, Vallo de Castro J, Vague J (1986) Association between adipose tissue distribution and non insulin dependent (Type II) diabetes. In: Vague J, Bjorntorp P, Guy-Grand B, Rebuffe-Scrive M, Vague P (eds) Metabolic complications of human obesities. Elsevier, Amsterdam, pp 77–84

Ward WK, Johnston CLW, Beard JC, Benedetti TJ, Halter JB, Porte D (1985) Insulin resistance and impaired insulin secretion in subjects with histories of gestational diabetes mellitus. Diabetes 34:861–869

Whitehead RG, Paul AA, Black AE, Wiles SJ (1981) Recommended dietary amounts for pregnancy and lactation in the United Kingdom. Food Nutr Bull [Suppl 5] 259–265

WHO (1985) Diabetes mellitus. WHO Tech Rep Ser 727. WHO, Geneva

4. Nutrition in Pregnancy

W. P. T. James and Ann Ralph

Introduction

The study of carbohydrate metabolism in pregnancy dominates this Colloquium together with questions relating to the problems of pregnant diabetic women. This chapter deals with neither of these two themes but seeks to explore whether there are general principles of nutrition in pregnancy which might be applicable to the problems covered by other contributors. As with other studies involving a nutritional component, the effect of a diet depends not only on the amount of specific nutrients eaten but on the individual's genetically determined response to that diet. Superimposed on this interaction is the physiological effect of pregnancy. Unfortunately we also have to recognize that a pregnant woman may deliberately change her diet and its effects are then modified by the different levels of the nutrient stores achieved in the prepregnant state. Only when one recognizes these different components of the problem will it be possible to assess the nutritional state of a pregnant woman in a meaningful way. This chapter illustrates some of these themes by reviewing evidence relating to protein needs, and vitamin and trace element metabolism in pregnancy.

The question of what constitutes an adequate diet and how to specify the nutrient needs of pregnancy has been a vexed question for both nutritionists and obstetricians for many years. Many conclusions are still being drawn on the basis of changes during pregnancy of the blood levels of circulating nutrients. There are also suggestions that good nutrition in the prepregnant state is of fundamental importance for the normal growth and development of the fetus based on indices of nutrient "deficiency" in early pregnancy. The problem is how to assess the validity of these propositions in the absence of a coherent approach to nutrient requirements in pregnancy.

The recent investigations of energy requirement in pregnancy have been assessed in another chapter (Chap. 3) and will not be considered further here. Although there have been many new studies on energy requirements in pregnancy, no comparable effort has been put into the issue of protein requirements. In part this stems from the fact that energy rather than protein requirements proved to be the major development in thinking in the early 1980s and so the re-evaluation of protein needs has been neglected.

Protein Requirements in Pregnancy

The assessment of protein requirements during pregnancy illustrates very simply one method by which nutrient needs can be assessed. First, from a series of body compositional studies Hytten and Leitch (1971) estimated that in the four quarters of pregnancy, i.e. during sequential 10-week phases, there is an average daily gain in body protein of 0.64, 1.84, 4.76 and 6.10 g protein. The total protein requirement estimated from analysis of body composition amounts to about 925 g if the total weight gain during pregnancy is taken to be 12.5 kg with the delivery of a 3.3-kg infant.

Table 4.1. Protein accumulation (g) during pregnancy

	Trimester		
	1st	2nd	3rd
Maternal			
Blood	10	100	135
Uterus	30	90	166
Breasts	12	65	81
	(52)	(255)	(382)
Fetal			
Fetus	1	150	440
Placenta	3	55	100
Amniotic fluid	0	2	3
	(4)	(207)	(543)
TOTAL	56	462	925

From Hytten and Leitch (1971)

   This accumulation of protein occurs differentially in different tissues and the pattern also varies with time during pregnancy (Table 4.1). Thus, the maternal increase in protein dominates the first trimester with a total of 52 g protein accumulated. In contrast, only about 4 g of protein is stored in the fetus, placenta and amniotic fluid. By the end of the second trimester the increase for fetal and maternal tissues in this time amounts to 203 g. The rapidly growing fetus dominates the demand for protein in the third trimester and explains the rapidly increasing total protein requirement, with a further 336 g accumulated compared with only 127 g in maternal tissues. Although these values for protein needs can only be considered as approximate, they illustrate the usefulness of the indirect body compositional approach to the assessment of protein requirements.
   A second classic approach is to study protein needs during pregnancy by monitoring nitrogen balance. In the second half of pregnancy it has been observed that the apparent retention of protein is about 50% greater than that predicted from the estimated nitrogen accumulation in fetus, placenta, maternal tissues and blood. The difference between the two estimates is about 330 g protein, i.e. equivalent to about 1.6 kg of lean body mass. Thus from N balance data one might consider that about 650 g of extra protein was needed for the second half of pregnancy rather than 462 g. Although similar N balance studies have not been conducted during the first half of pregnancy, the N balance data

imply an additional protein need of at least 400 g on top of the 925 g already estimated from body compositional studies. But for this to be true would require that the set of calculations based on body compositional studies were substantially in error. To obtain consistency one would then have to assume that the estimates of fat storage during pregnancy had been overestimated. Analyses of N balance data suggest that the amount of additional N accumulated per kilogramme weight gain in the second half of pregnancy amounts to a gain of about 12% protein. This is the figure one would expect from the body composition of the growing fetus and this therefore lends some support to the estimates based on N balance.

On the basis of these very incomplete analyses, the 1981 WHO/FAO/UNU Committee considered that it would be more appropriate to take the classic 925 g figure rather than erring on the "safe side" and taking the higher value. This judgement stemmed probably from two considerations. First, N balance studies are notoriously difficult to conduct and inaccuracies automatically tend to inflate the figure for nitrogen retention: losses in the collection of faeces, skin, hair and sweat may readily occur and this leads to an underestimate of true excretion rates, whereas the food measured as N ingested could easily fail to account for small amounts left uneaten. Both errors therefore tend to enhance the apparent N retention. The second consideration was more pragmatic in that to inflate the figure further would presuppose that protein deficiency in pregnancy could readily occur if pregnancy in reality required such a high demand for protein. Yet, there seemed very little clinical or epidemiological evidence to support the idea of a widespread problem of protein deficiency.

Given the choice of the lower figure, this then has to be amplified by 30% to allow for the full two standard deviation range of observed weight gain in pregnancy. The value is then further amplified by a theoretical estimate that only 70% of the absorbed protein is deposited in the tissues, the rest being catabolized. In all, this amounts to an additional allowance of 6 g protein/d throughout pregnancy or, as estimated, 1.2 g, 6.1 g and 10.7 g protein allowance per day in the three trimesters. This value is the additional increment of highly digestible protein which needs to be added to the allowance of the normal, non-pregnant woman. This latter figure was increased in 1981 to 0.75 g/kg per d so with a 55-kg woman becoming pregnant the new value for the requirement for a totally digestible "ideal" protein now amounts to about 0.86 g/kg per d.

Further allowances then have to be made for the digestibilities of different proteins which may fall from 95% for animal protein to values as low as 75% for vegetable protein in a diet with a high fibre content. This, in a 55-kg woman, means that the protein allowance needs to be increased to about 1 g/kg per d for a mixed protein source consumed in a diet containing moderate amounts of fibre. This value neglects any adjustment for the amino acid composition. In theory, net protein accretion will increase the requirements for essential amino acids substantially. Thus, in new tissue deposition about 50% of the amino acids have to be in the essential form whereas in adult non-growing women only about 84 mg/kg per d are required in a total of 600 mg/kg per d of total protein, i.e. 14%. Given an increment in the protein allowance from 0.75 to 0.86 g/kg per d it is evident that the theoretical proportion of essential amino acids in the whole diet will need to amount to about 19%. The 1981 Committee did not comment on this because there were no specific studies on the amino acid requirements of the pregnant woman and further research is needed to determine these. Nevertheless, it is clear that with a protein allowance of 1 g/kg per d a relatively inactive 55-kg woman with an energy need of 1800 kcal/d would require a protein/energy ratio of 12.2%. In practice, most diets contain 12%–13% protein and the proteins have more than 30% of their content as essential amino acids. It therefore does not seem likely that selective amino acid deficiency or protein deficiency will be a problem unless pregnant women consume an unusual diet.

Direct Assessment of Nutritional Status

Physicians may object to this tortuous course of theoretical analyses based on combining a host of different measures. Why not assess pregnant women's needs for protein by a more direct measure, monitoring, for example, the classic indices of protein nutritional state, e.g. the circulating levels of plasma albumin, transferrin, thyroxin-binding pre-albumin and retinol-binding protein (Shetty et al. 1979)? Unfortunately this is not possible because in pregnancy there are considerable changes in the circulating concentration of plasma proteins which will probably prove to be of profound significance. Certainly, the synthesis of hepatic export protein is under hormonal control and the marked effect of sex hormones on liver metabolism is evident in early pregnancy well before the growth of either the maternal tissues or the fetus and can constitute a major drain on the resources of protein. We thus have to conclude that the classic markers of inadequate protein intake are useless in pregnancy and one is therefore forced back to a policy of indirect measures.

One simple example of the changes in classic markers of protein metabolism is that of albumin metabolism. Plasma albumin falls in concentration by up to 25% in the first 6–20 weeks of pregnancy, but one can infer from sequential measurements of plasma volume that the total mass of circulating albumin increases once more in later pregnancy (Hytten and Chamberlain 1980). Thus, Tuttle et al. (1985) observed a 25% increase in intravascular albumin mass from the 14th week to the 35th week of pregnancy and inferred that there had been an appreciable increase in the hepatic synthesis of albumin. Yet the mass of circulating plasma proteins can be adjusted by modulating the proportion of total body albumin which circulates in the intravascular and extravascular compartments (James and Coward 1981). Thus, the initial fall and the subsequent rise in intravascular albumin mass could reflect simply an initial reduction in the lymphatic return of albumin from the extravascular tissues to be followed later in pregnancy by a progressive contraction of the extravascular mass.

Hønger (1968) has studied this in late pregnancy by monitoring the turnover of [131]-I-labelled albumin and demonstrated that the synthesis rate and fractional catabolic rate of albumin were unchanged in pregnancy. Furthermore, if one recalculates his data it becomes clear that the total mass of body albumin in the pregnant state is 221 g at 35 weeks of pregnancy compared with 236 g in the non-pregnant controls. A shift has occurred in albumin which is significantly reduced in the extravascular compartment with a rise in proportion of total albumin within the circulation itself. This shift is analogous to that seen in response to a fall in hepatic synthesis on a low protein diet (James and Hay 1968). In the case of pregnancy, however, the effects are probably produced by slow changes in vascular perfusion and interstitial colloid pressure. The control of the re-entry of albumin is little understood but in practice the fall in plasma albumin concentrations will lead to a concomitant drop in those nutrients, e.g. zinc and calcium, which are bound to albumin. These changes do not signify anything other than what appears to be a physiological response to the expansion in plasma volume.

Iron Requirements in Pregnancy

These have been repeatedly assessed and reviewed at intervals (see, for example, Bonnar and Goldberg 1969). The net requirement during pregnancy for iron has been estimated as approximately 0.5 g but during the course of blood volume expansion in early pregnancy there is a further heavy demand for iron, e.g. for haemoglobin synthesis. This amounts to about a further 0.5 g iron which has to be drawn from stores. However, unless there is heavy blood loss during delivery this can subsequently be re-used for covering the normal iron requirements of the woman and the additional demands for lactation.

The concentration of plasma iron often drops during pregnancy as the blood volume expands but the degree of fall is likely to depend on the availability of iron stores and on the degree to which the intestine can adapt its iron-absorbing mechanism. Nevertheless, one might expect a fall in all the circulating elements as the blood volume expands; the maintenance of blood concentrations must therefore signal an increase in the total plasma mass of the protein or nutrient.

A slow, progressive decline in free iron could, in theory, be responsible for the sustained rise in plasma transferrin concentration, hepatic transferrin synthesis being readily induced as iron availability in the liver declines. Since, however, transferrin synthesis is also induced in a variety of stress states, it is by no means clear that it is the iron status per se rather than the hormonal changes of pregnancy which induce these changes. Thus, in Table 4.2 there is a rise in transferrin levels despite there being no decline in serum iron in these pregnant Spanish women.

Table 4.2. Typical haematological changes and iron status of non-pregnant and pregnant females in Europe

	Non-pregnant	Pregnant, trimester		
		1st	2nd	3rd
Haemoglobin (g/dl)	13.9±1	12.6±1	11.9±1	12.5±1
Mean red cell volume (fl)	93.0±3	89.0±4	89.0±6	91.0±6
Mean corpuscular haemoglobin (g/dl)	33.0±1	34.0±1	33.0±2	33.0±1
Serum iron (μmol/l)	17.0±5	17.0±5	16.0±6	14.0±6
Transferrin (g/l)	30.0±5	32.0±5	42.0±8*	49.0±8*
Ferritin μg/l	45.0±34	28.0±19	14.0±16*	7.0±4*
Albumin (g/l)	46.0±4	45.0±3	40.0±3	41.0±2
Plasma folic acid (nmol/l)	12.0±4	13.5±5	12.0±5	12.4±9
Red cell folic acid (nmol/l)	1030.0±244	1809.0±894	1513.0±600	1383.0±663

*$P < 0.01$. Data simplified from cross-sectional studies on Spanish women (Zamorano et al. 1985)

It would seem reasonable to infer that a state of iron deficiency is common in pregnancy since transferrin saturation with iron does decline, indicating tissue iron depletion. A more sensitive index, and one which does not respond to stress as such, is the measurement of serum ferritin which below 10–15 μg/l indicates that there are no iron stores available in the marrow and other tissues for additional haemoglobin synthesis. About 30% of premenopausal women living in Northern Europe have serum ferritin concentrations below 15 μg/l and those who do have higher concentrations show a progressive decline in serum ferritin throughout pregnancy as haemopoiesis is stimulated and iron is transported to the placenta.

Given this progressive decline in serum iron and in the iron saturation of transferrin, the question arises as to how the growing fetus manages to obtain enough iron. Recent evidence has shown that the placenta has receptors for transferrin which increase markedly as pregnancy progresses. Iron-loaded transferrin is preferentially bound to yield iron for onward transport into the fetus. Thus there is a mechanism whereby the hepatic synthesis of the transport protein is induced in pregnancy and allows the transport of iron to the placenta where the abundance of receptors and the avidity of the growing fetus allows iron to pass from the mother to the child. The apoferritin is released back into the maternal circulation as the iron is transferred to the fetus (Baker et al. 1985). So effective is the selective channelling of iron that in experimental animals attempts to chelate the circulating iron lead to a fall in iron uptake by the liver but no effect on iron transfer to the placenta (Wong et al. 1987). There does therefore seem to be a very well-developed mechanism whereby maternal stores are drained of iron with selective transfer of this nutrient to the growing fetus.

Studies with iron supplementation of pregnant women have shown that 200 mg of elemental iron given daily can not only maintain haemoglobin levels but prevent the fall in serum iron and limit the decline in serum ferritin. The concentration of transferrin still increases (Puolakka 1980) so the increased hepatic synthesis of transferrin does seem to be a response to the pregnant state and not to iron deficiency per se.

Plasma Vitamin Concentrations

In Hytten and Chamberlain's summary of the physiological changes in pregnancy they emphasized the distinction between the responses of the water-soluble and fat-soluble vitamins (Hytten and Chamberlain 1980). Whereas the lipid-soluble vitamins tend to rise in association with the increase in circulating lipoprotein concentrations, the water-soluble vitamin concentrations tend to fall. Thus, there tends to be a fall in ascorbic acid, plasma folate, vitamin B_6 and biotin which some have ascribed to simple physiological dilution rather than to any specific changes. The response, however, seems to vary from study to study. This explains one of the principal difficulties in assessing nutrition during pregnancy: in many, if not in most, societies there is a strong cultural pressure to alter food intakes during pregnancy so that comparing the blood concentrations of pregnant and non-pregnant women may simply yield results which reflect the dietary practices during pregnancy in a particular culture rather than any physiological response to pregnancy. The increased physiological demand for a nutrient, e.g. folic acid, may also readily be met on some diets but not on others. Thus it is noteworthy that in a Spanish study conducted in Madrid (Table 4.2) the authors noted the high frequency of iron and folic acid deficiency in reports on nutritional deficiencies in pregnancy but found in their studies no change in folic acid concentrations. This probably reflects the much higher intake of vegetables rich in folic acid in Spain compared, for example, with Aberdeen where folate deficiency is common. Indeed, in the Spanish studies red cell folate actually increased. Perhaps dietary folate intakes were increased or more erythrocytes rich in folate during the early phase of their life span were being synthesized in women on an adequate diet.

Despite these changes there was a reduction in the total folate-binding capacity of the plasma (Zamorano et al. 1985) and this paralleled the fall in plasma vitamin B_{12}. It is not clear that these changes should be designated as a sign of deficiency since there may be marked increases in all three of the B_{12} transport proteins, transcobalamines (Fernandez-Costa and Metz 1982). Transcobalamine II is considered to be a transport protein which delivers vitamin B_{12} to peripheral tissues so if the peripheral transfer includes the placenta (as seems likely, see below), then the actual plasma concentrations in the maternal blood can be misleading. The maintenance of the plasma folic acid concentration, despite plasma dilution and the rise in red cell folate with a decline in total and unsaturated folate-binding capacity in pregnancy, cannot be explained without a clearer understanding of the mechanisms of vitamin transport through the plasma.

Placental Transfer of Water-Soluble Vitamins

Baker and his colleagues have done much to assess the concentration of water-soluble vitamins in well-nourished and malnourished mothers (Baker et al. 1981). By comparing the vitamin concentrations in maternal and neonatal blood (Table 4.3) Baker was able to establish that the concentrations of thiamine, riboflavin, nicotinic acid, pantothenic acid, vitamins B_6 and B_{12}, biotin and folate are all higher in neonatal blood than in the mother's circulation. The differences are substantial, i.e. with a neonatal/maternal ratio of about 6 or more for vitamin B_{12} and thiamine. Analyses of the placental concentrations of vitamins suggest a remarkable accumulation of folic acid, vitamin B_6 and nicotinic acid whereas the concentrations of the other vitamins were often less than those in either maternal or neonatal blood (Table 4.3). This suggests a combination of active transport into the placenta from the maternal blood and selective mechanisms for passing the vitamins on into the neonate. The basis for these differences in concentration rates are unknown but one might expect to discover eventually a biological explanation for the differences between the vitamin ratios. The special transport mechanisms can be demonstrated by in vitro perfusions of human placentae. For example, Dancis et al. (1985) showed that riboflavin was transferred by an active transport mechanism at a rate equivalent to that of glucose, the riboflavin being transported with the fetal circulation intact, whereas that retained by the placenta was metabolized, i.e. about 33%–75% was converted to the flavin mononucleotide. This transport system is not a high-capacity system as for glucose but a very effective way of concentrating the vitamin in the fetal circulation.

Table 4.3. Transport gradients for water-soluble vitamins

| | Ratio to maternal blood concentration | | | |
| | Well-nourished mother | | Malnourished mother | |
	Placental	Neonatal	Placental	Neonatal
Thiamine	0.11	2.0	0.16	4.3
Riboflavin	0.05	1.3	0.17	3.3
Nicotinic acid	16.1	1.5	26.7	1.9
B_6	23.3	1.7	48.4	1.8
Pantothenic acid	0.1	1.9	—	—
Biotin	0.8	1.4	—	—
Folic acid	5.5	2.0	10.9	3.0
B_{12}	0.3	3.5	0.4	2.4

Recalculated from average data on maternal and neonatal blood values and concentration in placental tissue given by Baker et al. (1981). Mothers were classified as malnourished for each individual vitamin where their blood values were below the normal range established by the same authors. No mothers were found with either biotin or pantothenic acid deficiency. The maternal concentrations in the malnourished category were by definition abnormally low but they had placental concentrations which were not significantly different from normal for thiamine, riboflavin, nicotinic acid and vitamin B_6 and unchanged neonatal concentrations of riboflavin and nicotinic acid. This means that the increases in ratio in these cases reflect primarily the fall in maternal concentrations

The higher concentration of all the vitamins in neonatal blood implies a well-developed transport system by the placenta. This was confirmed by Baker who monitored the response to either oral or transmuscular vitamin loading during labour. From Table 4.3 one might expect selective uptake of nicotinic acid, vitamin B_6 and folate into the placenta. Baker tested this by giving large doses of these vitamins before delivery. Only a small increase in maternal nicotinic acid blood levels was achieved but still the placental and neonatal blood concentrations were normalized in "malnourished" mothers. There was also an astonishing rise in the placental concentration of vitamin B_6 to about four times the usual concentration. Similarly, folic acid was selectively concentrated to very high levels within hours of the oral or intramuscular dose of the vitamins. The placenta retained vitamin B_6 and folic acid even when blood concentrations were falling back to normal. These loading tests therefore amplify the significance of the special transport system which must be developed during placental growth.

Table 4.3 shows that when there are low concentrations of nicotinic acid and folic acid in the maternal blood the placental gradient is extraordinarily high. It is noteworthy that nicotinic acid is fundamental to the provision of nicotinamide adenine-dinucleotide (NAD) and the oxidative metabolism of cells, a greater proportion of nicotinic acid probably being derived from tryptophan during pregnancy since oestrogens induce tryptophan dioxygenase, the first enzyme in the transformation of tryptophan to nicotinic acid (Horwitt et al. 1975). It is perhaps no coincidence that vitamin B_6 is also concentrated by the placenta: this vitamin is the coenzyme for over 60 different decarboxylation and transamination reactions, one of which is involved in the conversion of tryptophan to nicotinic acid. Folic acid is also of fundamental importance to cell metabolism so it is tempting to suggest that these three vitamins share a common attribute with a long-standing evolutionary pressure to concentrate these vitamins in the placenta.

There may, however, be some general nutritional observations of relevance. Thiamine, pantothenic acid, riboflavin and biotin are found in a large variety of foods whereas nicotinic acid, folate and vitamin B_6 are not so widely distributed. Thus the more limited availability of sources of these vitamins as well as their key metabolic roles may have proved important selective pressures. Whatever the explanation, it is evident that the placental transport differs from vitamin to vitamin and in nearly all cases there is not only a higher concentration of the vitamin in the neonatal blood but the concentration gradient is accentuated when mothers have low circulating concentrations.

Despite these concentration systems, Baker et al. (1981) showed that neonatal blood levels do fall when mothers have inadequate concentrations of vitamin B_6, folic acid and vitamin B_{12}. This response has also been demonstrated experimentally although again it is evident that the degree of depletion seen in the offspring of rodents fed a diet deficient in vitamin B_6 is less than that observed in the mother (Stipanuk and Kuo 1984). Maternal biochemical evidence of vitamin B_6 deficiency in Hispanic teenagers living in California was not found to affect the mean placental weight, birthweight or Apgar scores of their infants to a significant extent although there was a modest reduction in placental weight and infant birthweight (Martner-Hewes et al. 1986). In another study (Schuster et al. 1984) no difference in birthweights was evident in mothers with a low concentration of plasma pyridoxal phosphate and again it was observed that cord plasma levels of pyridoxeal 5'-phosphate were sustained at levels about eight times higher than in maternal blood. A placental B_6 dependent enzyme, diamine oxidase, has been found to be reduced in maternal plasma (Martner-Hewes et al. 1986) in women with B_6 deficiency and the enzyme level increases in response to oral vitamin B_6 therapy so the lower circulating concentrations of B_6 of the malnourished mothers are clearly affecting the placenta. These data emphasize the powerful concentrating capacity of the human placenta for vitamins and their ability to buffer but not eliminate the effects of maternal malnutrition on the growing fetus.

Dietary Fibre

One component of the diet which has received even less attention than the vitamins and trace elements is dietary fibre, despite the widespread occurrence of constipation in pregnancy. This constipation may relate to the prolongation of gastrointestinal transit time during the second and third trimesters which is followed by a return to normal in the postpartum period. A distinction needs to be made, however, between the transit time in the small and large intestines, the latter dominating the overall transit time of food through the intestine. Lawson et al. (1985) monitored only the small intestinal transit by timing the appearance of breath hydrogen after the ingestion of the non-digestible carbohydrate lactulose.

The transit time from the mouth to caecum was increased from 75 min to 99 min in the first trimester and to 125 and 137 min in the second and third phases. They noted that other studies show that gall bladder volume increases and lower oesophageal sphincter pressure is decreased so the effect of pregnancy is a general one on smooth muscle and presumably hormonally related because similar but more modest changes are evident in the luteal phase of the ovulatory cycle. Colonic transit time is probably also prolonged as shown by marker techniques (Wald et al. 1982) and this will have the effect of increasing bacterial fermentation of the non-starch polysaccharides entering the colon, thereby reducing faecal bulk (Stephen et al. 1986). In addition, the longer residence time in the colon will mean that there is a greater opportunity for colonic water absorption to occur thereby exacerbating further the constipation.

Anderson (1986) has shown that many British women in an attempt to limit constipation change their diet with the aim of increasing its fibre, i.e. non-starch polysaccharide content. Unfortunately they often fail to do this but if a genuine increase in fibre intake is achieved, e.g. from an average intake of about 18 g to 27 g a day, then it is effective in treating constipation (Anderson and Whichelow 1985). In Britain 38% of women on a British diet complain of constipation during pregnancy whereas in Israeli women on a much higher vegetable and fruit diet only 18% have symptoms (Levy et al. 1971). This shows the importance of the prevailing normal diet in determining the prevalence of a nutritional problem in pregnancy.

Trace Elements

This topic has been reviewed recently (Campbell 1988). Originally the fall in plasma zinc concentrations was taken to signify a state of developing zinc deficiency as the placental mechanisms concentrate zinc for transfer from the mother to the fetus. This seemed particularly likely because there are no readily demonstrable zinc storage sites so that, as is the case with many water-soluble vitamins, one might expect rapid deficiency states to develop. Campbell has noted the concordant changes of plasma zinc and plasma albumin concentrations. Despite this decline, however, there is a twofold greater concentration of zinc in cord blood than in the maternal circulation so the concentration gradient presumably ensures that the fetus can accumulate the 60 mg of zinc which it needs, about a quarter of it being present in the liver. Again, as with some vitamins, placental concentrations are higher than either maternal or cord blood levels.

Copper provides a further example of how easy it is to misinterpret blood changes when assessing nutritional state. Plasma copper rises during pregnancy in line with the increase in caeruloplasmin levels, so it is not surprising that cord blood concentrations are less than those in the maternal circulation. The fetus appears to store copper readily in early pregnancy and creates a hepatic store amounting to about half the total body stores, thus allowing the newborn baby to survive for an appreciable time with the very low intakes of copper usually found in breast milk.

From her analyses of these and other trace elements, Campbell concluded that the combination of intestinal absorption and placental transport allowed adaptive changes to occur which ensured the adequate provision of the minerals needed for normal fetal growth.

Calcium

A further example of the extraordinary metabolic adaptation during pregnancy is that involved in calcium metabolism. Fraser and Kodicek (1970) in their original demonstration of the generation of the vitamin D hormone by the kidney excluded all other organs in their search for tissues with the 1-α-hydroxylating enzyme for the conversion of 25-hydroxyvitamin D to the dihydroxy form. They forgot, however, to assess the placenta which turned out to have its own enzyme (see Pitkin 1985). This has been demonstrated in human placental tissue which also has specific cytosolic binding proteins for $1,25(OH)_2D$, similar to the well-characterized intestinal receptor.

Two colonic binding proteins are demonstrable, a calcium-dependent ATPase and a vitamin D-dependent calcium-binding protein (CaBP). The latter protein responds to exogenous $1,25(OH)_2D$, but the link between intrinsic hydroxylation of 25 OHD and calcium transport by the placenta remains uncertain (Lester 1986). Nevertheless, the plasma calcium level in the fetus remains higher than that found in maternal plasma through an active colonic transporting mechanism which appears to be finely regulated. During the course of pregnancy maternal parathormone levels increase, presumably to enhance both bone mobilization and intestinal uptake. This is needed to cope with the transport of calcium to the fetus. A much higher calcitonin concentration is found in the fetus and this presumably reflects the response of the fetus to the prevailing high levels of plasma calcium.

Conclusions

One of the themes that is beginning to emerge from nutritional studies on pregnancy is the profound metabolic adaptation which occurs. Classic approaches to assessing nutritional states are therefore inappropriate and there is a need to look more closely at the special problems of defining nutritional adequacy in pregnancy (Table 4.4).

Table 4.4. Potential approach to assessing the additional nutrient needs of pregnancy

---

1. Specify additional amount of nutrient deposited in new tissue
2. Estimate additional nutrient metabolized to achieve tissue deposition
3. Assess any specific adaptive mechanisms in the pregnant state, e.g.
   (a) enhanced absorption
   (b) selective channelling of absorbed nutrient to fetus
   (c) preferential maternal depletion with enhanced transfer to fetus

---

Given the variety of adaptive changes with increased secretion of hepatic transport proteins, the development of selective receptor sites on the placenta, the extraordinary variety of nutrient-concentrating systems in the placenta and the dual role of maternal and fetal hormones in controlling the provision of nutrients to the fetus, it is perhaps not surprising that substantial changes in maternal nutrition and weight gain are needed before appreciable effects are demonstrable on the fetus. This conclusion does not apply, however, to the very early phase of fetal life when the placenta is relatively rudimentary and the fetus more susceptible therefore to fluctuations in nutrient supply. Perhaps this physiological analysis emphasizes the need for an excellent nutritional state in the periconceptual period and early few weeks of pregnancy rather than later on in pregnancy when the unusual changes in circulating nutrient concentrations mislead by suggesting that pathological rather than physiological changes are occurring.

References

Anderson AS (1986) Dietary factors in the aetiology and treatment of constipation during pregnancy. Br J Obstet Gynaecol 93:245–249

Anderson AS, Whichelow M (1985) Constipation during pregnancy: dietary fibre intakes and the effect of fibre supplementation. Hum Nutr Appl Nutr 39A:202–207

Baker A, McArdle HJ, Morgan EH (1985) Transferrin cell interactions: studies with erythroid, placental and hepatic cells. In: Spik G, Montreuil J, Chrichton RR, Mazurier J (eds) Proteins of iron storage and transport. Elsevier, Amsterdam, pp 131–142

Baker H, Frank O, Deangelis B, Feingold S, Kaminetzky HA (1981) Role of placenta in maternal-fetal vitamin transfer in humans. Am J Obstet Gynecol 141:792–796

Bonnar J, Goldberg A (1969) The assessment of iron deficiency in pregnancy. Scott Med J 14:209–214

Campbell DM (1988) Trace element needs in human pregnancy. Proc Nutr Soc 47:45–53

Dancis J, Lehanka J, Levitz M (1985) Transfer of riboflavin by the perfused human placenta. Pediatr Res 19:1143–1146

Fernandez-Costa F, Metz J (1982) Levels of transcobalamins I, II and III during pregnancy and in cord blood. Am J Clin Nutr 35:87–94

Fraser DR, Kodicek E (1970) Unique biosynthesis by kidney of a biologically active vitamin D metabolite. Nature 228:764–766

Hønger PE (1968) Albumin metabolism in normal pregnancy. Scand J Clin Lab Invest 21:3–9

Horwitt MK, Harvey CC, Dahm CH (1975) Relationship between levels of blood lipids, vitamins C, A and E, serum copper compounds and urinary excretion of tryptophan metabolites in women taking oral contraceptive therapy. Am J Clin Nutr 28:403–412

Hytten FE, Chamberlain G (1980) Clinical physiology in obstetrics. Blackwell, Oxford

Hytten FE, Leitch I (1971) The physiology of human pregnancy, 2nd edn. Blackwell Scientific, Oxford

James WPT, Coward WA (1981) Metabolism of plasma proteins. In: Waterlow JC, Stephen JML (eds) Nitrogen metabolism in man. Applied Science Publishers, London, New Jersey, pp 457–473

James WPT, Hay AM (1968) Albumin metabolism: effect of the nutritional state and the dietary protein intake. J Clin Invest 47:1958–1972

Lawson M, Kern F, Everson GT (1985) Gastrointestinal transit time in human pregnancy: prolongation in the second and third trimesters followed by postpartum normalization. Gastroenterology 89:996–999

Lester GE (1986) Cholecalciferol and placental calcium transport. Fed Proc 45:2524–2527

Levy N, Lewberg E, Sharf M (1971) Bowel habit in pregnancy. Digestion 4:216

Martner-Hewes PM, Hunt IF, Murphy NJ, Swendseid ME, Settlage RH (1986) Vitamin B-6 nutriture and plasma diamine oxidase activity in pregnant Hispanic teenagers. Am J Clin Nutr 44:907–913

Pitkin RM (1985) Calcium metabolism in pregnancy and the perinatal period: a review. Am J Obstet Gynecol 151:99–109

Puolakka J (1980) Serum ferritin as a measure of iron stores during pregnancy. Acta Obstet Gynecol Scand [Suppl] 95

Schuster K, Bailey LB, Mahan CS (1984) Effect of maternal pyridoxine-HCl supplementation on the vitamin B-6 status of mother and infant and on pregnancy outcome. J Nutr 114:977–988

Shetty PS, Watrasiewic KE, Jung RT, James WPT (1979) Rapid-turnover transport proteins: an index of subclinical protein–energy malnutrition. Lancet II: 230–232

Stephen AM, Wiggins HS, Englyst HN, Cole TJ, Wayman BJ, Cummings JH (1986) The effect of age, sex and level of intake of dietary fibre from wheat on large bowel function in 30 healthy subjects. Br J Nutr 56:349–361

Stipanuk MH, Kuo S-M (1984) Effect of vitamin B_6 deficiency on cysteinesulfinate decarboxylase activity and taurine concentrations in tissues of rat dams and their offspring. Nutr Rep Int 30:667–679

Tuttle S, Aggett PJ, Campbell D, MacGillivray I (1985) Zinc and copper nutrition in human pregnancy: a longitudinal study in normal primigravidae and in primigravidae at risk of delivering a growth retarded baby. Am J Clin Nutr 41:1032–1041

Wald A, Van Thiel DH, Hoechstetter L et al. (1982) Effect of pregnancy on gastrointestinal transit. Dig Dis Sci 26:1015–1018

Wong CT, McArdle HJ, Morgan EH (1987) Effect of iron chelators on placental uptake and transfer of iron in rat. Am J Physiol 252:C477–C482

Zamorano AF, Arnalich F, Sanchez Casas E et al. (1985) Levels of iron, vitamin B_{12}, folic acid and their binding proteins during pregnancy. Acta Haematol 74:92–96

5. The Metabolic Basis for Birth Defects in Pregnancies Complicated by Diabetes Mellitus

N. Freinkel

By the beginning of the 1980s, perinatal mortality in pregnancies complicated by diabetes at Northwestern University Medical Center (Freinkel 1980) and several other clinics (Coustan et al. 1980; Jovanovic et al. 1980) had declined to levels that were beginning to approximate those of non-diabetic gravida. Thus, an incidence of about 2% was being observed. However, the increased frequency of birth defects associated with diabetic pregnancies had not changed (Soler et al. 1976; Pedersen 1977; Freinkel 1980; Mills 1982) and approximated the values that had persisted worldwide throughout the two to three decades in which the enhanced teratogenicity of diabetic pregnancies had been well documented (Mølsted-Pedersen et al. 1964; Kucera 1971). Indeed, during 1977 to 1981, birth defects were encountered in 4.9% of the pregnancies in our patients with "carbohydrate intolerance . . . with onset or first recognition during pregnancy" (i.e. gestational diabetes mellitus) and in 10.9% of those with known pregestational diabetes, whereas malformations were present in only 2.4% of the offspring of our concurrently enrolled gravida with normal glucoregulation (Simpson et al. 1983). Thus, in our Center, as elsewhere, congenital anomalies had become the leading cause of perinatal death in pregnancies complicated by diabetes, and represented the most compelling unresolved problem in this condition.

The basis for the diabetic embryopathy remained unexplained. However, certain important clues were beginning to emerge. Recognition that organogenesis takes place before the seventh week of gestation in the structures that are susceptible to diabetic embryopathy was becoming more widespread and highlighted the fact that the teratogenic event took place before there was awareness of pregnancy (Mills et al. 1979). As reviewed in detail elsewhere (Freinkel 1988), renewed efforts with animal models using streptozotocin (Deuchar 1977; Baker et al. 1981; Eriksson et al. 1982) rather than alloxan (Watanabe and Ingalls 1963; Endo 1966; Horii et al. 1966) as the diabetogenic agent clearly demonstrated that increased dysmorphogenesis could be replicated with experimentally induced diabetes and did not necessitate "diabetic genes". However, the animal experiments also underscored that genetic factors could influence the intrinsic susceptibility to the embryotoxic properties of "the diabetic state" (Goldman et al. 1985; Eriksson et al. 1986).

Estimates of glycosylated haemoglobin provided direct support for some relationship between the birth defects and metabolic events during early pregnancy. Thus, an association between markedly elevated values for glycosylated haemoglobin during the first trimester and malformations at birth were being reported in Europe (Leslie et al. 1978) as in the United States (Miller et al. 1981). However, the invocation of faulty maternal metabolism in the pathogenesis of diabetic embryopathy still failed to identify the specific teratogenic factor(s). For example, alterations in maternal haemodynamics, hydration, neurohumoral activity, hormonal counter-regulation and other components of poor regulation could, of themselves, affect uterine perfusion and thereby limit development of the conceptus during the tenuous early postimplantation period. Thus, more precise assessments of underlying events necessitated in vitro studies.

Studies with Rat Embryo Culture

Efforts in our laboratory were initiated in 1980 to test the proposition that aberrant fuels of maternal origin might be implicated directly, i.e. Freinkel's hypothesis that fuels and fuel-related products pharmacologically may modify phenotypic gene expression in the newly forming and differentiating cells of the conceptus and thereby modify programmed development ("fuel-mediated organ teratogenesis") (Freinkel 1980, 1981). We used outbred Charles River rats (Crl:CD®[SD]BR) and the whole embryo culture technique of New (1978) for our endeavours. This method enabled us to monitor the progression of embryogenesis in the postimplantation rat embryo from day 9.5 to day 11.5 of development (midnight of the night of mating is designated as day 0 of embryo development; the subsequent 24 h are considered the first day of gestation).

The culture precisely replicates the developmental events that occur during the same 48-h interval in the rat embryo in vivo (New 1978), i.e. the progression of the embryo from the presomite, headfold stage, and a total protein content of approximately 5 μg to the 26–29 somite stage, full neurulation and a protein content of about 150 μg. Attempts to explant the rat embryo for culture at earlier stages of development result in an increased incidence of spontaneous malformations, presumably due to increased fragility and excisional trauma (Cockroft 1984); embryo growth no longer replicates in vivo patterns when culture is extended beyond 11.5 d, presumably because the larger size of the conceptus compromises adequate diffusion and nutrient delivery (New 1978). The 48-h period from day 9.5 to day 11.5 of development in the rat embryo roughly corresponds to days 18 to 28 of human pregnancy and encompasses the interval during which such devastating consequences of faulty neural tube closure as anencephaly, meningomyelocele or spina bifida may be engendered.

For our initial experiments, we examined the dysmorphic potential of individual components of the "diabetic state" by appropriately modifying the culture medium. In our hands (Freinkel et al. 1983a, b, 1984, 1986) as in the prior pioneer studies of Cockroft and Coppola (1977) and Sadler (1980a), supplementation of the culture medium with "high glucose" elicited growth retardation and such developmental abnormalities during 48 h of culture as fusion of anterior and posterior neural folds, microcephaly and faulty formations of eyes, somites, vasculature, heart etc. The failure to replicate the dysmorphogenesis with equimolar isosmotic additions of hexoses such as sorbitol, fructose, inositol or galactose (Freinkel et al. 1984) documented the specificity of glucose. In keeping with pharmacological mechanisms, the effects of "high glucose" displayed clear concentration dependencies. Thus, during the period of these studies (1980–1982), isosmotic additions of 12 mg/ml D-glucose during culture from day 9.5 to day 11.5 of development elicited minor lesions in 49% and major lesions in 23% of the embryos. By contrast, supplementation of culture mediums with 9 mg/ml D-glucose elicited only 5.1% major and 17.8% minor lesions; 6 mg/ml resulted in only a 2.2% incidence of minor lesions and no major lesions; and 3 mg/ml evoked no discernible malformations (Freinkel et al. 1986). Exposure to "high glucose" for shorter periods disclosed that the dysmorphic properties of hyperglycaemia in the rat embryo were confined to the developmental period preceding the formation of 12–16 somites. Similar temporal limits to the embryotoxic effects of "high glucose" have also been observed by others (Sadler 1980a; Garnham et al. 1983; Cockroft 1984). Indeed, Cockroft (1984) has reported that substantially smaller amounts of glucose suffice to elicit dysmorphogenesis in the cultured rat embryo when the exposure is initiated at day 9.0 rather than day 9.5 of development, i.e. at the primitive streak to neural plate stage of embryogenesis.

However, diabetes is not a disorder of only a single fuel; multiple fuels may be disturbed. Thus, simultaneous and independent in vitro studies with mouse embryos (Horton and Sadler 1983; Horton et al. 1985) and with rat embryos (Lewis et al. 1983; Freinkel et al. 1986) indicated that supplementations of culture mediums with D,L-β-hydroxybutyrate can also retard growth and effect malformations. With ketones, as with glucose, the dysmorphic effects were shown to be dose-dependent and the lesions were of increasing severity as the concentration of ambient β-hydroxybutyrate was increased. Our laboratory was the first to suggest that additive and/or synergistic interactions between fuels can occur as part of "fuel-mediated organ teratogenesis" (Lewis et al. 1983). By combining subteratogenic amounts of glucose with subteratogenic amounts of β-hydroxybutyrate during 48-h culture of embryos from Charles River Crl:CD®(SD) BR rats, we elicited a devastating synergy of dysmorphogenesis. Amounts of D-glucose and D,L-β-hydroxybutyrate which caused no major lesions when tested individually produced a 27.7% incidence of major lesions by day 11.5 of development when added in combination (Lewis et al. 1983; Freinkel et al. 1986).

As yet, the possibilities of additive and/or synergistic interactions with other fuels which also may be disturbed in poorly regulated diabetes (e.g. amino acids, free fatty acids, triglycerides) remain to be evaluated. However, certain additional facets of the "diabetic state" have displayed definite teratogenic capabilities. For example, hyperosmolarity has been shown to synergize the dysmorphic properties of "high glucose" in embryo culture (Cockroft and Coppola 1977; Cockroft 1984) and we have noted that the capacity of serum from streptozotocin-diabetic rats to induce malformations in cultured embryos (Sadler 1980b) may parallel their net content of "somatomedin inhibitor(s)" (Cockroft et al. 1981; Freinkel et al. 1986). Sadler et al. (1986) have obtained growth retardation and teratogenesis in cultured mouse embryos by adding purified "somatomedin inhibitor" (of molecular weight 940) isolated from the serum of streptozotocin-diabetic rats. Thus, the presently available findings from rodent whole embryo culture have provided compelling evidence that diabetic embryopathy may be mediated in multifactorial fashion and that "fuel-mediated organ teratogenesis" is contributory (Freinkel et al. 1986; Freinkel 1988).

Clinical Extrapolation

The above clinical and laboratory observations prompted worldwide efforts to diminish the incidence of diabetic embryopathy by improving maternal diabetes regulation during early embryogenesis via intensification of preconceptional and periconceptional management (Pedersen and Mølsted-Petersen 1979; Freinkel 1980; Steel et al. 1980; Fuhrmann et al. 1983; Mills et al. 1983; Ballard et al. 1984; Fuhrmann et al. 1984). Special "prepregnancy clinics" for IDDMs were established and prospective studies were initiated to test the validity of the putative "metabolism–birth defect" relationships. Initial reports from East Germany were completely corroborative; in two consecutive series from 1977–1981 (Fuhrmann et al. 1983) and 1981–1983 (Fuhrmann et al. 1984), the incidence of birth defects in the offspring of diabetic mothers in East Germany was reduced to that of non-diabetic women when intensification of diabetes regulation was initiated prior to pregnancy whereas birth defects remained four- to five-fold more frequent when the same level of diabetes control was deferred until 8 or more weeks of pregnancy. Others have reported similar salutory effects of preconceptional intensification of diabetes control, although the limited number of patients in these series has precluded assessment of statistical significance (Steel 1985; Goldman et al. 1986).

By contrast, the recent experiences in National Institutes of Health-sponsored multicentre study have introduced some complexities (Mills et al. 1988). Herein, birth defects were encountered in 4.9% of the pregnancies of women with pregestational diabetes who were enrolled for observations prior to day 21 of pregnancy ("early entry") compared with birth defects in 2.1% of the women with normal glucoregulation enrolled at comparably early time-points, and 9.0% in women with known diabetes in whom observations commenced after day 21 of pregnancy ("late entry"). However, the seeming benefits of "early entry" were not clearly correlated with glycaemic control; levels of glycosylated haemoglobin or plasma glucose during organogenesis (as assessed by measurements secured from 5 weeks after the last menstrual period onward) were not significantly different in the mothers from the "early entry" group whose offspring had birth defects than in those whose offspring did not (Mills et al. 1988).

Although the multicentre study was not designed to test the effects of "tight" diabetes control per se, and more detailed scrutiny of the data has indicated that levels of glycosylated haemoglobin were actually higher in those "early entry" mothers whose offspring had the most serious birth defects (i.e. "severe or fatal", or "seriously handicapping"), the seemingly conflicting findings highlight the limitations of our existing knowledge concerning diabetic embryopathy. For example, as of April 1988 (a) the precise teratogen(s) have not been identified in any study; (b) *none* of the published reports have included measurements of multiple fuels so that the possibility of teratogenic effects via additive and/or synergistic fuel interactions cannot be evaluated; and (c) none have provided sufficiently detailed temporal documentation to assess the possibility of changing levels of susceptibility at different time-points in *early* organogenesis. Thus, definitive conclusions concerning precise therapeutic end points must be deferred pro tem. However, several of our more recent animal studies, summarized below, may have relevance for some of these unresolved questions.

The "Honeybee Syndrome" and Implications for Periconceptional Management of Diabetes

While testing hexoses other than glucose for dysmorphogenic potential in rat embryo culture, we found (Freinkel et al. 1983b, 1984) that the epimer of D-glucose, D-mannose, has extraordinary embryotoxicity during the period in which the postimplantation rat conceptus is wholly dependent upon glycolysis (Shepard et al. 1970; Tanimura and Shepard 1970; Neubert et al. 1971) (i.e. before about day 10.8 of development). Addition of as little as 1.5 mg/ml mannose to growth culture mediums containing 1.2 mg/ml glucose during that interval caused retarded embryo growth and gross dysmorphogenesis (Freinkel et al. 1983b, 1984). The added mannose did not modify the total "uptake" of hexoses (glucose plus mannose) but reduced glycolysis (i.e. formation of lactic acid) by about 20%. Such dysmorphic and metabolic actions were not seen when D-mannose was added to growth culture after about day 10.8. Moreover, we were able to diminish the teratogenicity of D-mannose before day 10.8 either by adding more glucose to the culture medium and thereby restoring lactic acid production to normal, or by culturing the conceptuses in a higher O_2 atmosphere to reduce their glycolytic dependence (Freinkel 1983b, 1984). Accordingly, we have ascribed most of the dysmorphogenic properties of mannose to the ability of this hexone to impair glycolytic flux during the period of glycolytic dependence in the postimplantation rat conceptus.

We have now shown that the glycolytic inhibition is due to a relative immaturity in the mechanisms for processing mannose-6-P in the conceptus of this time (Freinkel N, Passonneau JF, Lewis NJ, Akazawa S, Gorman L, Gutierrez J, unpublished observations). Comparably toxic actions of mannose had been observed previously only in the honeybee (von Frisch 1928; Staudenmayer 1939) and also attributed to an inhibition of glycolysis (Sols et al. 1960). We have designated this phenomenon as the "Honeybee Syndrome" (Freinkel et al. 1983b, 1984) and suggested a generic usefulness for the term to describe a transitory period in the life of the early postimplantation embryos during which there is inordinate teratogenic vulnerability to *any* agent capable of even mild interruptions of glycolysis.

The manifest sensitivity of the rodent embryo to interrupted glycolysis during the period of glycolytic dependence prompted our suggestion that the glucopenia of simple hypoglycaemia might exert similar teratogenic actions (Freinkel et al. 1985). To examine this premise under conditions which approximated clinical events, we tested the effects of brief periods of hypoglycaemica in the intact pregnant rat (Buchanan et al. 1986). We administered 60-min infusions of insulin on either day 9.5 or day 9.75 of gestation by square-wave delivery to effect circumscribed periods of hypoglycaemia in conscious mothers. To control for potential teratogenic effects of the insulin per se, we also infused similar amounts of insulin into paired "control" pregnant rats but "clamped" them at normoglycaemia by the concurrent administration of glucose.

The insulin infusions produced mean maternal insulin levels of 290–318 μU/ml throughout the 60-min interval on day 9.5 or 9.75 (Buchanan et al. 1986). In the absence of exogenous dextrose, plasma glucose levels fell rapidly from preinfusion levels of approximately 140–145 mg/dl to values of 40–45 mg/dl at the end of the 60 min. All mothers remained conscious and responsive to tactile stimuli throughout this period of hypoglycaemia. Plasma glucose levels were then restored to preinfusion levels with exogenous glucose within 20 min after the insulin was stopped. In the pair-matched euglycaemic "control" animals, the "glucose-clamping" preserved plasma glucose at preinfusion levels throughout the 60-min period of insulin infusion. Hysterotomy was performed on day 11.6 of gestation to evaluate the effects of the insulin infusions on the subsequent development of the embryos. Mean litter size and total resorbed conceptuses were not significantly different in the "hypoglycaemic" and "euglycaemic" groups. However, morphometric examinations disclosed significantly lower values for crown–rump length and somite number in the embryos from the "hypoglycaemic" group, and compositional analyses revealed significant diminutions in the total embryo content of protein and DNA. Moreover, dysmorphic changes were present on day 11.6 in 12 of the 275 embryos from the "hypoglycaemic" mothers but in only one of the 281 embryos from the "euglycaemic" mothers.

The lesions were not confined to isolated litters; malformations were present in embryos from three of the 10 mothers rendered hypoglycaemic on day 9.5 and five of the 10 mothers rendered hypoglycaemic on day 9.75 (Buchanan et al. 1986). Clearly, insulin itself was not the cause of the dysmorphogenesis since plasma insulin levels had not been different in the "euglycaemic" than in the "hypoglycaemic" mothers. Moreover, daily food intakes and weight gains had been similar in both groups so that differences in maternal nutrition cannot be invoked to explain the developmental abnormalities. It would therefore seem likely that the growth retardations and malformations resulted from the briefly diminished availability of glucose to the embryo during periods of glycolytic dependency (Buchanan et al. 1986).

However, the possibility that maternal counter-regulatory responses to the hypoglycaemia may have contributed to the manifest embryotoxicity cannot be excluded. Thus, an additional experimental approach has been employed to examine the developmental consequences of intracellular glucopenia in the embryo in vivo during the period of glycolytic dependence. The evanescent selective embryotoxicity of mannose in the embryo (Freinkel et al. 1983b, 1984) has provided us with a unique tool for such in vivo efforts (Buchanan et al. 1985). As summarized above, D-mannose can disrupt the growth and development of the early postimplantation rat conceptus by blocking glycolysis while the conceptus is still wholly dependent upon aerobic glycolysis. By contrast, later embryos and fetuses and adult rats are essentially unaffected by similar concentrations of mannose since they can metabolize mannose fully and utilize mannose and glucose interchangeably. Thus, mannose can be used in vivo to perturb metabolism specifically in the early postimplantation embryos without causing untoward effects in mothers. Moreover, the rapid disappearance of mannose from the circulation in the rat [$t\frac{1}{2}$ approximately 17 min; (Buchanan et al. 1985)] enables the perturbation to be instituted in a precisely timed fashion.

For the initial application of this novel approach to experimental teratogenesis, we delivered mannose into conscious, unrestrained pregnant rats by equilibrium infusions during the 12-h interval encompassing the establishment of the neural plate and the early fusion of the neural folds, that is day 9.5–10.0 of embryo development (Buchanan et al. 1985). Control pregnant animals were infused with equimolar amounts of glucose. The infused mannose effected plasma mannose levels of 168±7 and 188±5 mg/dl over the course of the infusions; concurrent plasma levels of glucose declined from 145±3 mg/dl preinfusion to 64±3 mg/dl during the last 3 h of the 12-h infusion period. Resultant plasma mannose/glucose ratios ranged from 2.1±0.1 at 1 h to 2.9±0.1 after 9 h of infusion so that mannose in vivo, as in vitro, could effectively compete with glucose for phosphorylation by hexokinase. The infusion of mannose did not disturb any aspect of maternal wellbeing (including brain metabolism as judged by the constancy of maternal rectal temperature). However, at hysterotomy 36 h later on day 11.6, all of the embryos from the mannose-infused mothers displayed generalized growth retardation, and 8.9% of them had specific dysmorphic changes (Buchanan et al. 1985). The studies provided further in vivo evidence that impaired growth and malformations may occur following transitory interruption of glycolysis in the early postimplantation embryo and then these phenomena may be triggered independently of any manifest disruption of homeostasis in the mother.

We have used the mannose infusion technique for more recent attempts (Weigensberg et al. 1988) to document the temporal variations in the vulnerability of the early postimplantation embryo to "fuel-mediated organ teratogenesis". Herein, we have infused mannose into pregnant rats for 12 h on day 8.5–9 of gestation, that is with the embryo at the primitive streak stage, or on day 9.5–10, that is with the embryo at the presomite headfold stage. The experiments were designed to see whether the developmental consequences of metabolic perturbations are different at these two phases of embryogenesis. Control rats were given no infusions at all or infused with equimolar amounts of glucose. The 8.5- and 9.5-day infusions of mannose produced similar plasma levels of mannose and glucose in the mother at both time points. However, at hysterotomy and examination of the embryos on day 11.6, manifest growth delay was far more pronounced in the embryos from the mothers which had been infused with mannose on day 8.5, and the incidence of malformations was eightfold greater. The heightened malformations in the embryos from the 8.5-day infused mothers consisted principally of microencephaly and faulty neural tube fusions. Thus developing neural structures may be inordinately vulnerable to metabolic interruption far earlier than hitherto suspected, and perhaps, maximally so even before the headfold is formed (Weigensberg et al. 1988).

The above exquisite sensitivity of the rodent embryo to glucose deprivation during the period of glycolytic dependence has now been confirmed in vitro in three separate laboratories with whole embryo culture under conditions of hypoglycaemia (Akazawa et al. 1987; Ellington 1987; Sadler and Hunter 1987). By contrast, similar degrees of hypoglycaemia do not seem to have teratogenic actions during later phases of embryogenesis in the rat when oxidative metabolism via the Krebs cycle has supervened, and alternative sources of fuel fulfilment are operative [i.e. from about day 10.8 of development onward (Buchanan and Sipos 1987)].

Comparable data with regard to metabolic dependencies in the early postimplantation human conceptus are not available. Thus, we do not know whether an analogous phase of dependence upon aerobic glycolysis ever obtains as part of normal human embryogenesis. However, if human patterns replicate those that have been described in rodents, and the developmental timetables are similar, the postimplantation human embryo may also be dependent upon uninterrupted access to normal ambient glucose during the interval in organogenesis which extends from the formation of the primitive streak (on about day 16–18 of gestation), to the closure of the anterior neural pore (on about day 24–25 of gestation). Moreover, the relative vulnerabilities may also vary at different times during that short-lived interval. Within that framework, some caveats concerning insulin therapy during the first 3 to 4 weeks of human pregnancy may not be inappropriate (Freinkel et al. 1985; Buchanan et al. 1986; Freinkel 1988).

It has now been documented that intensive insulin therapy cannot be instituted without concomitant increases in the frequency of hypoglycaemic reactions (The DCCT Research Group 1987). Moreover, the limitations of subjective awareness of hypoglycaemia (Sussman et al. 1963) have been underscored by the recent finding that sympathetic activation in response to hypoglycaemia progressively diminishes with improvement in glycaemic control (Heller et al. 1987). Indeed, hypoglycaemic unawareness seems to develop with increased frequency in the very tightly regulated diabetic patient (Amiel et al. 1988). For the moment therefore, until we know more about the metabolic dependencies of the early human postimplantation conceptus, some caution appears to be indicated in periconceptional programmes of insulin treatment. "Near normalization" (that is, regulation to levels of glycosylate haemoglobin which are slightly above the upper limits of normal), rather than "full normalization" (that is regulation to levels of glycosylated haemoglobin which are within two standard deviations of mean values for the reference laboratory), may well constitute the most prudent periconceptional therapeutic goal for those who, like the author, favour "meticulous control" at all other time-points in pregnancies complicated by diabetes mellitus.

General Summary

The past few years have generated important new insights concerning the pathogenesis of diabetic embryopathy. The expectation that we may be on the threshold of resolving this last enigmatic aspect of pregnancies complicated by diabetes seems well founded. However, in planning or interpreting future clinical efforts, certain lessons from existing animal studies may be useful. Firstly, it is apparent that no single parameter of the diabetic state can be viewed in isolation in attempts to correlate diabetic embryopathy with maternal "control"; dose–response relationships must be viewed in the context of multiple fuel interactions. Secondly, the entire early postimplantation period cannot be regarded as a fixed interval during which vulnerability to "fuel-mediated organ teratogenesis" remains constant; metabolic documentation must include more temporal stratifications. Thirdly, awareness of changing metabolic dependencies in the conceptus must be incorporated into therapeutic efforts; treatment strategies must acknowledge the theoretical possibility that "over-therapy" may be as harmful as "under-therapy" during that transitory phase of embryogenesis in which a full metabolic repertoire has not yet been established and glycolytic dependence may obtain. And finally, any attempts to extrapolate global experiences to the individual patient, or even to a single racial or ethnic group, must be tempered by the appreciation that there may be genetic differences in the susceptibility to "fuel-mediated organ teratogenesis" and to diabetic embryopathy.

Acknowledgement—This work was supported in part by Research grants DK–10699, HD–19070, RR48 and Training Grant DK–07169 from the National Institutes of Health.

The author is indebted to the following colleagues who have collaborated in various phases of the studies cited above: Shoichi Akazawa, Thomas Buchanan, David L, Cockroft, Paco Garcia-Palmer, Lisa Gorman, Nancy Jo Lewis, Boyd E. Metzger, Janet V. Passonneau, Lawrence S. Phillips, Mary Potaczek, Sanford I. Roth, Joyce K. Schemmer, George E. Shambaugh III, Robert Sobel and Marc Weigensberg.

The excellent assistance of Rebecca Jones and Carole Herhold in the preparation of this manuscript is also gratefully acknowledged.

References

Akazawa S, Akazawa M, Hashimoto M et al. (1987) Effects of hypoglycaemia on early embryogenesis in rat embryo organ culture. Diabetologia 30:791–796

Amiel SA, Sherwin RS, Simonson DC, Tamborlane WV (1988) Effect of intensive insulin therapy on glycemic thresholds for counterregulatory hormone release. Diabetes 37:901–907

Baker L, Egler JM, Klein SH, Goldman AS (1981) Meticulous control of diabetes during organogenesis prevents congenital lumbosacral defects in rats. Diabetes 30:955–959

Ballard JL, Holroyde J, Tsang RC, Chan G, Sutherland JM, Knowles HC (1984) High malformation rates and decreased mortality in infants of diabetic mothers managed after the first trimester of pregnancy (1956–1978). Am J Obstet Gynecol 148:1111–1118

Buchanan TA, Sipos GF (1987) The teratogenic effects of brief maternal insulin-hypoglycemia in the rat are limited to early organogenesis. 69th Annual Meeting of the Endocrinology Society, Indianapolis, IN, 10–12 June, Abstract no. 323

Buchanan T, Freinkel N, Lewis NJ, Metgzer BE, Akazawa S (1985) Fuel-mediated teratogenesis. Use of D-mannose to modify organogenesis in the rat embryo in vivo. J Clin Invest 75:1927–1934

Buchanan TA, Schemmer JK, Freinkel N (1986) Embryotoxic effects of brief maternal insulin-hypoglycemia during organogenesis in the rat. J Clin Invest 78:643–649

Cockroft DL (1984) Abnormalities induced in cultured rat embryos by hyperglycaemia. Br J Exp, Pathol 65:625–636

Cockroft DL, Coppola PT (1977) Teratogenic effects of excess glucose on head-fold rat embryos in culture. Teratology 16:141–146

Cockroft DL, Freinkel N, Phillips LS, Shambaugh GE (1981) Metabolic factors affecting organogenesis in diabetic pregnancy. Clin Res 29:577A

Coustan DR, Berkowitz RL, Hobbins JC (1980) Tight metabolic control of overt diabetes in pregnancy. Am J Med 68:845–852

DCCT Research Group: Diabetes Control and Complications Trial (DCCT) (1987) Results of feasibility study. Diabetes Care 10:1–19

Deuchar EM (1977) Embryonic malformations in rats, resulting from maternal diabetes: preliminary observations. J Embryol Exp Morphol 41:93–99

Ellington SKL (1987) Development of rat embryos cultured in glucose-deficient media. Diabetes 36:1372–1378

Endo A (1966) Teratogenesis in diabetic mice treated with alloxan prior to conception. Arch Environ Health 21:492–500

Eriksson UJ, Dahlström E, Larsson KS, Hellerström C (1982) Increased incidence of congenital malformations in the offspring of diabetic rats and their prevention by maternal insulin therapy. Diabetes 31:1–6

Eriksson UJ, Dahlström E, Lithell HO (1986) Diabetes in pregnancy: influence of genetic background and maternal diabetic state on the incidence of skeletal malformations in the fetal rat. Acta Endocrinol (Suppl 277): 66–73

Freinkel N (1980) The Banting Lecture 1980: Of pregnancy and progeny. Diabetes 29:1023–1035

Freinkel N (1981) Pregnant thoughts about metabolic control and diabetes. N Engl J Med 304:1357–1359

Freinkel N (1988) Diabetic embryopathy and fuel-mediated teratogenesis: lessons from animal models. Horm Metab Res (in press)

Freinkel N, Metzger BE, Cockroft D et al. (1983a) Inquiries into maternal metabolism: past, present and future – A progress report from the Northwestern University Diabetes in Pregnancy Center. In: Proceedings of the 11th Congress of the International Diabetes Federation, Nairobi, Kenya, 10–17 November 1982. (EN Mngola, ed.) Excerpta Medica, Amsterdam, pp 423–427

Freinkel N, Lewis NJ, Akazawa S, Gorman L, Potaczek M (1983b) The "honeybee syndrome": teratogenic effects of mannose during organogenesis in rat embryo culture. Trans Assoc Am Physicians 96:44–55

Freinkel N, Lewis NJ, Akazawa S, Roth SI, Gorman L (1984) The honeybee syndrome – implications of the teratogenicity of mannose in rat embryo culture. N Engl J Med 310:223–230

Freinkel N, Dooley SL, Metzger BE (1985) Care of the pregnant woman with insulin-dependent diabetes mellitus. N Engl J Med 313:96–101

Freinkel N, Cockroft DL, Lewis NJ et al. (1986) The 1986 McCollum Award Lecture. Fuel-mediated teratogenesis during early organogenesis: the effects of increased concentrations of glucose, ketones, or somatomedin inhibitor during rat embryo culture. Am J Clin Nutr 44:986–995

Fuhrmann K, Reiher H, Semmler K, Fischer F, Fischer M, Glöckner E (1983) Prevention of congenital malformations in infants of insulin-dependent diabetic mothers. Diabetes Care 6:219–223

Fuhrmann K, Reiher H, Semmler K, Glöckner E (1984) The effect of intensified conventional insulin therapy before and during pregnancy on the malformation rate in offspring of diabetic mothers. Exp Clin Endocrinol 83:173–177

Garnham EA, Beck F, Clarke CA, Stanisstreet M (1983) Effects of glucose on rat embryos in culture. Diabetologia 25:291–295

Goldman AS, Baker L, Piddington R, Marx B, Herold R, Egler J (1985) Hyperglycemia-induced teratogenesis is mediated by a functional deficiency of arachidonic acid. Proc Natl Acad Sci USA 82:8227–8231

Goldman JA, Dicker D, Feldberg D, Yeshaya A, Samuel N, Karp M (1986) Pregnancy outcome in patients with insulin-dependent diabetes mellitus with preconceptional diabetic control: a comparative study. Am J Obstet Gynecol 155:293–297

Heller SR, Macdonald IA, Herbert M, Tattersall RB (1987) Influence of sympathetic nervous system on hypoglycaemic warning symptoms. Lancet II: 359–363

Horii K, Watanabe G, Ingalls TH (1966) Experimental diabetes in pregnant mice. Prevention of congenital malformations in offspring by insulin. Diabetes 15:194–204

Horton WE Jr, Sadler TW (1983) Effects of maternal diabetes on early embryogenesis. Alterations in morphogenesis produced by the ketone body, B-hydroxybutyrate. Diabetes 32:610–616

Horton WE Jr, Sadler TW, Hunter ES III (1985) Effects of hyperketonemia on mouse embryonic and fetal glucose metabolism in vitro. Teratology 31:227–233

Jovanovic L, Peterson CM, Saxena BB, Dawood MY, Saudek CD (1980) Feasibility of maintaining normal glucose profiles in insulin-dependent pregnant diabetic women. Am J Med 68:105–112

Kucera J (1971) Rate and type of congenital anomalies among offspring of diabetic women. J Reprod Med 7:61–70

Leslie RDG, Pyke DA, John PN, White JM (1978) Haemoglobin A_1 in diabetic pregnancy. Lancet II: 958–959

Lewis NJ, Akazawa S, Freinkel N (1983) Teratogenesis from β-hydroxybutyrate during organogenesis in rat embryo organ culture and enhancement by subteratogenic glucose. Diabetes 32 (Suppl): 11A

Miller E, Hare JW, Cloherty JP et al. (1981) Elevated maternal hemoglobin A_{1c} in early pregnancy and major congenital anomalies in infants of diabetic mothers. N Engl J Med 304:1331–1334

Mills JL (1982) Malformations in infants of diabetic mothers. Teratology 25:385–394

Mills JL, Baker L, Goldman AS (1979) Malformations in infants of diabetic mothers occur before the seventh gestational week. Implications for treatment. Diabetes 28:292–293

Mills JL, Fishl AR, Knopp RH et al. (1983) Malformations in infants of diabetic mothers: problems in study design. Prev Med 12:274–286

Mills JL, Knopp RH, Simpson JL et al. (1988) Lack of relation of increased malformation rates in infants of diabetic mothers to glycemic control during organogenesis. N Engl J Med 318:671–676

Mølsted-Pedersen L, Tygstrup I, Pedersen J (1964) Congenital malformations in newborn infants of diabetic women. Lancet I:1124–1126

Neubert D, Peters H, Teske S, Köhler E, Barach H-J (1971) Studies on the problem of "aerobic glycolysis" occurring in mammalian embryos. Naunyn Schmiedebergs Arch Pharmacol 268:235–241

New DAT (1978) Whole-embryo culture and the study of mammalian embryos during organogenesis. Biol Rev 53:81–122

Pedersen J (1977) The pregnant diabetic and her newborn. Problems and management. Williams & Wilkins Company, Baltimore

Pedersen J, Mølsted-Pedersen L (1979) Congenital malformations: the possible role of diabetes care outside pregnancy. In: Pregnancy, metabolism, diabetes and the fetus. CIBA Foundation Symposium No. 63. Excerpta Medica, Amsterdam, pp 265–271

Sadler TW (1980a) Effects of maternal diabetes on early embryogenesis. I. The teratogenic potential of diabetic serum. Teratology 21:339–347

Sadler TW (1980b) Effects of maternal diabetes on early embryogenesis. II. Hyperglycaemia-induced exencephaly. Teratology 21:349–356

Sadler TW, Hunter ES III (1987) Hypoglycemia: how little is too much for the embryo? Am J Obstet Gynecol 157:190–193

Sadler TW, Phillips LS, Balkan W, Goldstein S (1986) Somatomedin inhibitors from diabetic rat serum alter growth and development of mouse embryos in culture. Diabetes 35:861–865

Shepard TH, Tanimura T, Robkin MA (1970) Energy metabolism in early mammalian embryos. Symp Soc Dev Biol 29:42–58

Simpson JL, Elias S, Martin AO, Palmer MS, Ogata ES, Radvany RA (1983) Diabetes in pregnancy, Northwestern University series (1977–1981) I. Prospective study of anomalies in offspring of mothers with diabetes mellitus. Am J Obstet Gynecol 146:263–270

Soler NG, Walsh CH, Malins JM (1976) Congenital malformations in infants of diabetic mothers. Q J Med 45:303–313

Sols A, Cadenas E, Alvarado F (1960) Enzymatic basis of mannose toxicity in honey bees. Science 131:297–298

Staudenmayer T (1939) Die Giftigkeit der Mannose für Bienen und andere Insekten. Z Vergleich Physiol 26:644–668

Steel JM (1985) Prepregnancy counseling and contraception in the insulin-dependent diabetic patient. Clin Obstet Gynaecol 28:553–568

Steel JM, Parboosingh J, Cole RA, Duncan LJP (1980) Prepregnancy counseling: a logical prelude to the management of the pregnant diabetic woman. Diabetes Care 3:371–373

Sussman KE, Crout JR, Marble A (1963) Failure of warning in insulin-induced hypoglycemic reactions. Diabetes 12:38–45

Tanimura T, Shepard TH (1970) Glucose metabolism by rat embryos in vitro. Proc Soc Exp Biol Med 135:51–54

von Frisch VK (1928) Versuche über den Geschmackssinn der Bienen. Naturwissenschaften 16:307–315

Watanabe G, Ingalls TH (1963) Congenital malformations in the offspring of alloxan-diabetic mice. Diabetes 12:66–72

Weigensberg M, Sobel R, Garcia-Palmer F, Freinkel N (1988) Temporal differences in vulnerability to "fuel-mediated organ teratogenesis." Diabetes (Suppl 1): 85A

6. Diabetes in Pregnancy: Genetic and Temporal Relationships of Maldevelopment in the Offspring of Diabetic Rats

U. J. Eriksson, J. Styrud and R. S. M. Eriksson

Introduction

The aetiology of the dysmorphogenesis (Miller 1946; Naeye 1965; Kucera 1971) and embryo–fetal wastage (Pedersen 1977; Pedersen and Mølsted-Pedersen 1982; Sutherland and Pritchard 1986) found in the offspring of diabetic mothers is unknown (Freinkel 1980; Mills 1982). To study this problem we have used a rat model in which female rats are made manifestly diabetic with streptozotocin 1–4 weeks prior to mating with non-diabetic males (Eriksson et al. 1980). The animals are an outbred substrain of Sprague–Dawley albino rats, which was originally imported from Zentralinstitut für Versuchtiersucht (Hanover, FRG) to a Swedish commercial breeding institution in 1962 (Anticimex/ALAB, Sollentuna, Sweden). In 1982 the colony was moved to our Department in Uppsala (hence, these animals are denoted U rats) and the Swedish breeder re-imported new outbred Sprague–Dawley rats from the original colony in Hanover (called H rats in the following; see also Fig. 6.1).

Despite their common origin, the effect of maternal diabetes on fetal

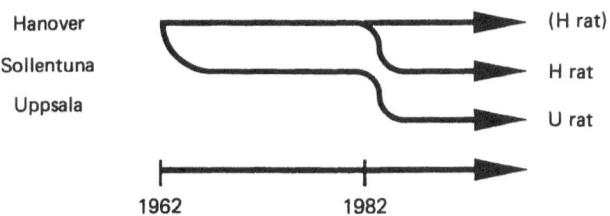

Fig. 6.1. Geographical and genetic interrelationships between the U and H rats of Sprague–Dawley origin.

development in these two substrains of rats is quite different (Eriksson et al. 1982, 1983a, 1986). When maternal diabetes is induced in the U rats prior to gestation we find skeletal malformations in 15%–20% of the liveborn offspring. About two-thirds of these are micrognathia (underdevelopment of the lower jaw, see Fig. 6.2a) and about one-third are sacral dysgenesis (underdevelopment of the sacral and lumbar vertebrae and absence of tail, see Fig. 6.2b). These two malformations are rarely seen in the same fetus.

In normal U rats we occasionally see liveborn fetuses without tails (less than 1%), whereas we have never found micrognathia in the offspring of a non-diabetic U rat. Furthermore, we have failed to detect any skeletal malformations in H offspring, regardless of whether or not the mother is diabetic (Fig. 6.3).

The skeletal malformations in the U offspring are dependent upon the maternal diabetic state, since the induction of diabetes with alloxan produces a similar malformation rate and insulin treatment of diabetic U rats (one daily subcutaneous dose of 4–8 IU Novo Ultralente Insulin) reduces the malformation rate by 75% (Eriksson et al. 1982) (Fig. 6.3).

We have also found a relationship between one of the malformations and the zinc levels of the offspring of U rats. Manifest diabetes (MD) changes the trace metal levels in the offspring; in particular the fetal zinc content is decreased by about 25% (Eriksson 1984). By feeding pregnant, non-diabetic U and H rats a zinc-depleted diet we reduced the fetal levels of this trace metal to levels comparable with those found in MD offspring. In the zinc-depleted normal (N) (U) fetuses we then found some malformations of the sacral dysgenesis type, whereas no malformations were seen in the offspring of H rats given the same diet (Styrud et al. 1986) (Fig. 6.4).

Supplementing the pregnant MD (U) rats with extra zinc in the drinking water did not alter the rate of skeletal malformations in the offspring, indicating that the decreased zinc concentration in the MD (U) fetuses did not correspond to lowered levels in the mother (Eriksson 1984).

Genetic Predisposition

To further characterize the genetic component of the malformations in the offspring of diabetic (U) rats we evaluated the fetal outcome in U and H rats and in hybrids between them (Eriksson 1988). We cross-mated U and H rats, and also used an F_1 hybrid (of U and H rats), to investigate whether the predisposition of the U strain towards congenital malformations in diabetic pregnancy was primarily associated with the genome of the mother or with the genetic composition of the conceptus.

In the normal rats, we found no malformations and only 3%–5% resorptions (Table 6.1). Induction of diabetes in the mother led to increased resorption rates in all groups. The MD(H) mothers showed the lowest incidence of resorptions among the diabetic rats (8%–9%) and produced no malformed fetuses in a U × H cross-mating combination. This was in contrast to the MD(U/H) and MD(U) rats (carrying U/H offspring) who displayed high resorption rates (16%–21%) and some malformations (3%–5%, see Table 6.1), indicating the occurrence of a

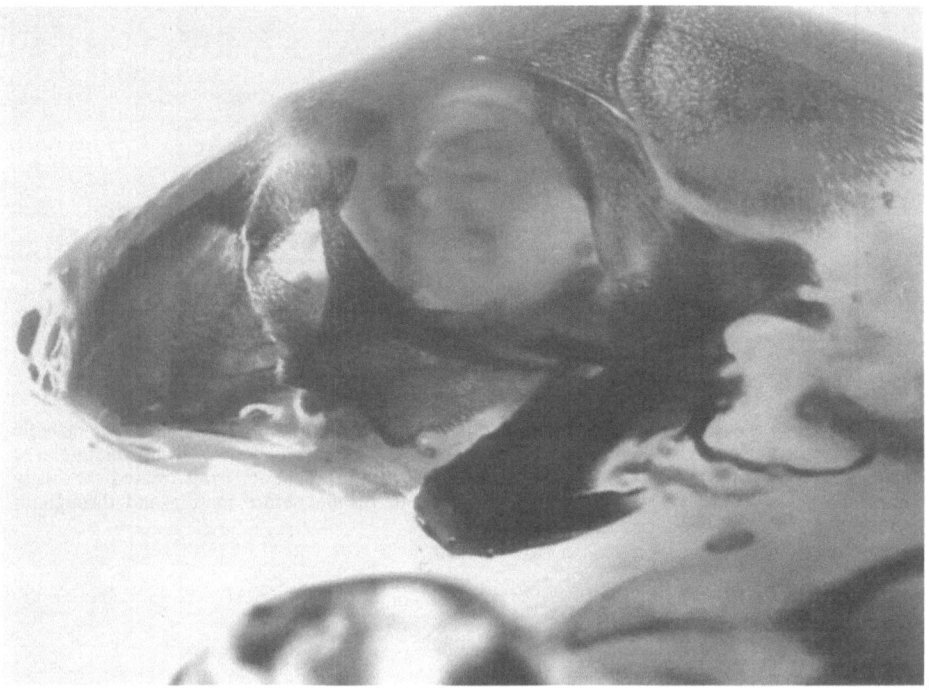

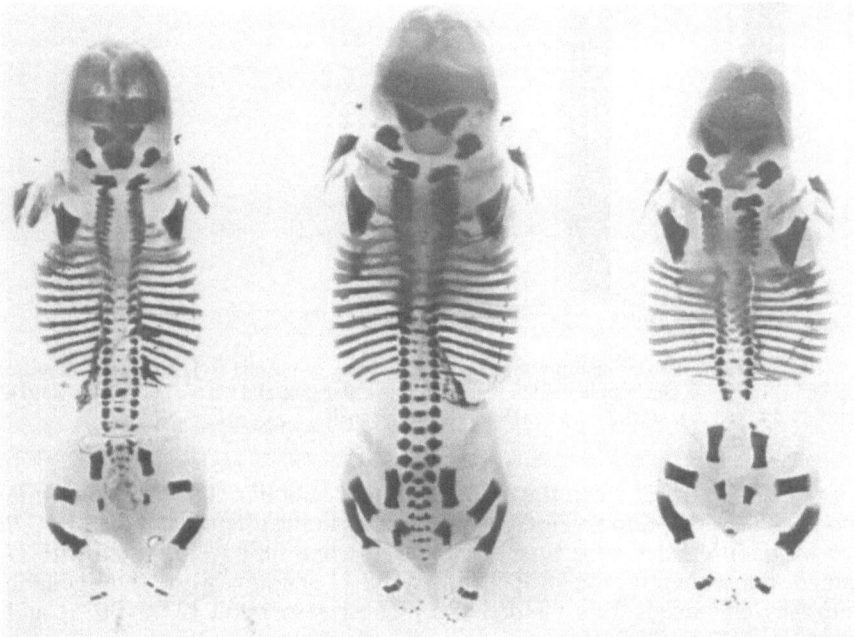

Fig. 6.2. a Head of a fetus of a manifestly diabetic U rat, displaying micrognathia. Stained with Alizarin Red S. **b** Offspring of manifestly diabetic U rats. The two fetuses to the left and right show sacral dysgenesis of varied severity. Stained with Alizarin Red S.

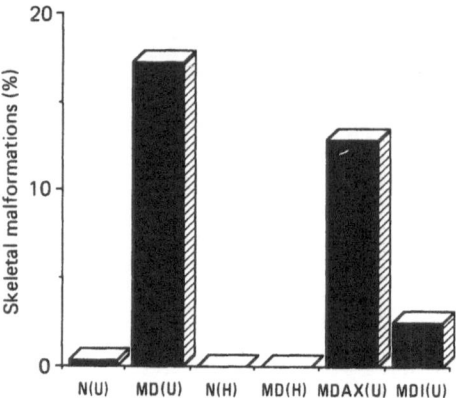

Fig. 6.3. Incidence of skeletal malformations in the offspring of normal (N) and manifestly diabetic (MD) rats of the U and H substrains. The MDAX(U) rats were made diabetic with alloxan instead of streptozotocin (used in all other MD groups). MDI(U) denotes diabetic U rats treated with daily subcutaneous injections of long-acting Novo Ultralente Insulin before mating and throughout gestation. Each group contains 10–40 pregnancies.

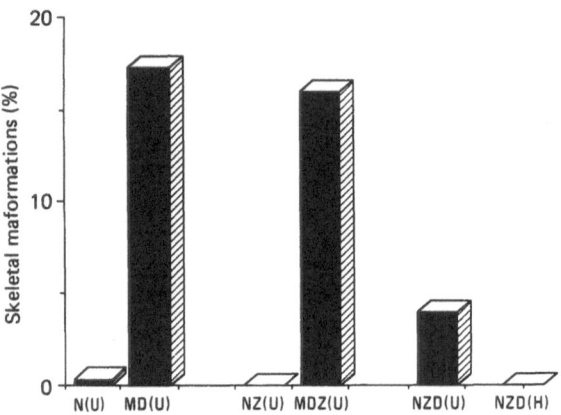

Fig. 6.4. Incidence of skeletal malformations in the offspring of normal (N), manifestly diabetic (MD) U and H rats, with zinc supplement in their drinking water (NZ and MDZ) and subjected to a zinc-deficient diet (NZD). Each group contains 8–40 pregnancies.

teratogenic environment when the diabetic mother contains 50% or more of the U genome. The resorption and malformation rates in the offspring of the MD(U/H) and MD(U) females were further increased when they were mated with U males and, consequently, the proportion of the U genome in the fetal genetic makeup was enhanced. This yielded the highest resorption (23%–30%) and malformation (17%–19%) rates in the diabetic groups and also implies an aetiological role for the fetal genome in the maldevelopment of the offspring of diabetic pregnancy. The importance of the maternal–fetal genome for the induction of malformations has been observed before. In the offspring of mice the

Table 6.1. Fetal outcome on gestational day 20 in normal (N) and manifestly diabetic (MD) rat mothers of the H, U and F_1 hybrid (U/H) type

Mother[a,b] (type)	Fetus (type)	Resorptions (%)	Malformations (%)
N (H)	H/H[c]	3	0
N (H)	U/H[d]	3	0
N (U/H)	U/H[e]	5	0
N (U)	U/H[f]	5	0
N (U)	U/U[g]	3	0
MD (H)	H/H[c]	9	0
MD (H)	U/H[d]	8	0
MD (U/H)	U/H[e]	21	5
MD (U/H)	75U/25H[h]	30	19
MD (U)	U/H[f]	16	3
MD (U)	U/U[g]	23	17

[a] Each group contains 4–19 pregnant rats.
[b] The data are compiled from Eriksson et al. (1985) and Eriksson (1988).
[c] H male×H female.
[d] U male×H female.
[e] (U/H) male×(U/H) female.
[f] H male×U female.
[g] U male×U female.
[h] U male×(U/H) female.

rate of corticosteroid-induced cleft palate has been shown to be largely dependent upon the strain used for the experiment (Fraser and Fainstat 1951). The teratogenic susceptibility to corticosteroids may be associated with both the genotype of the pregnant mice (Goldman 1984; Pratt 1984) and that of their embryos (Marsk et al. 1971). A high-sucrose diet induced different rates of embryonic maldevelopment in control, diabetic, Cohen diabetic and Cohen non-diabetic rats, reflecting different levels of genetic susceptibility (Zusman and Ornoy 1986). It has been suggested that in human pregnancy the incidence of neural tube defects in the fetus partially depends on the parental HLA-types (Schacter et al. 1979). Against this background, our findings would support the notion that both a maternal condition (at least 50% U genome and MD) and a fetal condition (at least 50% U genome) are necessary for the development of congenital malformations (and increased resorption rate) in this diabetic rat model. The precise biochemical nature of these conditions, e.g. the number of altered genes in the U genome, is not predictable from the present study.

Our results in the rat model would be in concert with the notion of maternal diabetes acting as a co-teratogen rather than a teratogen, as recently suggested by McCarter and collaborators (1987).

Teratogenic Period

The time period for the embryonic susceptiblity to malformations in human diabetic pregnancy has been estimated to be before the seventh week after conception (Mills et al. 1979), which would roughly correspond to the period before day 13–14 of gestation in the rat. In a previous attempt to delineate the period of maximal teratogenic susceptibility we used streptozotocin-diabetic U rats which received a long-acting insulin therapy (one daily subcutaneous injection of 4–8 IU Novo Ultralente Insulin) with periods of 2 d of interruption of treatment at various times during gestation (Eriksson et al. 1983a). The study indicated that the period during which fetal malformations resulted, if insulin therapy was discontinued, occurred very early, and partly before the implantation of the rat blastocyst on gestational days 4–5. This finding prompted us to perform a new study, using implanted osmotic mini pumps (ALZET 2002; ALZA, Palo Alto, CA, USA) filled with short-acting insulin (Novo Actrapid Human, 500 IU/ml) to regulate more precisely the glucose homeostasis of pregnant diabetic U rats (Eriksson et al. 1988a). Removal or reinsertion of pumps marked the beginning or end of a 2- or 4-d interruption period (Fig. 6.5).

In this recent study, fetal resorptions occurred in all interruption groups, but malformations were found only in animals which had had insulin withdrawal on

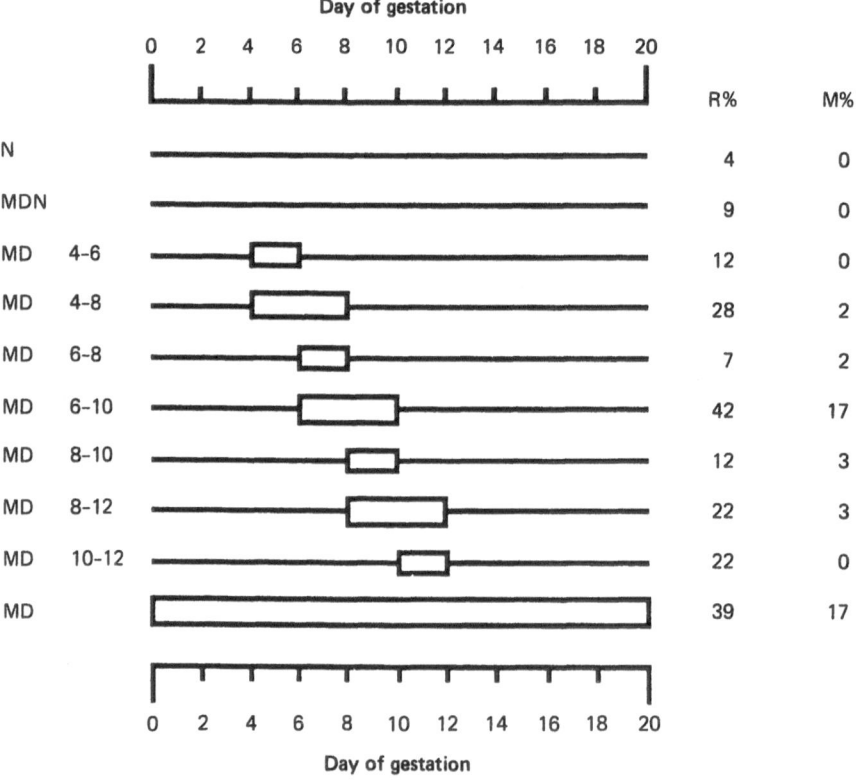

Fig. 6.5. Schedule for interruption of insulin therapy with implanted osmotic mini pumps (ALZET 2002), charged with short-acting Novo Actrapid Human Insulin, in U rats. N and MD denote normal and manifestly diabetic U rats, the latter group without any insulin treatment. MDN rats are MD rats with continuous insulin (pump) therapy before and throughout pregnancy, MD x–y are MD rats without insulin therapy on gestational days x–y, as indicated by horizontal bars in the figure (□). R% and M% are the rates of resorption (of all implantations) and malformation (of all viable fetuses) in the different groups, all of which contain 8–10 pregnant U rats.

gestational days 6–8, 8–10, 4–8, 6–10 and 8–12 or in MD rats with no insulin therapy during pregnancy. Both the highest resorption rate (42%) and the highest malformation rate (17%) were found in the animals subjected to insulin withdrawal during gestational days 6–10 (Fig. 6.5). It is noteworthy that the malformation rate in the MD 6–10 group (17%) exceeded that of the MD 6–8 and MD 8–10 groups combined (2%+3%). This suggests that a predisposing period of maternal metabolic imbalance is necessary for the development of congenital malformations.

Since manifestly diabetic U rats receiving no insulin treatment showed similar resorption (39%) and malformation rates (17%, see Fig. 6.5) as the MD 6–10 group, this study suggests that a teratogenic period occurs during days 6–10 in diabetic rat pregnancy, a time period corresponding to postconceptional weeks 2–4 in human gestation.

In view of the different methods employed to regulate and monitor the diabetic state in the previous (Eriksson et al. 1983a) and present (Eriksson et al. 1988a) investigations, the results may be complementary, rather than contradictory. The long-acting Ultralente Insulin used in the previous study would be expected to exert effects for some time after the termination of its administration (and to have a slow onset of action after resumption of treatment), whereas the surgical removal or reinsertion of osmotic pumps charged with short-acting insulin rapidly resulted in insulin deficiency or normalization of glucose levels respectively in the diabetic rats in the present study. The limits of the period of insulin withdrawal therefore were defined more concisely in the present than in the previous study, and the control of the glucose homeostasis in the diabetic pump-bearing rats was probably superior to that of the rats on injection therapy. The findings in a recent study of insulin-treated, spontaneously diabetic BB/E rats subjected to a 2-d interruption scheme support the results of the present investigation (Eriksson et al. 1988b). In the BB/E rat study, congenital malformations were found only when the therapy was withdrawn on gestational days 6–8 and 8–10 (Eriksson et al. 1988b). In another investigation, a diabetogenic dose of streptozotocin (SZ) was injected into pregnant albino rats on either gestational day 6 or day 12. Defects in skeletal ossification and fusion of vertebrae were only found in the fetuses of the former group, in which the anomalies disappeared if the pregnant rats were treated with insulin (Baker et al. 1981). The combined findings of the present and previous studies would, again, delineate pregnancy days 6–10 in the diabetic rat as a period of maximal teratological susceptibility.

The pathogenesis of the malformations in the present study is not clear. The developing embryos were subjected to maternal serum levels of about 30 mmol/l glucose and 1–4 mmol/l B-hydroxybutyric acid in utero. These levels do not cause major dysmorphogenesis in rodent embryos subjected to in vitro culture (Cockroft and Coppola 1977; Horton and Sadler 1983; Lewis et al. 1983). This may indicate that the malformations found in vitro and in vivo are pathogenetically different, e.g. that some other change(s) in the maternal environment occur(s) in addition to increased glucose and B-hydroxybutyric acid levels, which produce malformations in vivo. We have preliminary support for this view, since MD(U) rats with increased rates of embryonic malformations and resorptions show a more pronounced disturbance in maternal lipid and amino acid levels than do MD(U) rats with few embryonic malformations and resorptions (Eriksson et al., to be published).

The temporal relationships between the in vitro culture (gestational day 9 to day 10 or 11) and the in vivo teratogenic period (days 6–10, as outlined above) should also be considered, especially in conjunction with our finding that the malformation/resorption rates were much elevated when an interruption of insulin treatment on days 8–10 was preceded by interruption also on days 6–8 (see Fig. 6.5). When Sadler (1980) cultured mouse embryos in diabetic rat serum, he showed that the younger embryos (two to three somites at the start of culture) were more vulnerable than the older embryos (four to six somites at the start of culture). Likewise, Freinkel and collaborators (Chap. 5) have recently shown that rat embryos in vivo are markedly more susceptible to mannose infusion to the mother on day 8 compared to day 9 of gestation. In line with these results, we were unable to detect any in vitro difference in susceptibility towards raised levels of glucose and B-hydroxybutyric acid between cultured U and H embryos (Eriksson 1988), despite the marked in vivo difference between the embryonic development of these two substrains.

Organ Maldevelopment

Diabetes in the mother has been reported to be associated with growth disturbances of several fetal organs (Hultquist and Olding 1981). Organomegaly affecting the heart in fetuses of diabetic mothers has been reported (Miller 1946; Sheehan et al. 1986) whilst other organs, i.e. brain, lungs and kidneys, have been suggested to be smaller than normal in these infants (Cardell 1953; Gellis and Hsia 1959; Naeye 1965). In the present study we have investigated the growth of the brain, lungs, liver, heart, pancreas and kidneys in the fetuses of manifestly diabetic (U) rats.

Methods

Four normal (N) and four manifestly diabetic (MD) rats of the U strain were mated with normal males and killed on gestational day 20. The fetuses were quickly dissected out, weighed and inspected for resorptions and malformations. Two viable non-malformed fetuses were randomly chosen from each uterine horn and from each of these the brain, lungs, liver, heart, pancreas and kidneys were dissected out and weighed, minced with scissors, transferred into pre-weighed plastic tubes, freeze-dried and re-weighed. The samples were hydrolysed in 1 ml 0.5 M NaOH, ultrasonically disrupted for 10–15 s (20 kHz, 60 W), left at 4°C overnight and subsequently used to estimate organ contents of DNA (Kissane and Robins 1958; Hinegardner 1971) and protein (Lowry et al. 1951).

Results and Discussion

The maternal serum glucose concentration and maternal kidney weights were elevated in the MD rats compared to the N rats on gestational day 20, as expected (29.9 ± 1.4 mmol/l vs 4.5 ± 0.4 mmol/l; 2.6 ± 0.1 g vs 1.6 ± 0.1 g, $P<0.001$).

Similarly the resorption and malformation rates were increased in the MD litters compared to the N offspring (Table 6.2), whereas the fetal body weight was decreased and placental weight increased in the MD fetuses (Table 6.3). The weights of the malformed (MD) fetuses and their placentas did not differ from those of the non-malformed (MD) fetuses (Table 6.3).

In general, organs of MD fetuses weighed less and had lower content of protein and DNA than the corresponding N fetal organs (Table 6.4). Furthermore, the MD fetal organs showed similar or lower fractional weight (organ weight/fetal weight), similar or higher dry/wet weight ratio and similar protein/DNA ratio (Fig. 6.6), compared to N fetal organs.

Table 6.2. Fetal outcome on gestational day 20 in four normal (N) and four manifestly diabetic (MD) rat mothers

Mother	No. of implants	No. of resorptions	Per cent resorptions (of implants)	No. of viable fetuses	No. of malformed fetuses	Per cent malformed fetuses (of viable fetuses)
N	55	0	0	55	0	0
MD	53	12	23	41	6	15

Table 6.3. Fetal and placental weights on gestational day 20 in the offspring of four normal (N) and four manifestly diabetic (MD) rat mothers and in all malformed fetuses (MD$_{malf}$, all of MD mothers)

Mother[a]	Body weight (g)	Placental weight (g)
N[b]	3.69±0.06	0.52±0.01
MD[c]	2.56±0.13***	0.63±0.03***
MD$_{malf}$[d]	2.36±0.13***	0.63±0.04**

[a] Data are expressed as mean±SEM. Significances: **$P<0.01$ vs N, ***$P<0.001$ vs N (Student's two-tailed t-test, Ostle 1961).
[b] $n=8$ (no. of uterine horns with at least one viable fetus).
[c] $n=7$ (no. of uterine horns with at least one viable fetus).
[d] $n=7$.

There were some exceptions to this rule, the most notable being the MD fetal heart, which weighed the same as the N fetal heart, had slightly lower protein and DNA contents (Table 6.4) and showed increased volume and dry/wet weight ratio, as well as unchanged protein/DNA ratio (Fig. 6.6). This indicates that the fetal heart in the diabetic rat pregnancy is hyperplastic but not hypertrophic. Another fetal organ with a deviating weight pattern was the kidney. The fetal MD kidney showed decreased weight, decreased protein and DNA contents as well as decreased volume fraction. The dry/wet weight and protein/DNA ratios were increased, and these findings would indicate hypoplasia and cellular hypertrophy in the fetal kidneys in diabetic rat pregnancy. In line with a previous set of experiments, demonstrating pulmonary immaturity in MD offspring (Tydén et al. 1980; Eriksson et al. 1983b), the volume fraction was decreased and the dry residue (dry/wet weight ratio) increased in the lungs of these fetuses (Fig. 6.6).

Table 6.4. Weight, protein content and DNA content of different organs of fetuses of four normal (N) and four manifestly diabetic (MD) rats on gestational day 20

Organ[a]	Type	Weight (mg)	Protein (mg)	DNA (μg)
Brain	N[b]	111 ±2	9.7±0.3	630±46
	MD[c]	55 ±5***	4.7±0.4***	556±47***
Lung	N	90 ±2	7.6±0.3	912±34
	MD	55 ±5***	4.7±0.4***	556±47***
Liver	N	172 ±6	19.5±0.7	1637±75
	MD	95 ±5***	11.6±0.8***	1128±88***
Heart	N	12.5±0.6	1.7±0.1	92± 4
	MD	12.0±0.6	1.5±0.1*	76± 4*
Pancreas	N	12.9±0.8	2.7±0.1	101± 6
	MD	9.6±0.5**	1.9±0.2**	73± 7*
Kidney	N	20.1±0.1	2.1±0.1	219±10
	MD	11.6±1.4***	1.2±0.1***	108±11***

[a] Data are expressed as mean±SEM. Significances: *$P<0.05$ vs N, **$P<0.01$ vs N, ***$P<0.001$ vs N (Student's two-tailed t-test, Ostle 1961).
[b] $n=16$.
[c] $n=14$.

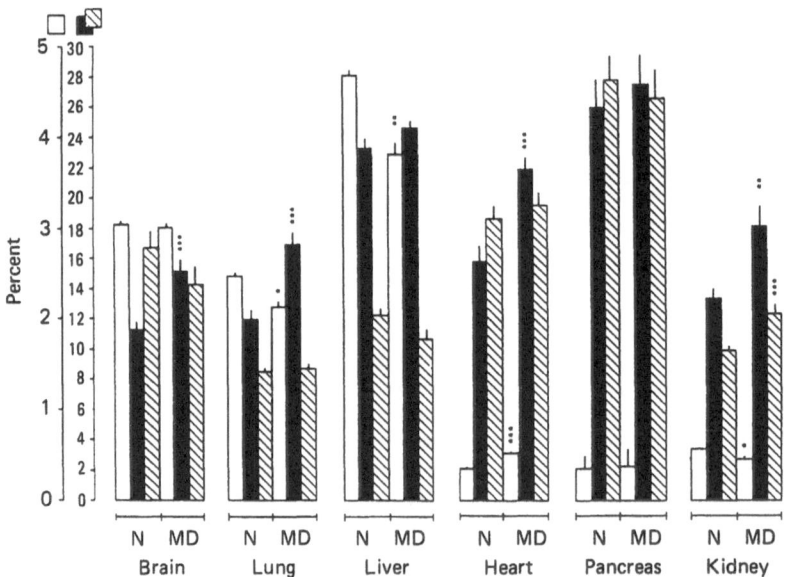

Fig. 6.6. Organ development in the offspring of four normal (N) and four manifestly diabetic (MD) rats on gestational day 20; organ wet weight as percentage of fetal wet weight (□), organ dry weight as percentage of organ wet weight (■) and organ protein/DNA ratio (▨). All N bars represent 16 observations, all MD bars 14 observations. Data are expressed as mean±SEM. Significant difference vs corresponding N parameter is depicted (*$P<0.05$, **$P<0.01$, ***$P<0.001$, Student's two-tailed t-test, Ostle 1961).

The fetal brain showed increased dry/wet weight ratio, and a trend towards decreased protein/DNA ratio, possibly signifying retarded development.

The malformed fetuses of MD rats showed analogous weight and protein–DNA contents to the non-malformed MD offspring.

The mechanisms causing altered growth and development of a number of fetal organ systems when the mother is diabetic are not known. The rat model presented here may serve as a tool for future research into this field, especially for investigating the different growth responses of the fetal heart and kidney when the mother is diabetic. Of special aetiological interest is that these changes occur in a hyperglycaemic but *not* a hyperinsulinaemic environment (Eriksson et al. 1980).

Conclusions

The present data support a role for both the maternal and the fetal genome in the maldevelopment of the offspring in diabetic pregnancy.

The teratogenic interval occurs early in pregnancy, corresponding to postconceptional weeks 2–4 in human gestation, a finding which strongly supports the current clinical view of the importance of optimal metabolic control of the mother at the time of conception.

While the results of the studies suggest that a disturbed trace metal handling (primarily of zinc), as well as altered maternal metabolism of carbohydrates, lipids and amino acids, are of importance for the induction of malformations and resorptions, the exact interplay between these and other possible teratogenic agents remains to be established.

Maternal diabetes in the rat causes heart hyperplasia without cellular hypertrophy and kidney hypoplasia with cellular hypertrophy in the offspring. This model for diabetic pregnancy may be of value in the search for the aetiological factors underlying the anomalies found in animal and human offspring of diabetic mothers.

Acknowledgements. These investigations were supported by the Swedish Medical Research Council (Grant no. 12X–7475), The Expressen Prenatal Research Foundation, The Swedish Diabetes Association, The Nordic Insulin Fund, The Novo Industri A/S, The Swedish Hoechst Diabetes Fund and The Juvenile Diabetes Foundation.

References

Baker L, Egler JM, Klein SH, Goldman AS (1981) Meticulous control of diabetes during organogenesis prevents congenital lumbosacral defects in rats. Diabetes 30:955–959

Cardell BS (1953) The infants of the diabetic mothers. J Obstet Gynaecol Br Emp 60:834–853

Cockroft DL, Coppola PT (1977) Teratogenic effects of excess glucose on headfold rat embryos in culture. Teratology 16:141–146

Eriksson UJ (1984) Diabetes in pregnancy: retarded fetal growth, congenital malformations and feto-maternal concentrations of zinc, copper and manganese in the rat. J Nutr 114:477–486

Eriksson UJ (1988) Importance of genetic predisposition and maternal environment for the occurrence of congenital malformations in offspring of diabetic rats. Teratology 37:365–374

Eriksson UJ, Andersson A, Efendic S, Elde R, Hellerström C (1980) Diabetes in pregnancy: effects on the fetal and newborn rat with particular regard to body weight, serum insulin concentration and pancreatic contents of insulin, glucagon and somatostatin. Acta Endocrinol (Copenh) 94:354–364

Eriksson UJ, Dahlström E, Larsson KS, Hellerström C (1982) Increased incidence of congenital malformations in the offspring of diabetic rats and their prevention by maternal insulin therapy. Diabetes 31:1–6

Eriksson UJ, Dahlström E, Hellerström C (1983a) Diabetes in pregnancy: skeletal malformations in the offspring of diabetic rats after intermittent withdrawal of insulin in early gestation. Diabetes 32:1141–1145

Eriksson UJ, Tydén O, Berne C (1983b) Development of phosphatidyl glycerol biosynthesis in the lungs of fetuses of diabetic rats. Diabetologia 24:202–206

Eriksson UJ, Dahlström VE, Styrud J (1985) Metabolically determined teratogenesis: malformations and maternal diabetes. Biochem Soc Trans 13:79–82

Eriksson UJ, Dahlström VE, Lithell HO (1986) Diabetes in pregnancy: influence of genetic background and maternal diabetic state on the incidence of skeletal malformations in the fetal rat. Acta Endocrinol (Copenh) 112(Suppl 277):66–73

Eriksson RSM, Thunberg L, Eriksson UJ (1988a) Diabetes in pregnancy: effects of interrupted insulin treatment on the fetal outcome of the pregnant rat. (submitted for publication)

Eriksson UJ, Bone AJ, Turnbull DM, Baird JD (1988b) Timed interruption of insulin therapy in diabetic BB/E rat pregnancy: effects on maternal metabolism and fetal outcome. (submitted for publication)

Fraser FC, Fainstat T (1951) Production of congenital defects in the offspring of pregnant mice treated with cortisone. Pediatrics 8:527–533

Freinkel N (1980) Of pregnancy and progeny. Diabetes 29:1023–1035

Gellis SS, Hsia DYY (1959) The infant of the diabetic mother. Am J Dis Child 97:1–41

Goldman AS (1984) Biochemical mechanism of glucocorticoid- and phenytoin-induced cleft palate. Curr Top Dev Biol 19:217–239

Hinegardner RT (1971) An improved fluorometric assay for DNA. Anal Biochem 39:197–201

Horton WE Jr, Sadler TW (1983) Effects of maternal diabetes on early embryogenesis. Alterations in morphogenesis produced by the ketone body, B-hydroxybutyrate. Diabetes 32:610–616

Hultquist GT, Olding LB (1981) Endocrine pathology of infants of diabetic mothers. Acta Endocrinol (Copenh) (Suppl 241) 97:1–202

Kissane JM, Robins E (1958) The fluorometric measurement of deoxyribonucleic acid in animal tissues with special reference to the central nervous system. J Biol Chem 233:184–188

Kucera J (1971) Rate and type of congenital anomalies among offspring of diabetic women. J Reprod Med 7:61–70

Lewis NJ, Akazawa S, Freinkel N (1983) Teratogenesis from B-hydroxybutyrate during organogenesis in rat embryo organ culture and enhancement by subteratogenic glucose. Diabetes 32 (Suppl 1): 11A

Lowry OH, Rosenbrough NJ, Farr AL, Randall RJ (1951) Protein measurement with the folin phenol reagent. J Biol Chem 193:265–275

Marsk L, Theorell M, Larsson KS (1971) Transfer of blastocysts as applied in experimental teratology. Teratology 4:494 (Abstract)

McCarter RJ, Kessler II, Comstock GW (1987) Is diabetes mellitus a teratogen or a co-teratogen? Am J Epidemiol 125:195–205

Miller HC (1946) The effect of diabetes and prediabetic pregnancies on the fetus and newborn infant. J Pediatr 29:455–461

Mills JL (1982) Malformations in infants of diabetic mothers. Teratology 25:385–394

Mills JL, Baker L, Goldman AS (1979) Malformations in infants of diabetic mothers occur before the seventh gestational week. Implications for treatment. Diabetes 28:292–293

Naeye RL (1965) Infants of diabetic mothers: a quantitative morphologic study. Pediatrics 35:980–988

Ostle B (1961) Statistics in research, 2nd edn. Ames, Iowa State University Press

Pedersen J (1977) The pregnant diabetic and her newborn, 2nd edn. Munksgaard, Copenhagen

Pedersen JF, Mølsted-Pedersen L (1982) Early growth delay predisposes the fetus in diabetic pregnancy to congenital malformation. Lancet I: 737

Pratt RM (1984) Hormones, growth factors, and their receptors in normal and abnormal prenatal development. In: Kalter H (ed.) Issues and reviews in teratology, vol. 2. Plenum Press, New York, pp 189–217

Sadler TW (1980) Effects of maternal diabetes on early embryogenesis. I. The teratogenic potential of diabetic serum. Teratology 21:339–347

Schacter B, Muir A, Gyves M, Tasin M (1979) HLA-A,B compatibility in parents of offspring with neural-tube defects of couples experiencing involuntary fetal wastage. Lancet I: 796–799

Sheehan PQ, Rowland TW, Shah BL, McGravey VJ, Reiter EO (1986) Maternal diabetic control and hypertrophic cardiomyopathy in infants of diabetic mothers. Clin Pediatr 25:266–271

Styrud J, Dahlström VE, Eriksson UJ (1986) Induction of skeletal malformations in the offspring of rats fed a zinc-deficient diet. Ups J Med Sci 91:29–36

Sutherland HW, Pritchard C (1986) Increased incidence of spontaneous abortion in pregnancies complicated by maternal diabetes mellitus. Am J Obstet Gynecol 155:135–138

Tydén O, Berne C, Eriksson UJ (1980) Lung maturation in fetuses of diabetic rats. Pediatr Res 14:1192–1195

Zusman I, Ornoy A (1986) The effects of maternal diabetes and high sucrose diets on the intrauterine development of rat fetuses. Diab Res 3:153–159

7. Diabetes Mellitus and Infertility

J. M. Randall, A. Hesham and A. A. Templeton

Introduction

It has long been thought that diabetes mellitus may impair female fertility (Macnaughton 1976). However, objective data are lacking (Sobel et al. 1986). Nonetheless it is likely that the introduction of insulin therapy has improved fertility by decreasing the incidence of amenorrhoea in diabetic women (Gilbert and Dunlop 1949). Certainly prior to the introduction of insulin in 1923, amenorrhoea was common among women with uncontrolled diabetes and accounted for the very low fertility rates observed at that time (Skipper 1933).

In the absence of contemporary data there is a strong case for a population-based survey of diabetic women and we report in this chapter our preliminary findings following a review of the literature and consideration of the usual factors which play a role in the aetiology of infertility. These include endocrine problems leading to defective ovulation, tubal disease interfering with oocyte pickup and unexplained infertility encompassing the areas of fertilization, gamete transport and implantation.

Endocrine Abnormalities and Defects of Ovulation

The menarche appears to be delayed when diabetes is present in the prepubertal female (Berquist 1954; Sterky 1963; Schriock et al. 1984) and this may indicate some derangement of the hypothalamic–pituitary–gonadal axis (Cicognani et al. 1978). Similarly it has been suggested that the menopause occurs prematurely in women with diabetes (Berquist 1954). Menstrual disorders have been reported in up to 30% of insulin-treated diabetic women (Berquist 1954; Trzeciak 1978), and the onset of the diabetes seems to be an important precipitating factor (Djursing et al. 1982).

In diabetic women in their reproductive years defects of the hypothalamic–pituitary–gonadal axis have been reported (Djursing 1987) and these include decreased basal prolactin secretion with a decreased prolactin response to metoclopramide (Djursing et al. 1983). These authors concluded that this was probably due to increased dopaminergic inhibitory activity on the lactotrophs.

In well-controlled diabetic women who are menstruating regularly basal gonadotrophin levels and the gonadotrophin response to gonadotrophin-releasing hormone (GnRH) have been reported as normal (Djursing et al. 1984), although Distiller et al. (1975) reported an inverse relationship between serum glucose levels and the luteinizing hormone (LH) response to GnRH, indicating the possibility that pituitary function was sensitive to circulating glucose levels. In addition there is evidence from animal studies that in the presence of diabetes there may be a pituitary hypothalamic insensitivity to circulating steroids and that these effects may be partially reversed by insulin treatment (Calvo et al. 1984).

Abnormalities of sex steroid secretion have also been reported in insulin-dependent diabetes mellitus (IDDM). Djursing et al. (1985) found raised androstenedione and testosterone levels in the presence of normal serum oestradiol. The elevated androgen levels were found exclusively in regularly menstruating women and the authors concluded that the source was ovarian. Hirsutism or menstrual disturbance did not occur, possibly because these changes were paralleled by changes in sex-hormone-binding globulin.

Djursing (1987) has suggested that amenorrhoea in the diabetic woman is caused by augmented dopaminergic inhibition of gonadotrophin excretion. Despite low follicle-stimulating hormone (FSH) and basal oestradiol levels (Djursing et al. 1985), there is a normal FSH response to GnRH. In addition there are abnormalities of LH pulsatility, and also the LH responsiveness to GnRH is blunted (Djursing et al. 1983). Dopamine blockade can, however, increase FSH levels (Djursing et al. 1985).

Problems of Oocyte Pick-up

The major causes of infertility among females include pelvic problems which affect oocyte pick-up and gamete transfer. These changes are most commonly postinfective or endometriotic. In a recent review of 405 women who underwent laparoscopy for infertility, 58% had primary infertility and 42% secondary infertility. Endometriosis occurred more commonly among women with primary infertility, i.e. in 64 (27.5%), compared with those with secondary infertility, i.e. in 22 (12.8%). Postinfective changes on the other hand were more common in the 172 women with secondary infertility ($n=67$, 39%) than in the 233 women with primary infertility ($n=61$, 25.5%) (Mahmood and Templeton, unpublished).

Although it has long been accepted that those with diabetes are more prone to infection (Younger 1965), the sites of infection are predominantly the urinary tract, the respiratory system and the skin. No specific defects in host defence have been reported among diabetic women and there are no data to confirm that the incidence of pelvic infection is more common in diabetic women. Nevertheless there has been a considerable increase in the incidence of pelvic infection both generally and at our hospital since the late 1960s. This is perhaps best documented in the studies of one of the most important sequelae of pelvic infection namely tubal pregnancy. Several reports have shown an increase in the overall incidence of ectopic pregnancy (Westrom et al. 1981; Rubin et al. 1983) and a recent detailed study in Aberdeen has shown a fourfold increase since 1970 (Flett et al. 1988). A study of the incidence of tubal infection and ectopic pregnancy among the diabetic population would be worthwhile now that reasonable control data are available. Similarly, endometriosis appears to be increasing in incidence (although this may in part reflect the increased use of laparoscopy) but again there is no information available to determine whether or not diabetic women are particularly prone to this ill-understood condition.

Unexplained Infertility

Unexplained infertility accounts for up to 25% of the infertility clinic population (Templeton and Penney 1982). In a recent survey of 26 infertile couples where the female partners had diabetes, Steel and Johnstone (1986) found no abnormality after routine investigation in 13 (50%) which perhaps suggests a higher-than-expected incidence of unexplained infertility in this population. Problems may arise in the areas of sperm transport (Templeton and Mortimer 1982a; Stone 1983), sperm fertilizing ability (Aitken et al. 1982), sperm–egg interaction (Fishel et al. 1988) and implantation (Whittaker et al. 1983), but unfortunately these factors cannot be assessed easily by routine clinical investigation. Moreover it is not known whether diabetic women are more prone to difficulties in these areas. Up to 30% of morphologically normal fertilized oocytes have major chromosome abnormalities (Angell et al. 1986; Plachot et al. 1987; Papadopoulos et al., unpublished) and it would be of considerable interest to know if diabetic women are any more susceptible to problems of this nature. This is particularly relevant in view of the doubt expressed about the incidence of spontaneous abortion in diabetic women which is reviewed in the next chapter.

General features which may affect fertility such as disturbance of female sexuality have not been reported in patients either with or without neuropathy (Ellenberg 1984), although neuropathy plays a significant role in infertility among diabetic males.

Secondary Infertility

The problem of secondary infertility is one that is frequently underestimated both in statistical and personal terms. Diabetic women may by particularly vulnerable in this respect for two reasons. Firstly, as mentioned already, the major cause for secondary infertility in women is postinfective tubal adhesions and diabetic women may be more prone to pelvic infection. Secondly, the babies of many diabetic women are delivered by Caesarean section, e.g. the Caesarean section rate for diabetic women in Aberdeen Maternity Hospital between 1975 and 1986 was 37%. There is some evidence to suggest that post-Caesarean section pelvic infection is more common in diabetic compared with non-diabetic women (Diamond et al. 1986). Furthermore, in a review of our total obstetric population it has become apparent that fewer women delivered by Caesarean section have a further pregnancy when compared with those who have had a normal vaginal delivery. This finding is not associated with social or marital status and can only be partly attributable to age (M. H. Hall, personal communication). A study is underway to determine whether this obstetrical effect on family size is also present in women with diabetes.

It is concluded that there is no good evidence to suggest that regularly menstruating diabetic women are any less fertile than their non-diabetic counterparts. However, there are a number of reasons why they might be so, and particularly why secondary infertility might be more prevalent in this group.

Survey of Diabetic Women

In view of the relative lack of information regarding the epidemiology of infertility within the diabetic population, we conducted a postal questionnaire survey through the Aberdeen Royal Infirmary Diabetic Clinic. The questionnaires were sent to 100 insulin-dependent diabetic women, aged 25–35, who had been otherwise randomly selected from the Diabetic Clinic records. There was an 83% return including two questionnaires incompletely answered and therefore only 81 were available for statistical analysis. The demographical details of the sample were as follows: mean age of 31 years (range 25–35 years); an average age of onset of diabetes of 17 years (range 1–32 years); average duration of diabetes was 14 years (range 1–33 years); 15% were single, 75% married and 10% separated or divorced; the mean duration of the menstrual cycle was 29 d (range 16–40 d) and 82% of respondents described their menstrual pattern as very or fairly regular. One patient had amenorrhoea secondary to renal failure. The mean age of menarche for the group was 13.2 years (range 9–16 years).

Analysis of their current contraceptive practice is shown in Table 7.1. It was found that 20% of the patients had opted for a permanent method of contraception, namely either tubal occlusion or vasectomy and 26% were using the oral contraceptive pill.

Table 7.1. Results of a questionnaire sent to 100 diabetic women. Methods of contraception being used by the respondents (percentages in brackets)

	Number
None	15 (19)
Combined oral contraceptive	21 (26)
IUCD	12 (15)
Barrier (sheath/diaphragm)	12 (15)
Female sterilization	10 (12)
Male sterilization	7 (8)
Coitus interruptus	3 (4)
Hysterectomy	1 (1)

In response to enquiry regarding a possible history of infertility 13 (16%) of the respondents reported that they had experienced some difficulty in becoming pregnant (see Table 7.2). However, only two patients out of the whole group had experienced more than 2 years involuntary infertility and all 13 patients achieved pregnancy within the time span stated.

Table 7.2. Duration of subfertility in 13 respondents who reported difficulty with conception

Duration	No. of patients
6 months	4
9 months	5
1 year	1
18 months	1
2 years	1
3 years	1

Overall these preliminary results reveal no increased incidence of menstrual disturbances such as oligomenorrhoea or amenorrhoea in comparison with a normal non-diabetic population and they demonstrate that there is no obvious increase in the incidence of infertility within the group. The study group is to be expanded to include all female patients between the ages of 20 and 45 attending the Diabetic Clinic, but on these preliminary findings it appears that in contemporary practice in Aberdeen, diabetic women are at no greater risk of menstrual disturbance or infertility than non-diabetic women.

Male Infertility

The male factor is recognized as having a significant causal role in infertility. Clinical assessment and semen analysis are prerequisites for an adequate consultation with an infertile couple. A standard approach to the assessment of the male should include a full history with reference to relevant factors such as occupation, tobacco and alcohol consumption, drug history, testicular trauma and episodes of orchitis or venereal disease.

The endocrine status of the patient can be superficially assessed by observation of the general body build, hair distribution and presence or absence of gynaecomastia.

Seminal analysis should be performed on samples collected by masturbation into a clean non-spermotoxic container and analysis of volume, pH, sperm density, morphology and motility characteristics should be performed. The sample should be preceded by at least 4 d sexual abstinence and three samples should be assessed, as variation occurs both qualitatively and quantitatively. Male factors are attributed as the cause of infertility in about a third of all infertile couples (Hull et al. 1985).

Diabetic males have particular problems which may lead to infertility. The role of these factors and their contribution to infertility amongst diabetic males will now be discussed.

It is well established that diabetes can affect the male in several ways which are likely to diminish fertility. These are mainly secondary to associated vasculopathy and neuropathy (Fairburn et al. 1982a). Male reproductive endocrinology has also been investigated but the results are controversial; the pituitary responsiveness as assessed by LH response to GnRH has been reported as blunted (Distiller et al. 1975) or normal (Jensen et al. 1979), and FSH response as blunted (Distiller et al. 1975), normal (Wright et al. 1976) or increased (Jensen et al. 1979). Jensen also reported that testosterone levels were normal among diabetic men. Spermatogenesis has been studied by examining variations in ejaculate volume, sperm density and motility but there appear to be no definitive abnormalities (Sobel et al. 1986).

Impotence

It is well recognized that impotence occurs more frequently among diabetic men than among non-diabetic men and this has been attributed to autonomic nerve damage. Many diabetic men with otherwise normal cardiovascular reflexes present with erectile dysfunction. When such men are followed up prospectively many appear to develop further signs of autonomic neuropathy (Ewing et al. 1980). It could be anticipated that diabetic men may be more prone to sexual problems because of the stress of the chronic condition and also there is some evidence of increasing marital disharmony and other psychological disturbances (Campbell and McCulloch 1979). Inevitably these problems, set against a background of autonomic disturbance, may cause performance anxiety and a vicious circle can develop. The contribution of psychological factors to sexual dysfunction, particularly in diabetic men, cannot be underestimated.

Impotence occurs with a frequency of around 25% in diabetic men aged 30–35 years (Rubin and Babbott 1958) but it is well recognized that the incidence of erectile difficulties increases with age. McCulloch et al. (1980) found an incidence of impotence of 5.7% in diabetic men aged 20–24 years, which rose to 52.4% in men aged 55–59 years. In another study the overall incidence of impotence of diabetic men of all ages ranged from 40%–60% (Fairburn et al. 1982b). However, none of these studies has reported the incidence of sexual dysfunction in non-diabetic patients with chronic disease. Interestingly a similar rate of impotence was found in diabetic and non-diabetic men in one other study (Lester et al. 1980). Nevertheless, impotence, whether psychological or related to neuropathy or vasculopathy, appears to be an important factor in the fertility of diabetic men.

Retrograde Ejaculation

Retrograde ejaculation is the second major problem of sexual function which occurs among diabetic men. In this condition there is a disturbance of the ejaculatory process such that semen passes backwards into the bladder rather than into the urethra. The diagnosis is confirmed by examination of the postejaculatory urine. The prevalence of this ejaculatory disorder within the diabetic population has not been fully described. Kolodny et al. (1974) had two patients out of 175, whereas Fairburn et al. (1982b) found that over a third of their patients had some form of ejaculatory disorder. These authors suggested that there was considerable under-reporting of this particular problem.

Treatment of retrograde ejaculation may be attempted in two ways. Hotchkiss et al. (1955) reported recovery of spermatozoa from a postejaculatory urine specimen. The method, however, had a poor success rate due to the adverse physical and chemical properties of urine, particularly the effects of pH and osmolality on sperm viability and motility (Crich and Jequier 1978). Using modern sperm-washing techniques the method has been developed and with these improvements ensuing successful pregnancies have been reported (Zavos and Wilson 1984; Ingerslev 1985). An alternative approach to treatment is to bring about antegrade ejaculation by encouraging the patient to produce a masturbated semen specimen with a full bladder. It appears that the full bladder is more likely to cause the forward progression of the ejaculate into the urethra. Quite commonly with this technique a specimen of good quality is obtained (Crich and Jequier 1978). There are published reports of pregnancies using this method (Templeton and Mortimer 1982b). For those patients who find this method acceptable it provides a better chance of pregnancy than recovery of spermatozoa from the bladder.

In summary there appear to be no consistent effects of diabetes mellitus upon male endocrinology and spermatogenesis, although extragonadal problems, such as impotence and retrograde ejaculation, are frequent and affect fertility. Both these difficulties are probably under-reported and are major contributing factors to the subfertility of diabetic men.

Acknowledgements. Our thanks to Dr. Donald W. M. Pearson for help with the Diabetic Infertility Survey and for permission to study his patients.

References

Aitken RJ, Best FSM, Richardson DW et al. (1982) An analysis of sperm function in cases of unexplained infertility: conventional criteria, movement characteristics and fertilising capacity. Fertil Steril 38:212–221

Angell RR, Templeton AA, Aitken RJ (1986) Chromosome studies in human in vitro fertilisation. Hum Genet 72:333–339

Berquist N (1954) The gonadal function in female diabetics. Acta Endocrinol (Suppl) Copenh 19:1–20

Calvo JC, Baranao JLS, Tesone M, Charrean EH (1984) Hypothalamic hypophyseal–gonadal axis in the streptozotocin-induced diabetic male rat. J Steroid Biochem 20:769–772

Campbell IW, McCulloch DK (1979) Marital problems in diabetes. Practitioner 223:343–347

Cicognani A, Zappulla F, Bernardi F et al. (1978) Hypophyso gonadal function in the diabetic child. Acta Paediatr Scand 67:151–155

Crich JP, Jequier AM (1978) Infertility in men with retrograde ejaculation: the action of urine on sperm motility and a simple method for achieving adequate ejaculation. Fertil Steril 30:572–576

Diamond MP, Entmann SS, Salyer SL, Vaughn WK, Boehm FH (1986) Increased risk of endometriosis and wound infection after Caesarean section in insulin dependent diabetic women. Am J Obstet Gynecol 155:297–300

Distiller LA, Sagel J, Morley JE, Joffe BI, Seftel HC (1975) Pituitary responsiveness to luteinizing hormone releasing hormone in insulin dependent diabetes mellitus. Diabetes 24:378–380

Djursing H (1987) Hypothalamic-pituitary gonadal function in insulin treated diabetic women with and without amenorrhoea. Dan Med Bull 34:139–147

Djursing H, Nyholm NC, Hagen C, Carstensen L, Pedersen LM (1982) Clinical and hormonal characteristics in women with anovulation and insulin treated diabetes mellitus. Am J Obstet Gynecol 143:876–882

Djursing H, Hagen C, Nyholm HG, Carstensen L, Andersen AN (1983) Gonadotrophin responses to gonadotrophin releasing hormone and prolactin responses to thyrotropin-releasing hormone and metoclopramide in women with amenorrhoea and insulin treated diabetes mellitus. J Clin Endocrinol Metab 56:1016–1021

Djursing H, Carstensen L, Hagen C, Andersen AN (1984) Possible altered dopaminergic modulation of pituitary function in normal menstruating women with insulin dependent diabetes mellitus. Acta Endocrinol 107:450–455

Djursing H, Hagen C, Nyboe Andersen A, Svenstrup B, Bennett P, Mølsted Pedersen L (1985) Serum sex hormone concentrations in insulin dependent diabetic women with and without amenorrhoea. Clin Endocrinol 23:147–154

Ellenberg M (1984) Diabetes and female sexuality. Women and Health 9:75–79

Ewing DJ, Campbell IW, Clarke BF (1980) The natural history of diabetic autonomic neuropathy. Q J Med 49 (193):95–108

Fairburn CG, McCulloch DK, Wu FC (1982a) The effects of diabetes on male sexual function. In: Bancroft J (ed) Clinics in endocrinology and metabolism, vol 11 (3). WB Saunders, London, pp 749–767

Fairburn CG, Wu FC, McCulloch DK, Borsey DQ, Ewing DJ, Clarke BF, Bancroft JH (1982b) The clinical features of diabetic impotence: a preliminary study. Br J Psychiatry 140:447–452

Fishel S, Webster J, Faration B, Jackson P (1988) Place of GIFT in infertility services. Lancet I:470

Flett GMM, Urquhart DR, Fraser C, Terry PB, Fleming JC (1988) Ectopic pregnancy in Aberdeen 1950–1985. Br J Obstet Gynaecol (in press)

Gilbert JAL, Dunlop DM (1949) Diabetic fertility, maternal mortality and foetal loss rate. Br Med J 1: 48–51

Hotchkiss RS, Pinto AB, Kleegman S (1955) Artificial insemination with semen recovered from the bladder. Fertil Steril 6:37–42

Hull MGR, Glazener CMA, Kelly NJ et al. (1985) Population studies of causes, treatment and outcome of infertility. Br Med J 291:1693–1697

Ingerslev HJ (1985) Retrograde ejaculation: successful artificial homologous insemination. Lancet II:519

Jensen SB, Hagen C, Froland A, Pedersen PB (1979) Sexual function and pituitary axis in insulin treated diabetic men. Acta Med Scand (Suppl) 624:65–68

Kolodny RC, Kahn CB, Goldstein AA, Barett DM (1974) Sexual dysfunction in diabetic men. Diabetes 23:306–309

Lester E, Grant AJ, Woodroffe FJ (1980) Impotence in diabetic and non-diabetic out-patients. Br Med J 281:354–355

Macnaughton MC (1976) Abnormalities of menstruation. In: Walker J, MacGillivray I, Macnaughton MC (eds) Combined textbook of obstetrics and gynaecology. Churchill Livingstone, Edinburgh, pp 639–670

McCulloch DK, Campbell IW, Wu FC, Prescott RJ, Clarke BF (1980) The prevalence of diabetic impotence. Diabetologia 18:279–283

Plachot M, Junca A-M, Mandelbaum J, de Grouchy J, Salat-Baroux J, Cohen J (1987) Chromosome investigations in early life. II. Human pre-implantation embryos. Hum Reprod 2:29–35

Rubin A, Babbott D (1958) Impotence and diabetes mellitus. J Am Med Ass 168:498–500

Rubin GL, Peterson HB, Dorfman SF et al. (1983) Ectopic pregnancy in the United States. 1970 through 1978. J Am Med Ass 249:1725–1729

Schriock EA, Winther RJ, Traisman HS (1984) Diabetes mellitus and its effect on menarche. J Adolesc Health Care 5:101–104

Skipper E (1933) Diabetes mellitus and pregnancy: a clinical and analytical study. Q J Med 2:353–380

Sobel RJ, Liel Y, Glick SM (1986) Medical conditions leading to infertility. In: Insler V, Lunefied B (eds) Infertility in male and female. Churchill Livingstone, Edinburgh, pp 673–696

Steel JM, Johnstone FD (1986) Prepregnancy management of the diabetic. In: Chamberlain G, Lumley J (eds) Prepregnancy care: a manual for practice. John Wiley, Chichester, pp 165–182

Sterky G (1963) Diabetic school children. Acta Paediatr 144:5–39

Stone SC (1983) Peritoneal recovery of sperm in patients with infertility associated with inadequate cervical mucus. Fertil Steril 40:802–804

Templeton AA, Mortimer D (1982a) The development of a clinical test of sperm migration to the site of fertilisation. Fertil Steril 37:410–415

Templeton AA, Mortimer D (1982b) Successful circumvention of retrograde ejaculation in an infertile diabetic man. Case report. Br J Obstet Gynaecol 89:1064–1065

Templeton AA, Penney GC (1982) The incidence, characteristics and prognosis of patients whose infertility is unexplained. Fertil Steril 37:175–182

Trzeciak B (1978) The effect of diabetes mellitus upon the incidence of abnormal genital bleedings in women. Ginekol Pol 49:119–123

Westrom L, Bengtsson LPH, Mardh PA (1981) Incidence, trends and risks of ectopic pregnancy in a population of women. Br Med J 282:15–18

Whittaker PG, Taylor A, Lind T (1983) Unsuspected pregnancy loss in healthy women. Lancet I:1126–1127

Wright AD, London DR, Holder G, Williams JW, Rudd BT (1976) Luteinizing release hormone tests in impotent diabetic males. Diabetes 25:975–977

Younger D (1965) Infections and diabetes. In: White P (ed) Diabetes. Medical Clinics of North America. WB Saunders, Philadelphia, pp 1005–1013

Zavos PM, Wilson EA (1984) Retrograde ejaculation: etiology and treatment via the use of a new non-invasive method. Fertil Steril 42:627–632

8.   Epidemiology of Spontaneous Abortion in Insulin-Dependent Diabetic Women

N. C. Smith

Introduction

The first documentation of pregnancy in a diabetic woman was made by Bennewitz in 1826. No large series were published until the early 1900s but this is not surprising because the life expectancy after diabetes developed in the adult was 6 years and the fertility rate was at most 5% (Von Noorden 1882). Williams (1909) reported the outcome of 82 pregnancies in diabetic women from which there were 25 (30%) maternal deaths and only 30 live births, resulting in a total fetal wastage of 65%. An infant born alive to a diabetic mother was considered fortuitous and therapeutic abortion was often undertaken in those few unfortunate women who did fall pregnant. Abortion which occurred spontaneously was frequently regarded as a divine life-saving grace.

In 1921, Banting and Best discovered insulin and following its introduction, the life expectancy and health of the diabetic were greatly improved such that infertility was no longer a problem for the diabetic woman in her reproductive years. By the 1930s, clinical data on the pregnancy outcome of insulin-dependent diabetic women were accumulating rapidly and the perinatal mortality rate was reported in seven different series; by the late 1950s the outcome of a further 46 series of diabetic pregnancies had been published (Gellis and Hsia 1959). Many of these publications included spontaneous abortions and, reviewing these, Gellis and Hsia (1959) concluded that, although pregnancy failures were several times more common in patients with diabetes mellitus compared to normal women, this excessive loss occurred almost exclusively after 28 weeks' gestation so that the incidence of spontaneous abortion, prior to the period of viability, was not a serious problem.

Over the last three decades there has been a steady decline in the perinatal mortality rate and incidence of fetal malformations in the diabetic due to improved control of maternal hyperglycaemia before conception, during embryogenesis and throughout pregnancy, better obstetric and neonatal care and improved living standards. Consequently, the incidence of spontaneous abortion in diabetic women has assumed increasing prominence, and controversy still exists as to whether or not this is higher than in the normal population (Kalter 1987). It is the purpose of this review to speculate on the pathogenesis of spontaneous abortion in insulin-dependent diabetic women, to identify the problems of data collection and to review the larger epidemiological studies to determine if the incidence of spontaneous abortion is higher in diabetic compared to non-diabetic women and if it has changed over the years with better control of maternal blood glucose.

Pathogenesis of Spontaneous Abortion in Insulin-Dependent Diabetic Women

In non-diabetic women, around half of all clinically recognized first trimester abortions are chromosomally abnormal (Simpson and Bombard 1987). Anembryonic pregnancies account for about another 10% and these frequently have major abnormalities of karyotype (Fantel and Shepard 1987). The proportion of fetuses with major structural abnormalities is difficult to elucidate because many series include therapeutic abortions performed following ultrasound detection. Creasy et al. (1976) examined the pathology of 2607 spontaneous abortions: 804 had no identifiable fetus or sac but in the remainder, only 4% had structural malformations, half of which were neural tube defects.

There are no series which have completely documented the pathological, histological and karyotypical features of the products of conception following spontaneous abortion in diabetic women. This would be valuable information because the incidence of fetal abnormality in babies born to diabetic mothers is about three times that in the non-diabetic population. However, the described abnormalities are anatomical, as opposed to chromosomal, and disordered structure would be virtually impossible to identify in first-trimester products of conception. It is probable that a higher proportion of early pregnancy losses in diabetic women are due to fetal abnormality. Ultrasonic evidence of growth delay in the first trimester has been demonstrated in the pregnancies of diabetic women, especially if control has been poor around the time of conception (Pedersen et al. 1984). Such initial growth delay is associated with a higher risk of fetal abnormality (Pedersen and Mølsted-Pedersen 1981) and spontaneous abortion (Mantoni and Pedersen 1982).

It has been demonstrated clearly that improved control of maternal hyperglycaemia before conception and during embryogenesis reduces the fetal malformation rate (Miller et al. 1981). Hypoglycaemia tends to be more common than hyperglycaemia in the first trimester. However, higher glycosylated haemoglobin levels have been found in those diabetic women who abort compared to those who do not (Wright et al. 1983; Miodovnik et al. 1985). Recent work presented at this meeting by Hare and co-workers (1988) demonstrated a 33% risk of spontaneous abortion in 15 patients with HbA_1 values of 14% or more in the first trimester.

It seems highly likely, therefore, that the pathogenesis of the excess spontaneous abortion rate in diabetic women is directly attributable to poor glycaemic control which may result in initial growth delay and embryonic death with or without associated malformation. By ensuring good glycaemic control before and during early pregnancy, a reduction in the spontaneous abortion rate should ensue.

Problems of Data Collection and Analysis

In attempting to evaluate the incidence of spontaneous abortion in diabetic women, there are problems relating to definition, methods of detection and to the characteristics of the study population.

Definition

Most studies include all clinical losses up to 20 weeks gestational age, some up to 24 weeks and a few up to 28 weeks. Only one study has attempted to evaluate preclinical losses in diabetics by measuring serum human chorionic gonadotrophin (HCG) within 3 weeks of conception (Mills 1984). In the United Kingdom, legislation dictates that any fetus born dead at or after 28 weeks gestation is registered as a stillbirth and so any fetus born dead before this time is regarded as an abortion. The World Health Organization (1977) definition of spontaneous abortion is "loss of concepti weighing less than 500 g (which is approximately equal to 22 weeks completed gestation) irrespective of whether or not there is any sign of life". This can be applied easily and should be used universally so that comparisons can be made readily.

All studies include spontaneous abortions but many also include induced abortions performed because of the presence of diabetic complications or following prenatal diagnosis of fetal abnormality or intrauterine death. All may be related to the diabetes and therefore should be documented but defined clearly into separate categories.

Methods of Detection

The only certain method of detecting all abortions in diabetic women is to recruit subjects prepregnancy and evaluate prospectively. Most studies are retrospective, data being obtained from hospital admissions of referred diabetics, and so early losses in unbooked patients are frequently under-reported. Confirmation of pregnancy should be obtained by urinary or serum HCG assay and/or histological confirmation of trophoblast. Now that prepregnancy care of the diabetic is recognized internationally as being beneficial for both mother and fetus, detection of spontaneous abortion should be facilitated and the true incidence ascertained.

Characteristics of the Study Population

Many reports on the epidemiology of spontaneous abortion in diabetic women are from referral centres where the more badly controlled patients may be managed. Patients may not be seen until the second trimester and will not be referred if early spontaneous abortion has already occurred. Thus an unrepresentative study population can easily result. There are also many confounding variables which are rarely stated. These include age, parity, maternal compensation for previous losses, race and exogenous factors such as social habits and occupational toxins. However, to take account of these confounding variables and further subdivide the study population would result most often in meaningless data because few centres can accumulate sufficient numbers of pregnant insulin-dependent diabetic women in the first instance. The ideal study should be from a defined region, recruiting prepregnancy a representative sample of the population with matched controls.

The Frequency of Spontaneous Abortion

The true frequency of spontaneous abortion in the diabetic woman has yet to be established and there is considerable debate in the literature as to whether or not it is higher than in non-diabetic women. The debate revolves around the problems, already outlined, of devising a true epidemiological study. To compare the incidence of spontaneous abortion in diabetics with that of the normal population is also difficult because a flawless study recruiting non-diabetic women prospectively, before pregnancy, has never been achieved. Roman and Stevenson (1983) cite 10 studies of normal patients and found the average clinical spontaneous abortion rate to be 15%.

A historical review of spontaneous abortion in diabetic women was undertaken by Kalter (1987). Over 50 series published between 1950 and 1986 were cited and from a total of 8041 diabetic pregnancies the spontaneous abortion rate was found to average 10.0%. However, the majority of these studies did not specify the gestation interval covered or the time of first examination.

Table 8.1 lists the spontaneous abortion rates from those series in which the total pregnancy number was greater than 200 and these rates range from 4.0% to 14.2%. In the largest series of 1053 diabetic pregnancies accumulated over 34 years from 1951 to 1984 in Dublin (Drury 1986), the spontaneous abortion rate was found to be only 9.0%. However, in an earlier report of the series, Drury et al. (1977) stated that the referrals, which came from all over Ireland, occurred "at varying stages of gestation and sometimes far too late for effective management". It is likely therefore that significant under-reporting of all spontaneous abortions must have occurred. Such epidemiological problems are found with all the reports because the patients referred to the centres do not constitute all the diabetic pregnancies in the population under study and the catchment area is frequently ill-defined.

The reported rates over specific time intervals from Dublin and the Joslin Center in Boston, two of the biggest referral centres in the world, are

Table 8.1.   Abortion rates in insulin-dependent diabetic women from published series of more than 200 pregnancies

Authors	Total pregnancy number (%)	Therapeutic abortion rate (%)	Spontaneous abortion rate (%)
Pedowitz and Schlevin (1955)	246	2.5	10.8
Clayton (1956)	201	4.0	4.0
Gellis and Hsia (1959)	934	4.6	14.2
Komrower and Langley (1961)	213	—	9.4
O'Leary and Freda (1965)	256	—	13.3
Delaney and Ptacek (1970)	243	—	4.9
Crane and Wahl (1981)	214	—	12.1
Mølsted-Pedersen and Kuhl (1986)	223	4.0	7.9
Drury (1986)	1056	—	9.0

documented in Tables 8.2 and 8.3. Although the time intervals are not strictly comparable, it is quite clear that the spontaneous abortion rates have remained remarkably static compared with the perinatal mortality rates which have shown a dramatic decline with improvements in the obstetric and diabetic management of pregnant women and in the intensive care given to their newborn infants.

Table 8.2.   Spontaneous abortion rates reported from Dublin (Drury et al. 1977; Drury 1986)

Study period	Total pregnancies	Perinatal mortality rate	Spontaneous abortion rate
1951–1976	618	9.5%	8.4%
1977–1984	435	5.3%	9.9%
Total	1053	7.4%	9.0%

Table 8.3.   Spontaneous abortion rates reported from Joslin Clinic, Boston (Gellis and Hsia 1959; Kitzmiller et al. 1978)

Study period	Total pregnancies	Perinatal mortality rate (%)	Abortion rate (%) Therapeutic	Spontaneous	Total
1898–1922	115	30.0	not stated		24.3
1940–1950	471	18.9	4.9	11.1	15.0
1950–1956	463	15.3	3.8	11.8	15.6
1975–1976	162	3.1	4.3	12.9	17.2

It is of interest that more recently reported series, specifically addressing the question of spontaneous abortion in diabetic women, have reported higher rates. Wright et al. (1983) from Birmingham, England, reported a rate of 26% in 58 consecutive pregnancies and Miodovnik et al. (1984) in a long-term study of juvenile diabetics seen at the University of Cincinnati Medical Center, Ohio, found a rate of 30% in 132 pregnancies. Sutherland and Pritchard (1986) have published the only series where a total population was studied. These workers reported a spontaneous abortion rate of 17% from 164 pregnancies in the years 1956 to 1975, from the Grampian region of Scotland where all pregnant insulin-dependent diabetics are seen by a single team of physicians and obstetricians. From 1976 to 1987 a further 200 insulin-dependent diabetics have been managed and the spontaneous abortion rate has fallen to 13.5%. This fall has coincided with the introduction of prepregnancy care in 1976.

Conclusions

Although there are few reports in the literature which demonstrate that the incidence of spontaneous abortion in insulin-dependent diabetic women is higher than in the normal population, the association of poor glycaemic control with early growth delay and fetal abnormality in diabetic pregnancies is evidence of a pathological basis which is likely to lead to an increased risk of loss in the first and second trimesters. With the widespread practice of prepregnancy counselling a clear picture should emerge in the forthcoming years to demonstrate whether or not poor glycaemic control in early pregnancy increases the risk of spontaneous abortion.

References

Bennewitz HG (1826) Jahresberichte des Königlichen Poliklinischen Institutes der Universität zu Berlin, vol. 12. G. Reimer, Berlin, p. 23
Clayton SG (1956) The pregnant diabetic: a report on 200 cases. J Obstet Gynaecol Br Commonw 63:532–541
Crane JP, Wahl N (1981) The role of maternal diabetes in repetitive abortion. Fertil Steril 36:477–479
Creasy MR, Crolla JA, Alderman E (1976) A cytogenic study of human spontaneous abortions using banding techniques. Hum Genet 31:177–196
Delaney JJ, Ptacek J (1970) Three decades of experience with diabetic pregnancies. Am J Obstet Gynecol 106:550–556
Drury MI (1986) Management of the pregnant diabetic patient – are the pundits right? Diabetologia 29:10–12
Drury MI, Greene AT, Strong JM (1977) Pregnancy complicated by clinical diabetes mellitus. 49:519–552
Fantel AG, Shepard TH (1987) Morphological analysis of spontaneous abortuses. In: Bennett MJ, Edmonds DK (eds) Spontaneous and recurrent abortion. Blackwell, Oxford, pp 8–28
Gellis SS, Hsia DY-Y (1959) The infant of the diabetic mother. Am J Dis Child 97:1–41
Hare JW, Greene MF, Cloherty JP et al. (1988) First trimester glycaemic risk for major malformations and spontaneous abortions. Poster presentation at 4th Aberdeen International Colloquium on Carbohydrate Metabolism in Pregnancy and the Newborn
Kalter H (1987) Diabetes and spontaneous abortion. Obstet Gynecol 156:1243–1253
Kitzmiller JL, Cloherty JP, Younger MD et al. (1978) Diabetic pregnancy and perinatal morbidity. Am J Obstet Gynecol 131:560–580
Komrower GM, Langley FA (1961) The fate of the diabetic woman's child. Manchester Med Gaz 40:166–171
Mantoni M, Pedersen JF (1982) Fetal growth delay in threatened abortion: an ultrasound study. Br J Obstet Gynaecol 89:525–527

Miller E, Hare JW, Cloherty PJ et al. (1981) Elevated maternal haemoglobin A_{1C} in early pregnancy and major congenital anomalies in infants of diabetic mothers. N Engl J Med 304:1331–1334

Mills JL (1984) A prospective study of fetal losses in diabetic and control pregnancies from the third week post conception. Diabetes 33 (supplement):46A

Miodovnik M, Lavin JP, Knowles HC et al. (1984) Spontaneous abortion among insulin-dependent diabetic women. Am J Obstet Gynecol 150:373–376

Miodovnik M, Skillman C, Holroyde JC et al. (1985) Elevated maternal glycohemoglobin in early pregnancy and spontaneous abortion among insulin-dependent diabetic women. Am J Obstet Gynecol 153:439–442

Mølsted-Pedersen L, Kuhl C (1986) Obstetrical management in diabetic pregnancy: the Copenhagen experience. Diabetologia 29:13–16

O'Leary JA, Freda VJ (1965) Maternal blood group and fetal wastage in pregnant diabetics. Obstet Gynecol 26:695–697

Pedersen JF, Mølsted-Pedersen L (1981) Early growth delay detected by ultrasound marks increased risk of congenital malformation in diabetic pregnancy. Br Med J 283:269–271

Pedersen JF, Mølsted-Pedersen L, Mortensen HB (1984) Fetal growth delay and maternal hemoglobin A_{1C} in early pregnancy. Obstet Gynecol 64:351–352

Pedowitz P, Shlevin EL (1955) The pregnant diabetic patient. Am J Obstet Gynecol 69:395–404

Roman E, Stevenson AC (1983) Spontaneous abortion. In: Barron SL, Thomson AM (eds) Obstetric epidemiology. Academic Press, London, pp 61–87

Simpson JL, Bombard A (1987) Chromosomal abnormalities in spontaneous abortion: frequency, pathology and genetic counselling. In: Bennet MJ, Edmonds DK (eds) Spontaneous and recurrent abortion. Blackwell, Oxford, pp 51–76

Sutherland HW, Pritchard CW (1986) Increased incidence of spontaneous abortion in pregnancies complicated by maternal diabetes mellitus. Am J Obstet Gynecol 155:135–138

Von Noorden CH (1882) Die Zuckerkrankheit. Trans Obstet Soc Lond 24:256

WHO (1977) Recommended definitions, terminology and format for statistical tables related to the perinatal period. Acta Obstet Gynecol 56:247–253

Williams JW (1909) The clinical significance of glycosuria in pregnant women. Am J Med Sci 137:1

Wright AD, Nicholson HO, Pollock A et al. (1983) Spontaneous abortion and diabetes mellitus. Postgrad Med J 59:295–298

9.   Ultrasound Studies on Fetal Growth

J. Fog-Pedersen, L. Mølsted-Pedersen and S. Møller

The aim of this study has been to examine, by ultrasound scanning, the growth process that in the diabetic pregnancy quite often leads to fetal macrosomia and delivery of the typical big, fat "diabetes baby".

During the study we observed that some fetuses in early diabetic pregnancy, as judged from the crown–rump length, are smaller than normal (Pedersen and Mølsted-Pedersen 1979), and furthermore are at a higher risk of being malformed (Pedersen and Mølsted-Pedersen 1981). However, only three groups have confirmed the existence of an early growth delay (Tchobroutsky et al. 1985; Visser et al. 1985; Sutherland 1986) and a multicentre study in the United States has demonstrated only a minimal discrepancy between ultrasound age and menstrual age (J. L. Mills, personal communication).

In this chapter we will therefore first give our present view on the early growth delay and its consequences. Thereafter we will, on the basis of serial ultrasound measurements of fetal head and trunk, discuss growth in the second and especially the third trimesters. Our goals will be (a) to establish a population growth curve and observe when and how it deviates from normal, and to evaluate our ability to (b) pick out fetuses that are macrosomic and (c) pick out, as early in pregnancy as possible, fetuses that are in the process of developing macrosomia.

Early Growth Delay

Our study population comprises 201 insulin-dependent diabetic pregnancies. The mothers had given reliable information on regular menstrual cycles of 28–30-day (d) intervals, had not been using the pill during the last 3 months prior to pregnancy, had reported to the diabetes centre early enough to have at least one ultrasound examination showing a fetus with a CRL of 10–80 mm, normally equivalent to a menstrual age of 7 to 14 weeks, and were delivered of a singleton fetus of 1000 g or more.

For each CRL determination we calculated the discrepancy between fetal age as assessed from the CRL and the age from the first day of the last menstrual period (LMP) (Pedersen 1982). We use the term "early growth delay" for this discrepancy, which was on an average 4.2 d (Fig. 9.1).

We have various indications that poor diabetes control leads to early growth delay. Most prominent is that HbA_{1c} concentrations in the first trimester are significantly lower in mothers of normal-size fetuses than in mothers with too small fetuses (Pedersen et al. 1984). We also believe that diabetic control around the time of conception and in early pregnancy has improved during the 10 years this study has been running.

The series was therefore divided at LMP before or after 1 January 1980, which gives two groups of almost equal size. The first group (Fig. 9.1, upper panel) is almost identical to the series reported on 5 years ago (Pedersen et al. 1984). The dashed lines symbolize the 95% confidence interval in our control series, ±5.5 d (Pedersen 1982). Fetuses to the right of this range are therefore significantly smaller than normal. Forty per cent of the fetuses in the first half of the series were smaller than normal, and to this must be added the fact that within the normal range there is an obvious skewness.

It is beyond the scope of this chapter to discuss in more detail when this growth delay takes place. A postovulation delay has been observed in patients with basal body temperature measurements (Pedersen 1986), but it is not surprising that a delay in ovulation may occur in diabetic patients (Pedersen and Mølsted-Pedersen, unpublished). For practical purposes it is enough to state that there is in the early diabetic pregnancy a discrepancy between ultrasound age and menstrual age.

In the last half of the series (Fig. 9.1, lower panel) the number of significantly too small fetuses has fallen to 30%, but the distribution within the normal range is still skewed to the right, so that most, if not all, fetuses in early diabetic pregnancy are affected by some degree of growth delay, only today it is to a lesser extent than earlier in the series. The average growth delay has fallen from 5 d to 3½ d.

The number of malformed fetuses has also fallen dramatically, not only in this study but also in the whole Copenhagen series of insulin-dependent diabetic women. There were 10 malformed fetuses (10%) in the first half of the series (Table 9.1), mainly with cardiac and neural-tube defects. In the second half there were only three malformed babies (3%), but type and severity were unchanged. The high risk involved with significant growth delay has fallen from 21% to 6%. The figures are now fortunately very small, but early growth delay may still be a risk marker for congenital malformation (6% vs 1%).

We believe that this fortunate trend is a result of improved diabetes control. We also believe that the quality of the metabolic compensation explains the difference between our results and most others'. Other centres usually see their diabetic patients for the first time later in pregnancy, so that the subgroup of patients they do see early enough to measure CRL are specially motivated, and their regulation is probably better-than-average.

By contrast in Copenhagen we see, for traditional and geographical reasons, almost a complete cross-section of the pregnant diabetic population in the first trimester, including both the well-compensated patients and the less well compensated, who are likely to show significant early growth delay.

Table 9.2 shows that the babies in the early growth delay group at birth weigh 400 g less than those of normal size in early pregnancy, in spite of a greater gestational age. Their ultrasound age, which takes the early growth delay into account, however, is 4.5 d younger. Contrary to our earlier belief (Pedersen and

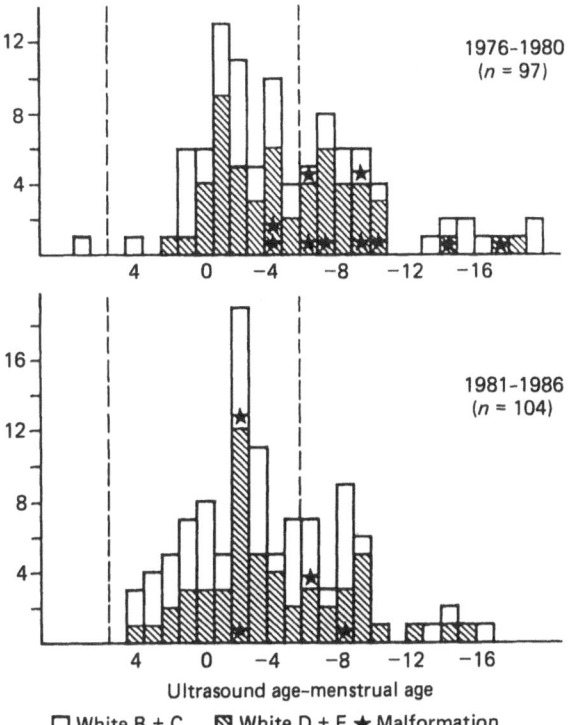

1976-1980
(n = 97)

1981-1986
(n = 104)

Ultrasound age-menstrual age

□ White B + C   ◪ White D + F ★ Malformation

Fig. 9.1. Distribution of differences between ages as assessed by ultrasound and by using menstrual data in 201 early diabetic pregnancies. *Dashed lines* indicate normal range (± 5.5 d). Series divided at last menstrual period before or after 1 January 1980.

Table 9.1. Incidence of severe congenital malformation (SM) related to fetal size (crown–rump length) in early pregnancy in the first and last half of a series

Early fetal size	SM before 1.1.1980	SM after 1.1.1980	Total
<6 d too small	2/58 (3%)	1/73 (1%)	3/131 (2%)
≥6 d too small	8/39 (21%)	2/31 (6%)	10/70 (14%)
Total	10/97 (10%)	3/104 (3%)	13/201 (6%)

Mølsted-Pedersen 1981) that this difference in ultrasound age could explain the observed birth weight difference, with this larger series we now assume that fetuses that are too small in early pregnancy also grow more poorly in the second and third trimesters, and that this is not just a manifestation of a genetic difference in growth potential.

A group of paediatricians has examined the infants of the first part of the study at 4 years of age. In the present context it is very interesting that they found the well-recognized slightly poorer psychomotor development of infants of diabetic mothers confined to those who were too small in early pregnancy (Petersen et al. 1988). Maybe, therefore, there is in the embryos which are subject to significant

Table 9.2. Clinical characteristics of pregnancy in 201 insulin-dependent diabetic women in relation to fetal size (crown–rump length) in early pregnancy

	Early fetal size	
	<6 d too small	≥6 d too small
No. of mothers	131	70
Mean birthweight (g)	3498	3102
Mean gestational age at birth (d)	255.4	259.0
Mean difference between menstrual age and "ultrasound age" in early pregnancy (d)	1.4	9.5
Mean "ultrasound age" at birth (d)	254.0	249.5

early growth impairment an analogy between induction of malformations and induction of tiny cerebral lesions.

Summary and Conclusions on Early Growth Delay

Our present view on the early growth delay can be summarized as follows:

1. The early growth delay, whenever it takes place, is a reality.
2. Early growth delay is the result of a less-than-optimal metabolic compensation.
3. Early growth delay is (or has been) a risk marker for congenital malformation.
4. Early growth delay is apparently followed by poorer fetal growth.
5. Early growth delay is followed by poorer postnatal psychomotor development.
6. Metabolic control at conception and in early pregnancy should be optimal so as to avoid early growth delay and its associated manifestations. Pregnancy should be planned.
7. Diabetic women should have an ultrasound scan for dating in the first part of pregnancy. Patient management throughout pregnancy should in the case of a discrepancy be guided by the ultrasound age rather than the menstrual age.

Fetal Growth in the Second and Third Trimesters

Growth of Head and Trunk

The following observations originate from a subgroup of the patients that were included in the first part of this chapter, namely those studied in the period 1 January 1976 to 1 January 1982. The subgroup includes 125 insulin-dependent diabetic women in whom apart from the CRL measurement(s) a total of 633 measurements of the biparietal diameter (BPD) and 533 measurements of abdominal circumference (AC) were obtained from week 12–14 until delivery. For comparison a control series of volunteers was studied in a similar longitudinal design, and over the same period of time. The composition of the control series has been described elsewhere (Pedersen 1986). All ultrasound measurements were obtained with a Nuclear Enterprises' (Edinburgh) Diasonograph, and by the same observer (JFP).

The CRL growth curve (in weeks 7–14) is convex to the right, whereas the growth curves of BPD and AC (in weeks 14–20) are convex to the left. A growth model common to all three parameters should therefore be s-shaped. Furthermore it should preferably be zero at the day of conception, whch would enable us to use the CRL measurements to define a common zero-point for all three curves, and thus correct for the early growth delay.

The Rossavik model (Rossavik 1982) will come up with such a curve. It has the formula $P=ct^{(k+st)}$ where P is the parameter, c is a coefficient mainly indicating growth rate in the first two trimesters, t is time calculated from the zero-point, s is a coefficient that reflects the changes in growth rate in the third trimester and k is a coefficient with a value relative to the dimension of the parameter.

To facilitate the handling of the early growth delay we rewrote the formula as follows: $P=c^{[k+s(t-t_0)]}$ where t is the time calculated from the first day of the last menstrual period.

In order to achieve a normal distribution, the observations were first subjected to logarithmic transformation, and the formula used for the estimation was therefore $\log P=\log C+[k+s(t-t_0)]\log(t-t_0)$. A t_0 of 14 was first chosen and the individual coefficients were estimated. From those a set of common coefficients was established and used to estimate individual t_0 values, and the cycle was repeated three times. The procedure was the same in the control and the diabetes series. Through this procedure all significant variation in CRL was transferred to t_0, which means that the fetuses had the same CRL growth curve but different t_0. In fact t_0-14 is the computer-estimated equivalent of the delay. The coefficients for the average growth curves are seen in the formulas in Tables 9.3 and 9.4.

Table 9.3. Longitudinal study of growth of fetal crown–rump length (CRL), biparietal diameter (BPD) and abdominal circumference (AC) in 101 control pregnancies (number of observations given in parentheses)

CRL (in mm) = $0.001642 \times A^{(2.4640-0.0003731 \times A)}$	($n=300$)
BPD (in cm) = $0.003177 \times A^{(1.9911-0.0008914 \times A)}$	($n=710$)
AC (in cm) = $0.004891 \times A^{(1.7126-0.0004718 \times A)}$	($n=581$)

A = days since first day of last period$-t_0$, t_0 being the individually estimated age correction. (t_0-14 is the computer estimated equivalent of the delay.)

There was no difference in the first trimester between the CRL curves from the normal and diabetic pregnancies. The BPD curves overlap almost completely and the difference never exceeds 0.3 mm (Fig. 9.2). This is not surprising, and in keeping with the observations by others (Murata and Martin 1973; Aantaa and Forss 1980; Ogata et al. 1980).

Table 9.4. Longitudinal study of growth of fetal crown–rump length (CRL), biparietal diameter (BPD) and abdominal circumference (AC) in 125 insulin-dependent diabetic pregnancies (number of observations given in parentheses)

CRL (in mm) = 0.0008598 × $A^{(2.6504-0.0008518 \times A)}$	($n=216$)
BPD (in cm) = 0.005095 × $A^{(1.9981-0.0008874 \times A)}$	($n=633$)
AC (in cm) = 0.003931 × $A^{(1.7441-0.0003728 \times A)}$	($n=533$)

A = days since first day of last period—t_0, t_0 being the individually estimated age correction. (t_0-14 is the computer estimated equivalent of the delay.)

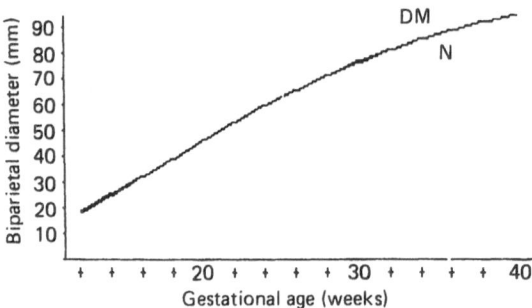

Fig. 9.2. Growth of biparietal diameter in normal (*N*) and diabetic (*DM*) pregnancy. Graphic representation of formulas given in Tables 9.3 and 9.4.

The average curve of AC deviates from normal from week 24 (Fig. 9.3). It is not surprising either, although it is a little earlier than observed by others (Ogata et al. 1980). There is a remarkably linear increase in the deviation from normal: one centimetre at 28 weeks, 2 cm at 32 weeks and 3 cm at 36 weeks. One would also have expected a small difference earlier than 24 weeks, but analysis of the raw data confirms that there is no difference. With more data it might be possible to tell whether the expected difference is hidden by an early-growth-delay-associated growth impairment.

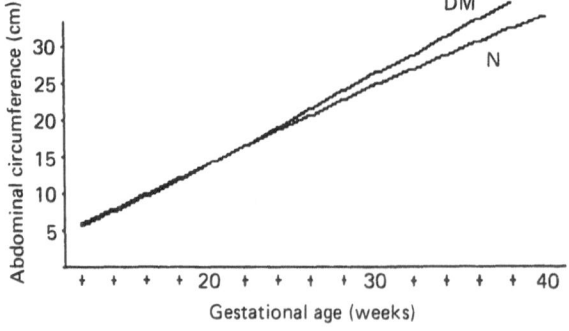

Fig. 9.3. Growth of abdominal circumference in normal (*N*) and diabetic (*DM*) pregnancy. Graphic representation of formulas given in Tables 9.3 and 9.4.

The Population Growth Curve

There are many formulas that try to estimate fetal weight from one or more ultrasound measurements. Two quite popular formulas, by Warsof et al. (1977) and Shepard et al. (1982), use BPD and AC (Table 9.5). They are constructed for non-diabetic pregnancies, and in order to evaluate their efficacy in diabetic pregnancy we extracted from the 125 fetuses 63 who had a set of BPD and AC measurements obtained within 7 d before delivery. We used the two formulas to estimate weight, and added to the estimates 40 g/d for the expected growth from the ultrasound exam until delivery. These weights were compared with the actual birthweights.

Table 9.5. Formulas for estimating fetal weight (FW) from biparietal diameter (BPD) and abdominal circumference (AC)

$\log_{10}$ (FW) = $-1.599 + 0.144$ (BPD) $+ 0.032$ (AC)
  -0.111 (BPD^2 × AC)/1000

(Warsof et al. 1977)

$\log_{10}$ (FW) = $-1.749 + 0.166$ (BPD) $+ 0.046$ (AC)
  -2.646 (AC × BPD)/1000

(Shepard et al. 1982)

The mean errors and standard deviations (Table 9.6) are slightly smaller than those reported recently by Benson et al. (1987) for diabetic pregnancies and slightly bigger than those reported for non-diabetic pregnancies (Hadlock et al. 1984). The Shepard formula had the smallest systematic error, and therefore was used to calculate weight. The resulting average growth curve for the fetus of a diabetic mother is shown in Fig. 9.4, together with a similar growth curve obtained from the 101 control pregnancies.

Table 9.6. Performance characteristics of current formulas for estimating fetal weight (mean ± SD) ($n=63$)

Formulas	Error (g)	Error (%)
Warsof et al.	-191 ± 342	-5.1 ± 9.8
Shepard et al.	-44 ± 345	-0.6 ± 10.3

It is noteworthy that the growth curve in the non-diabetic pregnancy is linear from week 32, without a late flattening. The daily weight gain in this period is 30 g, whereas the average weight gain from week 32 to 38 in an American growth standard is 29 g (Brenner et al. 1976). Eik-Nes et al. (1980) and Secher et al. (1986) have found similar linear population weight-for-gestational-age charts in two large series of ultrasound-dated pregnancies. Eik-Nes et al. (1980) concluded that the usual s-shape is produced by gestational ages that are incorrect. Another

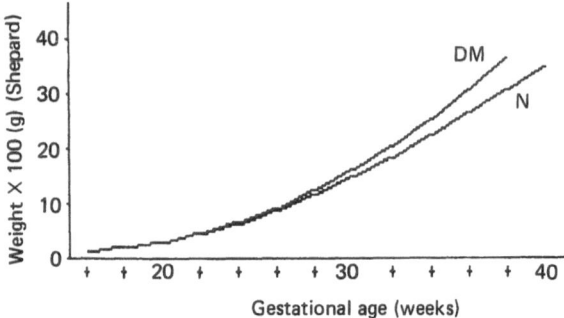

Fig. 9.4. Fetal growth in normal (*N*) and diabetic (*DM*) pregnancy. Weight estimated from biparietal diameter and abdominal circumference by formula of Shepard et al. (1982).

reason is that large fetuses tend to be delivered early, and therefore will be missing in late pregnancy.

In the diabetic pregnancy, growth from week 32 is also linear (Fig. 9.4), but of course steeper, the average daily weight gain being 40 g. Given the linear growth in the control pregnancies this finding is not surprising, but we are not aware of similar studies or of birthweight-for-gestational-age charts based on ultrasound-dated diabetic pregnancies that could confirm or question it.

It should be kept in mind that the Shepard formula, and similar ones, is based upon combined ultrasound and birthweight data, and therefore not necessarily valid for birth weights below 2000 g, where the amount of data is small. However, there is no reason to believe that the difference between the diabetes and control curves should not be estimated fairly reliably. With the described procedure and a larger number of pregnancies it should be possible also to define growth patterns for subgroups of diabetic pregnancies.

Detection of Manifest Macrosomia

Macrosomia has been defined absolutely as weight >4000 g (Elliott et al. 1982; Benson et al. 1987) or, better, relatively as birthweight above the 90th centile (Hadlock et al. 1985; Tamura et al. 1986). From Fig. 9.4 it is obvious, however, that the fetus of a diabetic mother on average will traverse several centile lines as pregnancy progresses, i.e. the older a fetus is, the higher will be its centile ranking. Instead an arbitrary cut-off line has been defined. It passes through 4000 g at 37 weeks, or 259 d, and has a slope of 40 g/d. This means that the line goes from 2600 g at 32 weeks to 4840 g at 40 weeks.

The figures in Table 9.6 indicate that we estimate fetal weight with a 95% confidence interval of ± 700 g (=± 2 SD). It is therefore not surprising that in utero diagnosis of macrosomia is found to be somewhat inaccurate (Tamura et al. 1986; Benson et al. 1987).

Addition of femur length to measurements of head and trunk would, because of the association between femur length and crown–heel length, improve prenatal estimates of fetal weight (Hadlock et al. 1984). However, this would not necessarily be an advantage in the diabetic pregnancy, where in fact the abdominal circumference may be a biologically more relevant parameter than weight.

Detection of Developing Macrosomia

The aim was to find the earliest 2-week period in which a reliable prediction of macrosomia as defined above can be made. (A 2-week period was considered the narrowest interval that would be realistic if patients were to be scheduled for an ultrasound study.) One could of course use the weight estimates, but since the BPD does not deviate from normal in diabetic pregnancy, it seems more rational to use only the abdominal circumference. In weeks 26 and 27 there were too many false-negative macrosomia predictions, but in weeks 28 and 29 a fairly reliable prediction could be achieved. Figure 9.5 shows the AC values from 47 fetuses who had an abdominal circumference measurement taken in the 28th or 29th week. If there was more than one measurement, the one closest to the centre of the interval was chosen. The solid line in Fig. 9.5 is the average AC growth curve, and the dashed line is just 1 cm above.

Fetuses who in week 28 or 29 have an abdominal circumference 1 cm or more above average have a likelihood of developing macrosomia of 15/19 or 77%, whereas fetuses with abdominal circumferences smaller than that have a likelihood of not becoming macrosomic of 27/28 or 96% (Table 9.7). Table 9.8 lists the cut-off values. The point of this is of course that if we can define a high-risk group as early as this, we have 10 weeks in which we could intensify therapy in an attempt to avoid, or at least lessen, the macrosomia.

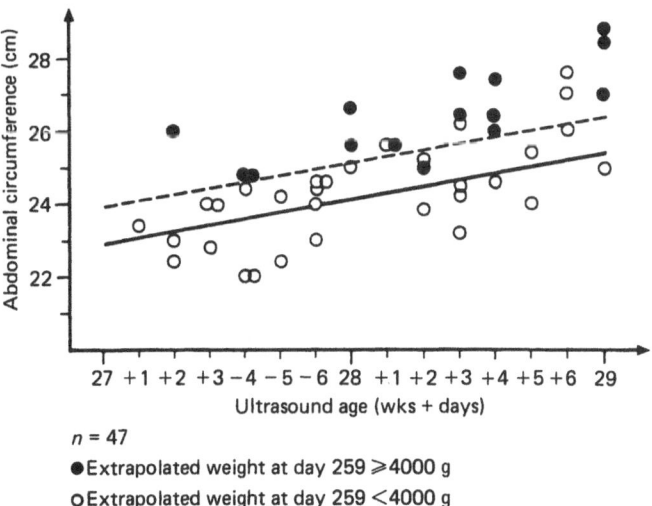

n = 47

● Extrapolated weight at day 259 ≥4000 g

○ Extrapolated weight at day 259 <4000 g

Fig. 9.5. Prediction of macrosomia for measurement of abdominal circumference (AC) in weeks 28 and 29. *Solid line* represents average curve of AC in diabetic pregnancy, *dashed line* is 1.0 cm above.

Table 9.7. Prediction of macrosomia from abdominal circumference (AC) measurements at week 28

	AC≥limit	AC<limit	Total
Macrosomia	15	1	16
No macrosomia	4	27	31
Total	19	28	47

Prevalence of macrosomia 16/47 (34%).

Table 9.8. Lower limit of abdominal circumference (AC) predictive of macrosomia

Ultrasound age[a] (weeks+days)	AC (cm)	Ultrasound age (weeks+days)	AC (cm)
27+1	24.1	28+1	25.3
+2	24.3	+2	25.5
+3	24.4	+3	25.7
+4	24.6	+4	25.9
+5	24.8	+5	26.0
+6	25.0	+6	26.2
28+0	25.1	29+0	26.4

[a] Ultrasound age defined from CRL determination in first trimester.

References

Aantaa K, Forss M (1980) Growth of the fetal biparietal diameter in different types of pregnancies. Radiology 137:167–169

Benson CB, Doubilet PM, Salzman DH (1987) Sonographic determination of fetal weights in diabetic pregnancies. Am J Obstet Gynecol 156:441–444

Brenner WE, Edelman DA, Hendricks CH (1976) A standard of fetal growth for the United States of America. Am J Obstet Gynecol 126:555–564

Eik-Nes SH, Persson P-H, Grottum P (1980) Revaluation of standards for human fetal growth. In: Eik-Nes SH (ed.) Ultrasonic assessment of human fetal weight, growth and blood flow. Thesis Malmö, Litos Reprotryk AB

Elliott JP, Garite TJ, Freeman RK et al. (1982) Ultrasonic prediction of fetal macrosomia in diabetic patients. Obstet Gynecol 60:159–162

Hadlock FP, Harrist RB, Carpenter RJ, Deter RL, Park SK (1984) Sonographic estimation of fetal weight. Radiology 150:535–540

Hadlock FP, Harrist RB, Fearneyhough TC, Deter RL, Park SK, Rossavik IK (1985) Use of femur length/abdominal circumference ratio in detecting the macrosomic fetus. Radiology 154:503–550

Murata Y, Martin CB (1973) Growth of the biparietal diameter of the fetal head in diabetic pregnancy. Am J Obstet Gynecol 115:252–256

Ogata ES, Sabaggha R, Metzger BE, Phelps RL, Freinkel N (1980) Serial ultrasonography to assess evolving fetal macrosomia. J Am Med Ass 243:2405–2408

Pedersen JF (1982) Fetal crown–rump length measurement by ultrasound in normal pregnancy. Br J Obstet Gynaecol 89:926–930

Pedersen JF (1986) Ultrasound studies in fetal crown–rump length in early normal and diabetic pregnancy. Dan Med Bull 33:296–304

Pedersen JF, Mølsted-Pedersen L (1979) Early growth retardation in diabetic pregnancy. Br Med J 1:18–19

Pedersen JF, Mølsted-Pedersen L (1981) Early fetal growth delay detected by ultrasound marks increased risk of congenital malformation in diabetic pregnancy Br Med J 283:269–271

Pedersen JF, Mølsted-Pedersen L, Mortensen HB (1984) Fetal growth delay and maternal hemoglobin A_{1c} in early diabetic pregnancy. Obstet Gynecol 64:351–352

Petersen MB, Pedersen SA, Greisen G, Pedersen JF, Mølsted-Pedersen L (1988) Early growth delay in diabetic pregnancy: relation to psychomotor development at age 4. Br Med J 296:598–600

Rossavik IK (1982) Patterns and principles of fetal growth. Thesis University of Oslo

Secher NJ, Hansen PK, Lenstrup C et al. (1986) Birthweight-for-gestational age charts based on early ultrasound estimation of gestational age. Br J Obstet Gynaecol 93:128–134

Shepard MJ, Richards VA, Berkowitz RL, Warsof SL, Hobbins JC (1982) An evaluation of two equations for predicting fetal weight by ultrasound. Am J Obstet Gynecol 142:47–54

Sutherland HW (1986) Methods of fetal monitoring and assessment of placental function in diabetic pregnancy. Acta Endocrinol 112 (Suppl 277):90–100

Tamura RK, Sabaggha RE, Depp R, Dooley SL, Socol ML (1986) Diabetic macrosomia: accuracy of third trimester. Obstet Gynecol 67:828–832

Tchobroutsky C, Breart GL, Rambaud DC, Henrion R (1985) Correlation between fetal defects and early growth delay observed by ultrasound. Lancet I:706–707

Visser GHA, Bekodam DJ, Muldeer EJH, van Ballegooie E (1985) Delayed emergence of fetal behaviour in type-1 diabetic women. Early Hum Dev 12:167–172

Warsof SL, Gohari P, Berkowitz RL, Hobbins JC (1977) The estimation of fetal weight by computer-assisted analysis. Am J Obstet Gynecol 128:881–892

10. Magnetic Resonance Imaging of the Feto-placental Unit

F. W. Smith

Introduction

The ability to assess metabolic change by non-invasive methods has long been sought after. Magnetic resonance imaging is a technique which shows considerable promise within this field, being a method for producing images of the body which are dependent upon the relationships of hydrogen protons in both water and fat.

Imaging of the human body using the phenomenon of nuclear magnetic resonance (NMR) has been introduced to more than 300 centres worldwide since the first clinical trial of the technique was started in 1980 at the University of Aberdeen (Edelstein et al. 1981; Smith et al. 1981a, b). Since 1980 it has been shown to be of diagnostic value in studying the brain (Bydder et al. 1982), abdomen and pelvis (Smith et al. 1981c, 1982; Smith 1986) and in paediatric practice (Levene et al. 1982; Smith 1983). More recently its potential for examining the normal fetus in utero has been demonstrated (Smith et al. 1983; Johnson et al. 1984; Smith et al. 1984), as well as abnormal pregnancy (McCarthy et al. 1985; Stark et al. 1985). The technique is free from hazard to both mother and fetus, relying not on ionizing radiations to produce an image, but on radiofrequency radiation which is harmless. The images are made up of information directly obtained from hydrogen atoms in the body and are more tissue-specific than X-ray computerized tomography (CT) images, which they closely resemble. The tissue specificity of the technique is due to the relationships of water to protein within different tissues and the hydrogen concentration in fat.

The potential use of this new imaging system in pregnancy is being explored and preliminary findings indicate that its images are more informative than those produced using ultrasound, but because the examination time is about four times longer than for ultrasound, it is not suggested that it replace ultrasound for the routine examination of the fetus. It is more likely to become a useful method for studying abnormal pregnancy and fetal body composition.

Physical Principles

The NMR phenomenon and the methods used for obtaining images using this technique are quite complex. Some of the phenomena can be explained only by quantum mechanics, but those relevant to a basic comprehension of the technique and sufficient for the appreciation of its applications in medicine may be understood using the principles of mechanics and magnetism.

To understand the underlying phenomenon, we should return to basic physics and chemistry. Each atomic nucleus is made up of nucleons, that is, protons and neutrons. (The one exception to this is the hydrogen atom, which consists of a single proton.) These nucleons rotate or "spin" about their axes. When pairs of protons or pairs of neutrons exist in the nucleus, they align in such a way that their spins cancel each other out, and such pairs are of no interest to us for this discussion. However, when a nucleus contains an unpaired proton or neutron or both, the nucleus will have a net spin (i.e. it will rotate on its axis). Because the nucleus has an electric charge, the spin corresponds to a current flowing about the spin axis; this in turn generates a magnetic field. The nucleus may, therefore, be considered a small bar magnet spinning on its axis.

In normal circumstances, these nuclei spin while pointing in a random direction, but when placed in a uniform static magnetic field, a portion of them will align with the field's lines of force. These spinning nuclei behave like tiny spinning tops or gyroscopes which, if tipped away from the vertical axis, will rotate about this axis in a motion known as precession. To make the nuclei precess around their axes, a smaller external electromagnetic field must be applied. This applied electromagnetic radiation must match the natural precessional frequency of the nuclei in the sample, hence the term nuclear magnetic resonance. This resonance frequency, often known as the Larmor frequency, is related mathematically to the externally applied magnetic field. The frequency is equal to the strength of the field measured in tesla (1 tesla = 10 000 gauss) multiplied by the gyromagnetic frequency, which is unique for each species of nucleus. Thus, for hydrogen protons in a 1-tesla field, the resonance frequency is 42.57 MHz. In the same field, the resonance frequencies of ^{31}P and ^{23}Na are 17.24 and 11.26 MHz respectively. These frequencies are far below those of X-rays and visible light, and are too weak to do any biological damage.

By choosing relevant frequencies, one can tune in to specific nuclei and observe their reactions. So far, all medical NMR images have been obtained with resonances from hydrogen nuclei (^1H). This is not only because hydrogen is abundant in the body, but also because it has a higher intrinsic NMR sensitivity than do other nuclei. ^{31}P is found in concentrations too low to image at present, but it is in sufficient quantity to be measured spectroscopically.

Several methods are available that use the NMR signal for image production. By manipulation of smaller electromagnetic fields around the static field, a number of different imaging techniques have been developed. Whether they use the projection reconstruction method used in X-ray CT or the sensitive-point, sensitive-line, steady-state free precession, or spin-warp methods, they all rely on measuring proton density (PD) and proton relaxation times (T_1 and T_2). Each of the different methods produces a slightly different type of image. Some rely purely on proton density, others purely on T_1 and T_2.

The different methods all rely on pulsed radiofrequency radiations of known strength, but they vary in the length of the pulse applied to manipulate the protons. The pulse sequence may also be varied (i.e. the intervals between pulses may be varied) to obtain useful data for image construction. The principles of the image production are simply explained. When the length of the applied radiofrequency is increased (so that the angle of precession is rotated through 90° and then stopped), the protons decay or relax, emitting the radiation they absorbed when they moved through 90°. The strength of this signal is a measure of the proton density of the section being examined. If a longer excitation pulse is used, the angle of precession can be moved through 180° (i.e. the spins are inverted). When the radiation is measured (specifically the length of time taken for the protons to return to equilibrium), the proton spin–lattice relaxation time or T_1 is measured.

T_1 varies from substance to substance, this variation depending on the relationship of the hydrogen atoms to their surroundings or molecular lattice. Short relaxation times exist where water (rich in hydrogen) is closely bound to proteins such as are found in muscles or liver, or in fat, which is also rich in hydrogen. Long relaxation times occur in fluids such as urine and cerebrospinal fluid and very short times occur in fat. Depending on the amounts of free and bound water in tissues, the T_1 will vary, allowing for good tissue discrimination and evaluation. The other important relaxation time is T_2 or the spin–spin relaxation time. Its magnitude depends on the magnetic interaction between nuclear spins during the relaxation of decay period. It therefore makes a significant contribution to the decay of the NMR signal. It may be measured specifically by applying a string of 180° pulses and recording the decaying emitted signal. T_2 is the main component of spin-echo images. Inversion recovery (IR) sequences have a number of advantages because they are sensitive to changes in both T_1 and T_2. The T_1 and T_2 signals are additive, thereby enhancing the contrast between different tissues. Because the decay characteristics of the IR signal are such that it falls to zero at the time of the 90° pulse for inverting pulse (TI) intervals, which are between 0.5 and 0.7 of the T_1 value of a particular tissue, when the repetition time (TR) value is greater than three times the T_1 value of the tissue, it is possible to select that value so as to suppress the signal from any chosen tissue (Smith and Sutherland 1988).

No reports of any adverse effect from the technique have been made. There are three areas of potential hazard; the static magnetic field, the rapidly changing electromagnetic fields and the radiofrequency radiation. The safe limits for all three are well above the levels employed by all currently available magnetic resonance imagers. The guidelines for imaging published by the National Radiological Protection Board lay down the safe limits and indicate that patients with cardiac pacemakers and ferromagnetic implants should be excluded. Whilst no evidence of any mutagenic effect has been reported in cell culture (Cooke and Morris 1981), dividing bacteria (Thomas and Morris 1981) or goats (Foster et al. 1983), it is advised that pregnancy in the first trimester should not be imaged unless that pregnancy is going to be terminated. However, in the second and third trimesters, when organogenesis is complete, no contraindication to imaging exists.

Patients and Methods

The imaging of pregnant patients in Aberdeen began in 1982 when a series of first-trimester pregnancies were examined prior to therapeutic termination of pregnancy to assess the feasibility of using NMR imaging (Smith et al. 1983). In 1984, following approval by the Ethical Committee and complying with the guidelines recommended by the National Radiological Protection Board (1983), imaging of second- and third-trimester pregnancies was started. Since this time, 117 pregnant patients have been examined (Table 10.1), 53 of the patients being examined on two or more occasions.

Table 10.1. Patients examined by magnetic resonance imaging (MRI) in pregnancy with associated complications and indications

Pregnancy condition	No. of patients
Mid-trimester abortion	9
Normal serial	29
Diabetes	24
Pre-eclampsia	6
Intrauterine growth retardation	5
Placental localization	10
Pelvimetry	16
Miscellaneous	18
Total number of patients	117
Total number of examinations	170

All examinations were performed using the University of Aberdeen NMR imager which uses a low field strength resistive magnet of 0.08 tesla (800 gauss) producing a resultant frequency of 3.4 MHz for the hydrogen proton. The "spin–warp" method of imaging is employed, using a pulse sequence of interleaved saturation recovery and inversion recovery pulses (TR = 1000 ms, TI = 200 ms). The inversion recovery pulse is preceded by adiabatic fast passage. For those requiring a more detailed description, the technique is fully documented elsewhere (Edelstein et al. 1980, 1981; Hutchison et al. 1980). The data needed to produce each set of images of a section are collected in just over 4 min (256 s); each section may be either 1.2 or 1.5 cm thick. These are interpolated to 256 × 256 for final presentation on a grey scale video display unit.

The principal aims of the study were to evaluate how well NMR imaging demonstrated maternal and fetal anatomy, and to determine normal fetal and maternal tissue characteristics by measuring T_1 at various stages of normal and complicated pregnancies.

Observations

The most striking feature of NMR images is the clarity with which different soft tissue structures are demonstrated. Unlike ultrasound and X-ray CT, no artefacts from bone or from bowel gas occur and maternal anatomy is invariably well demonstrated. Good definition of superficial tissues such as fat and muscle, as well as deep structures including bone, placenta, myometrium and cervix is obtained. This good definition is optimally demonstrated on the calculated T_1 images, where the contrast between the different tissues is best appreciated and structures with a short T_1 value, such as fat, appear dark grey, those with intermediate values appear light grey and those with long T_1 values, usually fluids, appear white. The proton density images are relatively featureless but are important because of the good spatial resolution seen at soft tissue/fluid and soft tissue/bone interfaces. The inversion recovery images demonstrate fat as white and are the most useful for measuring fat thickness. When TI intervals of between 300 ms and 500 ms are used, these will have the effect of suppressing the signal from long T_1 tissues such as fetal lung, allowing for the clear demonstration of the heart. Similarly, the basal ganglia of the brain may be visualized by suppressing the strong signal for unmyelinated brain. Using these long TI intervals has the effect of enhancing short T_1 tissues such as fat, enabling fetal subcutaneous fat measurements to be made.

Short IR sequences using TI values of below 200 ms suppress the signal from fat and, while this is useful when imaging the adult abdomen, its main value in imaging pregnancy is the reduction of artefact caused by maternal respiration or fetal movement (Fig. 10.1). A T_1-weighted image is available which is produced by subtracting the inversion recovery signal from the proton density signal giving an image which has the contrast resolution of the calculated T_1 image and is a useful general image.

In the first and second trimesters of pregnancy the fetus is best demonstrated on the proton density and D images. It is not well seen in the T_1 and inversion recovery images due to the presence of the relatively large volume of amniotic fluid, which has a long relaxation time and appears very similar to the fetus and placenta. The placental site is easily localized even when situated posteriorly, as shown in Fig. 10.2. After 26 weeks there is an improvement in the quality of the fetal images and fetal organs are recognizable. The poor detail due to excessive fetal movement occurs commonly at early gestations while after 26 weeks there is less movement with resultant improved image quality. It has been found that if the patient is imaged lying on her side, the fetus tends to be still allowing good quality images to be made. In the third trimester identification of the fetal brain, lungs, heart, liver, bowel, bladder, limbs and umbilical cord is possible. It has been found that for the best examination after about 22 weeks the patient should have sagittal imaging lying supine (one midline section is usually adequate to demonstrate fetal lie and placental site), followed by axial sections from the vertex to the rump, 4 cm apart.

Measurements of T_1 for various maternal and fetal tissues showed considerable variations which sometimes correlated with the stage of pregnancy. For example, T_1 of cervix progressively increases with advancing pregnancy and may reflect the increasing water content of the cervix during pregnancy. Conversely, T_1 of fetal brain decreases from mid-pregnancy (90 ms) until term (600 ms) and this fall has been found to continue after delivery. This fall in T_1 continues until the adult levels (225–300 ms) are reached, reflecting myelination of the central nervous system (Levene et al. 1982). All the other fetal organs are also well displayed and MRI may be used to study the normal and abnormal fetus (McCarthy et al. 1985; Smith 1985; Smith et al. 1985).

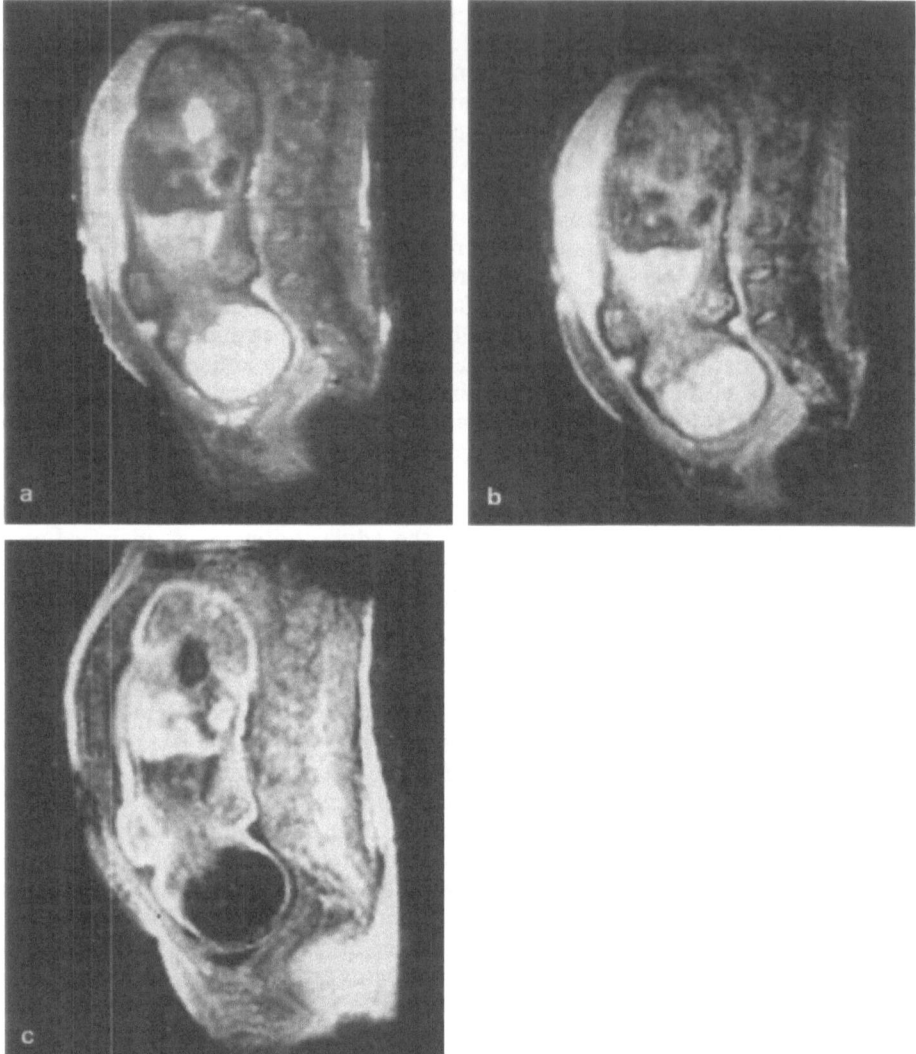

Fig. 10.1a–c.   Normal 38-weeks gestation fetus. Anterior placenta. Sagittal section. **a** Calculated T_1 image. Strong signal from long T_1 structures shown as white; placenta, brain, urinary bladder and lungs. Weak signal, dark grey, from liver and subcutaneous fat. **b** Inversion recovery TR 1000/TI 100 ms. The signal from subcutaneous fat is suppressed and in the fetus appears black, whilst it is not seen in the mother. Strong signal from placenta, brain and lung appears enhanced. **c** Inversion recovery TR 1000/TI 500 ms. The fetal and maternal fat signal is enhanced, appearing white. The strong signal from the placenta, brain and lung is suppressed with the result that the cardiac chambers are visible.

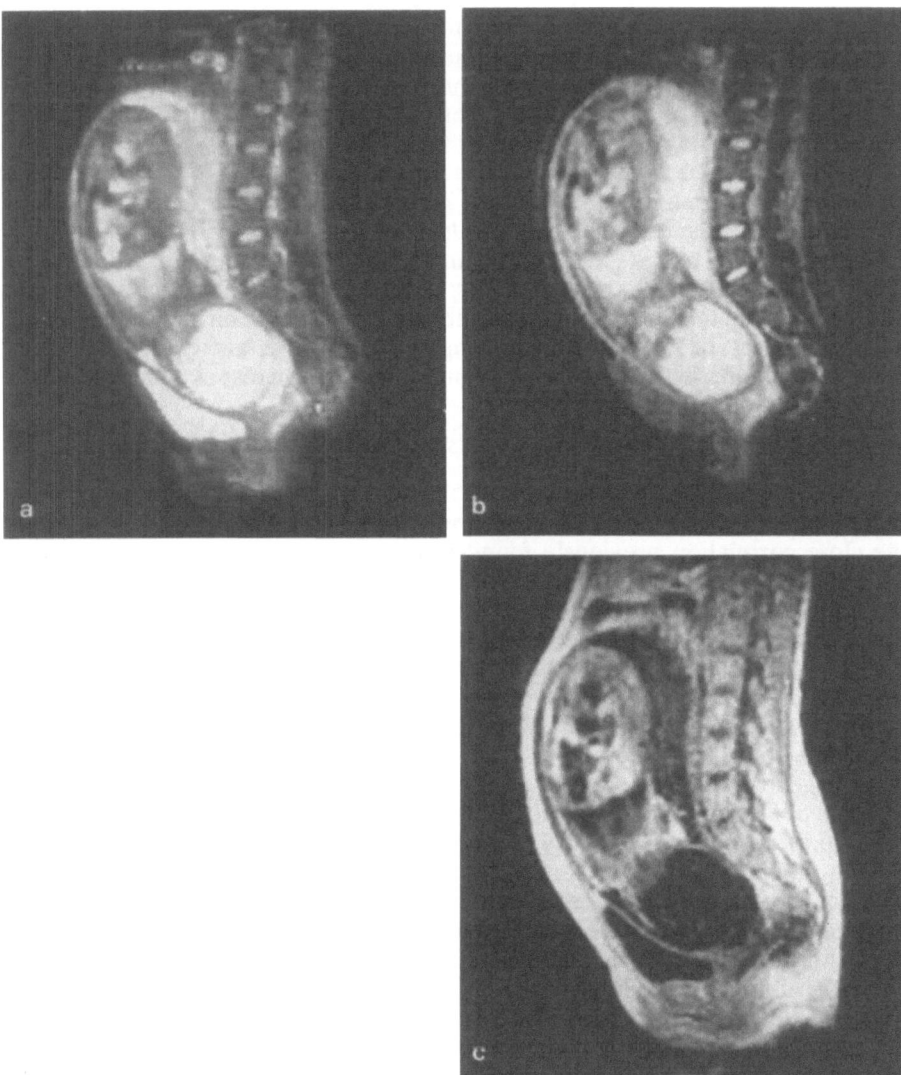

Fig. 10.2a–c. Growth-retarded 38-week gestation fetus. Posterior placenta. Sagittal section. **a** Calculated T_1. **b** Inversion recovery TR 1000/TI 100 ms. **c** Inversion recovery TR 1000/TI 500 ms. Ample maternal subcutaneous fat visualized using IR sequence 1000/500, but very little fetal fat seen. Other organs appear normal.

Fetal fat when present is easily identified and its thickness may be measured accurately after 32 weeks. Because of the short T_1 relaxation time of fat, which is due to the large amount of closely bound hydrogen protons in fat, it is well visualized on the T_1 and inversion recovery images, appearing almost black on T_1 images and white on inversion recovery (Figs. 10.1–10.3).

Magnetic resonance images comprise not only morphological detail but also physiological information in the form of T_1 and T_2 relaxation time measurements for the different tissues. When the T_1 values for the major organs are calculated, each organ is seen to have a relaxation time unique to it (Table 10.2). Because of this it is possible to make measurements of fetal subcutaneous fat in one of two ways. Either the thickness of the fetal subcutaneous fat can be measured directly from the images, or following the drawing of a region of interest on the computer screen around the fetus the computer can be asked to express as a percentage the amount of fat in that section.

Using the direct measurement method, nine normal fetuses and 14 with diabetic mothers have been studied. When the MRI measurements were compared with birthweight and neonatal skinfold calliper measurements, good correlation between the results was found. This finding was expected because of the close correlation previously found in adults between the measurement of subcutaneous fat using MRI and skinfold callipers (Hayse et al. 1985). In the normal fetus the subcutaneous fat is seen as a thin dark grey structure using T_1 images, and as a white structure using inversion recovery TR 1000/500 (Fig. 10.1). In four cases of intrauterine growth retardation it was not possible to visualize any fetal subcutaneous fat (Fig. 10.2), whilst in the fetus of the diabetic mother the fat was always seen and in gross macrosomia it was seen to be very thick (Fig. 10.3). In one case of polyhydramnios studied, where the fetus was grossly oedematous due to agenesis of the thoracic duct, the subcutaneous tissues were oedematous and free of fat, appearing very different from the normal and macrosomic fetuses (Fig. 10.4).

Using this method, nine normal fetuses and 14 with diabetic mothers were studied. Measurements of the subcutaneous fat thickness over the triceps, mid-thigh and subscapular area of the back were made from the magnetic resonance images in the 38th or 39th week of gestation and within 48 h of delivery using skinfold callipers. In the nine normal fetuses MRI measurements lay between 4.0 and 6.0 mm and in the 14 fetuses of diabetic mothers between 4.5 and 8.5 mm. In all cases close correlation with the skinfold thickness and birth weight was obtained.

In an effort to assess the accuracy of measuring the T_1 relaxation time of fetal fat and expressing it as a percentage of body composition a further 10 normal and 10 diabetic pregnancies have been studied during the 38th and 39th week of gestation. In this ongoing study, multiple transaxial sections through the fetus at 4-cm intervals are made. For each section a region of interest is drawn around the fetus and the computer is then asked to calculate the number of pixels (1 mm × 1 mm picture elements) that have a T_1 value of between 180 and 230 ms and to express this value as a percentage of the total number of pixels in the section. The range 180–230 ms has been chosen because from experience this is the range of values for fetal fat and is very different from the values obtained for muscle (Table 10.2). This calculation is made for each of the sections and the result expressed as an average of all the sections.

In the 10 normal pregnancies studied the total average percentage of fat per

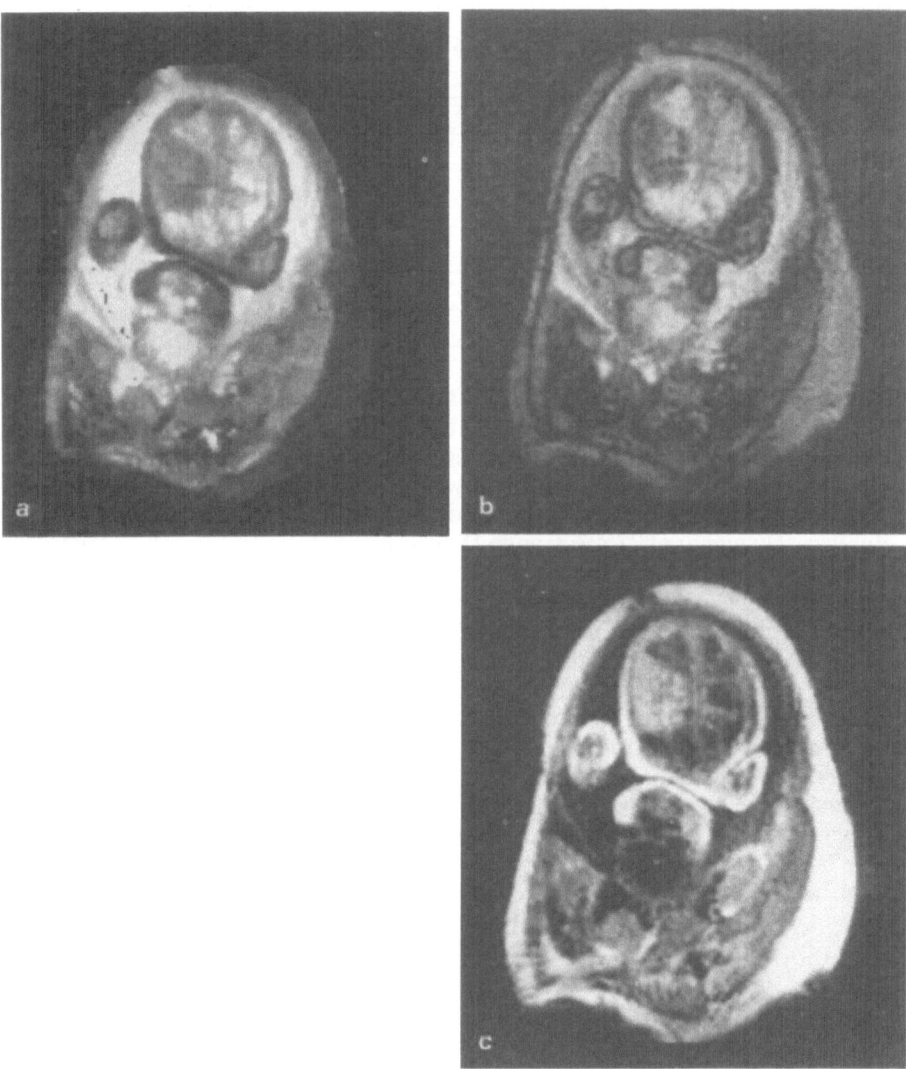

Fig. 10.3a–c. Macrosomic 38-week fetus of a diabetic mother, axial section. **a** Calculated T_1. **b** Inversion recovery 1000/100 ms. **c** Inversion recovery 1000/500 ms. Thick layer of subcutaneous fat visualized as white on the IR 1000/500 image and as dark grey on the calculated T_1 image.

Table 10.2.   Proton spin – lattice relaxation times (T_1) measured at 3.4 MHz for some fetal tissues, between 36 and 40 weeks gestation

Tissue	T_1 (ms) Average	Range
Brain	790	600–900
Lung	480	250–650
Liver	340	200–550
Muscle	350	250–450
Fat	200	180–230

fetus was 17% (range 11.8%–25.0%). The average birthweight was 3483 g (range 2940–4300 g), all babies lying between the 10th and 90th centiles for weight for gestation. The results obtained from the babies of diabetic mothers (all insulin dependent) showed the average birth weight to be higher than for the normal group, at 3872 (range 2840–5450 g) and the total average percentage of fat per fetus was also higher at 27.4% (range 15.6%–33.6%). Six of the babies lay within the 10th to 90th centiles for weight for gestation, three were above the 90th centile, having percentage fat values of 33.6%, 30.1% and 23.8%, and one below the 10th centile where the percentage fat was only 15.6%.

One baby suffering from intrauterine growth retardation had a percentage fat value of 3.6% and weighed 2600 g at delivery.

The values obtained for percentage of fetal fat by this method are by no means absolute. However, by studying a group of normal fetuses, a reference group has been obtained against which other potentially abnormal fetuses can be compared. The range of values for percentage of fat per fetus is large (11.8%–25.0%) but it has been possible to show definite differences between these normal babies and those large-for-dates babies of diabetic mothers and the single case of intrauterine growth retardation and good correlation with birthweight.

Discussion

NMR now offers an alternative to ultrasound and X-ray for imaging during pregnancy. Moreover, it uses no ionizing radiation and although several biological effects from radiofrequency and strong magnetic fields have been suggested, none have been realized at the levels in current use.

Accurate placental localization is possible, even when it is situated posteriorly. By using a combination of sagittal and axial images, precise location and lower margin can be determined. The relaxation time-dependent images, T_1 and inversion recovery are better than the proton density ones for demonstrating the placenta due to the long relaxation time of the placenta when compared with that of the uterus and fetus.

The absence of ionizing radiation means that patients may be imaged frequently throughout pregnancy, allowing for serial studies of fetal development. Measurement of fetal dimensions such as head, chest and abdomen

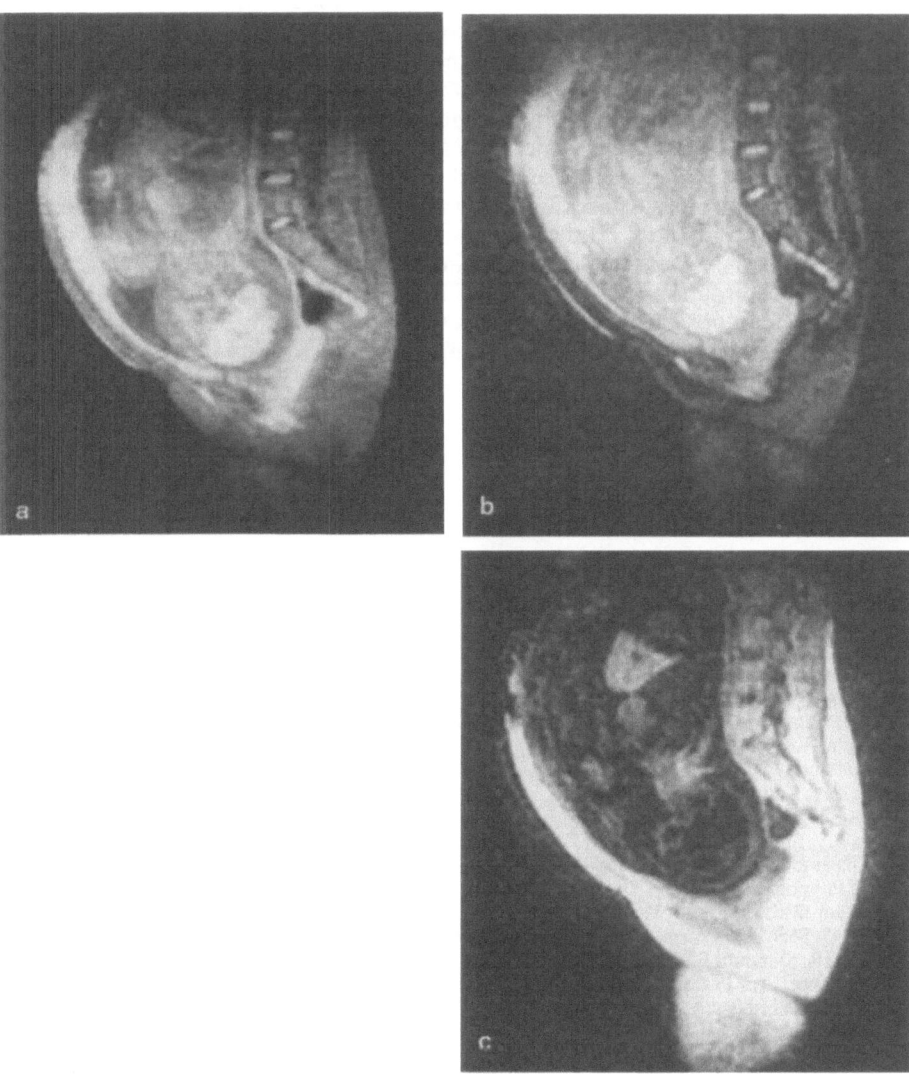

Fig. 10.4a–c. Hydroptic 38-week gestation fetus. Anterior placenta. **a** T_1 image. **b** Inversion recovery TR 1000/100 ms. **c** Inversion recovery TR 1000/TI 500 ms. Oedematous cheeks seen in T_1 image and there is no evidence of fetal subcutaneous fat. Compare with Fig. 10.3.

circumference are easily achieved and may be used as a means for estimating fetal size, weight and gestation. Alternatively fetal growth may be followed by measuring uterine size, a particularly easy procedure with NMR as all uterine dimensions are available on a single sagittal image.

The good soft tissue discrimination afforded by the technique allows for detailed study of both maternal and fetal tissues, the different T_1 signal received from the different tissues making for easy recognition of the uterus, placenta, amniotic fluid and fetus. Especially useful is the ability to measure fetal fat thickness which is of particular interest in pregnancies complicated by intrauterine growth retardation and diabetes. Thin or absent subcutaneous fat after 34 weeks has been observed in fetuses subsequently found to be growth retarded, while relative adiposity in fetuses of diabetic mothers correlates well with birth weight.

References

Bydder GM, Steiner RE, Young IR et al. (1982) Clinical NMR imaging of the brain: 140 cases. Am J Roentgenol 139:215–236

Cooke P, Morris PG (1981) The effects of NMI exposure on living organisms. II. A genetic study of human lymphocytes. Br J Radiol 54:622–625

Edelstein WA, Hutchison JMS, Johnson G, Redpath TW (1980) Spin-warp NMR imaging and applications to human whole-body imaging. Phys Med Biol 25:751–756

Edelstein WA, Hutchison JMS, Smith FW, Mallard JR, Johnson G, Redpath TW (1981) Human whole-body NMR tomographic imaging: normal sections. Br J Radiol 54:149–151

Foster MA, Knight CH, Rimmington JE, Mallard JR (1983) Fetal imaging by NMR: a study in goats. Radiology 149:193–196

Hayse PA, Smith FW, Soward PJ (1985) Distribution and quantification of human body fat using nuclear magnetic resonance imaging: comparison with a skinfold caliper method. Proceedings of the Physiological Society, Oxford, 11–13 July

Hutchison JMS, Edelstein WA, Johnson G (1980) A whole-body NMR imaging machine. J Phys [E] 13:947–955

Johnson IR, Symonds EM, Kean DM et al. (1984) Imaging the pregnant uterus with nuclear magnetic resonance. Am J Obstet Gynecol 148:1136–1139

Levene MI, Whitelaw A, Dubowitz V et al. (1982) Nuclear magnetic resonance imaging of the brain in children. Br Med J 285:774–776

McCarthy S, Filly RA, Stark DD, Calen PW, Golbus MS, Hricak H (1985) Magnetic resonance imaging of fetal abnormalities in utero: early experience. Am J Roentgenol 145:677–682

National Radiological Protection Board ad hoc Advisory Group on Nuclear Magnetic Resonance Clinical Imaging (1983) Revised guidance on acceptable limits of exposure during nuclear magnetic resonance clinical imaging. Br J Radiol 56:974–977

Smith FW (1983) The potential role of NMR imaging in pediatric practice. Pediatr Radiol 13:141–147

Smith FW (1985) The potential use of nuclear magnetic resonance imaging in pregnancy. J Perinat Med 13:265–276

Smith FW (1986) Magnetic resonance tomography of the pelvis. Cardiovasc Intervent Radiol 8:367–376

Smith FW, Sutherland HW (1988) Magnetic resonance imaging: the use of the inversion recovery sequence to display fetal morphology. Br J Radiol 61:338–341

Smith FW, Hutchison JMS, Mallard JR et al. (1981a) Oesophageal carcinoma demonstrated by whole body nuclear magnetic resonance imaging. Br Med J 282:510–512

Smith FW, Mallard JR, Hutchison JMS et al. (1981b) Clinical application of nuclear magnetic resonance. Lancet I:78–79

Smith FW, Mallard JR, Reid A, Hutchison JMS (1981c) Nuclear magnetic resonance tomographic imaging in liver disease. Lancet I:963–966

Smith FW, Reid A, Mallard JR, Hutchison JMS (1982) Nuclear magnetic resonance imaging of the pancreas. Radiology 142:677–680

Smith FW, Adam AM, Phillips WDP (1983) NMR imaging in pregnancy. Lancet I:61–62

Smith FW, MacLennan F, Abramovich DR, MacGillivray I, Hutchison JMS (1984) NMR imaging in human pregnancy: a preliminary study. Magnetic Resonance Imaging 2:57–64

Smith FW, Kent C, Abramovich DR, Sutherland HW (1985) Nuclear magnetic resonance imaging: a new look at the fetus. Br J Obstet Gynaecol 92:1024–1033

Stark DD, McCarthy SM, Filly RA, Hricak H, Paver JR (1985) Intra-uterine growth retardation: evaluation by magnetic resonance. Radiology 155:425–527

Thomas A, Morris PG (1981) The effect of NMR exposure on living organisms. I. A Microbial assay. Br J Radiol 54:615–621

11. The Placenta in Diabetes Mellitus

H. Fox

Introduction

During the past decade there have not been any dramatic advances in our knowledge or understanding of either the effects of diabetes mellitus on the human placenta or of the role, if any, played by the placenta in the fetal complications of diabetic pregnancies. There has, however, been an increasing, though still far from complete, consensus as to the abnormalities seen in the placenta of the diabetic woman, the functional effects of these changes and their relationship to the severity, and control achieved, of the diabetic state (Fox 1978; Haust 1981; Rushton 1984; O'Herlihy and O'Driscoll 1987; Desoye 1988).

This measure of limited agreement has stemmed from two factors. Firstly, it has been accepted generally that attempts to define the placental changes characteristic of diabetes mellitus must be based on studies which eliminate complicating factors capable of blurring the significance of any observed abnormalities: thus, cases with superimposed pregnancy-induced hypertension, pregnancies terminating in stillbirth and gestations complicated by abruptio placentae must be rigorously excluded as must placentas from women who have smoked cigarettes, taken drugs or abused alcohol during their pregnancies. Secondly, it has been recognized that to consider "diabetic pregnancy" as a single entity is far too simplistic an approach and efforts have therefore been made not only to discriminate between placentas from women with insulin-dependent diabetes mellitus and those from patients with gestational diabetes but also to consider separately placentas from the various subgroups, as defined in terms of the White classification, of insulin-dependent diabetics.

Morphology of the Placenta in Diabetes Mellitus

Macroscopic Appearances

The traditional belief that the placenta of the insulin-dependent diabetic is unusually bulky and oedematous is correct in only a very small minority of cases.

It is true that the average weight of the diabetic woman's placenta is slightly greater than is that of placentas from non-diabetic women (Thomson et al. 1969; Nummi 1972): the range of weights encountered is, however, wide and many placentas from diabetic women fall well within the normal placental weight range found in non-diabetic pregnancies. Placentas from women with gestational diabetes also show a tendency to be heavy though most are within normal weight limits: very heavy, oedematous placentas are not found in this group.

Apart from the tendency towards an increased weight the placentas of both insulin-dependent and gestational diabetic women are unremarkable to the naked eyes. Fetal artery thrombosis, a clinically unimportant lesion, occurs with increased frequency in these placentas but there is otherwise no excess of gross abnormalities. In particular, infarction is, in the absence of superimposed pregnancy-induced hypertension, not found with any greater frequency than in placentas from uncomplicated pregnancies.

Histological Findings

On light microscopy about 40% of third-trimester placentas from insulin-dependent diabetics have villi which show a normal degree of morphological maturity for the length of the gestational period (Fox 1969). In the remaining 60% the villous maturity is at odds with the length of the pregnancy, about half of these placentas having villi which are unduly immature and about half showing accelerated villous maturation. Villous oedema, albeit usually of mild degree, occurs with moderate frequency but villous vascularity is very variable: in many placentas the villi are normally vascularized but in some they are hypovascular and in yet others the villous vessels are unusually numerous, dilated and congested. Villous cytotrophoblastic cells are commonly numerous and unduly prominent whilst the trophoblastic basement membrane frequently shows a degree of focal or diffuse thickening. An increase in the number of villi which have undergone fibrinoid necrosis is a common finding. The fetal stem arteries are normal in most placentas from insulin-dependent diabetics but in about 25% an "obliterative endarteritis" is seen: no changes suggestive of a diabetic angiopathy are encountered in any part of the fetal–placental vasculature.

On histological examination occasional placentas from women with gestational diabetes are virtually normal but the majority show changes identical in character to those found in placentas from patients with insulin-dependent diabetes (Fox 1979). The pathological abnormalities tend to be less marked and to occur with decreased frequency compared with placentas from insulin-dependent diabetics but there is, nevertheless, a not inconsiderable degree of overlap, some placentas from gestational diabetics being histologically identical to those from women with long-standing severe insulin-dependent diabetes.

Ultrastructural Changes

Electron microscopy confirms the presence of many large cytotrophoblastic cells in the villi of the insulin-dependent woman's placenta (Jones and Fox 1976a): these are mainly of the intermediate type, showing a cytoplasmic complexity intermediate between that of the organelle-rich syncytiotrophoblast and that of the organelle-depleted resting cytotrophoblastic cell. Mitotic figures are occasionally seen in these cells whilst newly divided cytotrophoblastic cells with large pale ovoid nuclei are sometimes noted.

The villous syncytiotrophoblast appears fully viable in most areas but occasional small scattered foci of syncytial necrosis are encountered, these showing nuclear pyknosis, increased cytoplasmic density and loss of organelles. The syncytial rough endoplasmic reticulum tends to be moderately dilated and the cisternae contain electron-dense flocculent material. A normal, or sometimes increased, number of syncytial pinocytotic vesicles are present whilst there is commonly an increase in both the number and size of syncytial osmiophilic secretory droplets. The microvilli on the free surface of the villous syncytiotrophoblast are of normal size and shape and appear to be present in normal density.

The trophoblastic basement membrane is irregularly thickened, the membrane having both amorphous and fibrillary components and containing occasional dense granular inclusions and fine filaments. No evidence is seen of immune complex deposition or formation in the thickened areas of the membrane.

At the ultrastructural level placentas of gestational diabetics tend to show the same spectrum of changes as do those from insulin-dependent diabetics (Jones and Fox 1976b; Fox 1979): thus, focal syncytial necrosis, dilatation of syncytial endoplasmic reticulum, a normal or increased number of syncytial pinocytotic vesicles, an increased number of syncytial secretory droplets, focal basement membrane thickening and evidence of cytotrophoblastic proliferation are all encountered, sometimes to the same extent and degree as in placentas of insulin-dependent women.

Morphometric Studies

Morphometric techniques, which identify quantitative, rather than qualitative, changes within a tissue or organ have only recently been applied to the diabetic's placenta. Singer et al. (1981) studied a wide variety of quantitative parameters, at both light and electron microscopic levels, and were unable to show that placentas from diabetic women differed in any significant way from those of patients with uncomplicated pregnancies. Other morphometric studes have, however, yielded more positive results. Teasdale (1981) compared placentas from women having White's class A diabetes mellitus (gestational diabetes) with control placentas from non-diabetic women, estimating in each placenta the amount of parenchymatous tissue (i.e. the intervillous space, villous trophoblast and villous fetal vessels) and the quantity of non-parenchymal tissue (i.e. decidual and chorionic plates, villous connective tissue and perivillous fibrin), considering the parenchymal components to be those parts of the placenta concerned with materno-fetal exchange. The placentas from the class A diabetics were not significantly heavier than those from the controls but contained more parenchymal and villous tissue, were more cellular and had a greater surface area for materno-fetal exchange. Teasdale (1983) later studied placentas from mothers with White's class B diabetes mellitus and in this group placentas from babies of expected weight for gestational age differed from those of a control group only in showing a greater degree of villous vascularization. By contrast those placentas from unduly large infants were heavier than control placentas, had a significantly increased amount of non-parenchymal tissue, a moderate increase in parenchymal tissue and a moderately increased materno-fetal exchange area. In a subsequent study Teasdale (1985) examined placentas from patients with White's class C diabetes mellitus and demonstrated that, irrespective of fetal weight, these placentas were heavier than controls, showed a synchronous increase in both parenchymal and non-parenchymal tissues and had an increased area available for materno-fetal exchange.

Quantitative ultrastructural studies of the diabetic's placenta have been limited to a single report by Teasdale and Jean-Jacques (1986) that placentas from diabetic women, of all White classes, showed a significant increase in the density of microvilli on the free surface of the villous syncytiotrophoblast.

Immunopathology of the Placenta in Diabetes Mellitus

In placentas from insulin-dependent diabetics, staining for immunoglobulins shows a pattern which is qualitatively and quantitatively similar to that found in placentas from uncomplicated pregnancies (Galbraith and Faulk 1979; Galbraith et al. 1984): various complement components are distributed in a normal pattern in the diabetic's placenta but there is more marked deposition of C3 in the trophoblastic basement membrane, a more striking amount of C4 in villi showing fibrinoid necrosis and a greater quantity of Clq in the walls of the fetal stem vessels than in placentas from healthy women. Immunofluorescent staining for coagulation components shows plasminogen/plasmin in localized patches on the villous syncytiotrophoblast and fibrinogen/fibrin focally present in the trophoblastic basement membrane of the diabetic's placenta.

The immunopathological findings in placentas from gestational diabetics are similar to those noted in placentas from insulin-dependent diabetics, though tending, in general, to be less marked (Galbraith et al. 1981).

Relationship Between Placental Abnormalities, Severity of the Diabetic State and Degree of Diabetic Control

Jones and Fox (1976a) were unable to show any consistent correlation between the degree and extent of the abnormalities noted in placentas from women with insulin-dependent diabetes and the severity or duration of the maternal diabetic state. They also commented on their inability to demonstrate that the placental changes were any less marked in cases of well-controlled diabetes than in placentas from women with poor metabolic control. Further, Jones and Fox (1976b) showed that the placental changes in gestational diabetes were sometimes quantitatively identical to those in placentas from insulin-dependent diabetics.

This lack of correlation between the extent of placental structural change and the clinical severity of the diabetic state has also been noted in morphometric studies. Thus, Teasdale (1981, 1983, 1985) showed that the quantitative changes in placentas from women with severe insulin-dependent diabetes (White's class C) did not differ significantly from those in placentas from gestational diabetics (White's class A): he further noted that within a single well-defined group of insulin-dependent diabetics, those in White's class B, there was a markedly heterogeneous pattern of morphometric placental findings. Immunopathological studies (Galbraith and Faulk 1979; Galbraith 1979; Galbraith et al. 1984) have similarly failed to show that the changes noted in placentas from gestational diabetics are necessarily less marked or extensive than are those in placentas from women with insulin-dependent diabetes.

Björk and Persson (1982) used light microscopy of fresh unstained villous tissue to describe a range of villous abnormalities in placentas from women with insulin-dependent diabetes of varying severity, their findings being difficult to compare with those obtained by conventional light microscopy. They were, however, able to plot, in each individual case, the degree of diabetic control achieved throughout pregnancy and showed that no relationship existed between the extent of the placental changes and the level of blood glucose control achieved in late pregnancy: by contrast, there was a significant correlation between the presence of placental abnormalities and the degree of metabolic control attained in early gestation.

The definitive demonstration that the degree of metabolic control, at any stage of pregnancy, does not influence in any way the development of placental abnormalities in maternal diabetes mellitus has, however, come from a study by Laurini et al. (1987). These workers studied a group of insulin-dependent women (White classes B–D) who were treated by continuous subcutaneous insulin infusion. This form of control was instituted before conception in some of the patients, before the 16th week of gestation in others and, in the case of one woman, at the 23rd gestational week. Very tight metabolic control was achieved in all the patients but placental abnormalities, at both light and electron microscopic levels, were totally unrelated to either the degree of control of blood sugar levels or the stage of pregnancy at which rigid control was attained. Thus, quite severe lesions were found in the placentas of some women who were normoglycaemic in the periconceptual period and throughout pregnancy whilst there were no significant differences noted between placentas from patients in whom periconceptual control was achieved and those in whom control was attained postconceptually. Even more strikingly, placentas from some women whose hyperglycaemia was rigidly controlled throughout pregnancy by insulin infusion showed the same abnormalities as were found in placentas from the same women during previous pregnancies in which metabolic control was poor.

Pathogenesis of Placental Abnormalities in Diabetes Mellitus

None of the lesions found in the placenta of the diabetic woman are in any way specific to the diabetic state, though when taken together the spectrum of abnormalities forms a very characteristic pattern. There is, however, no single all-embracing pathogenetic hypothesis that can be evoked to explain this particular combination of findings. We have no knowledge of the factors which control the growth and rate of maturation of the villous tree and do not know therefore whether the abnormalities of villous maturation found in many placentas from diabetic women are due to a fault in fetal control mechanisms or to an intrinsic placental growth disturbance. It is worth noting, however, that the fully mature villous pattern, in which terminal villi predominate, is that which is most functionally efficient: accelerated maturation is therefore not a manifestation of "placental senescence" but represents a compensatory mechanism which allows for the more rapid achievement of optimal transfer capacity. The mechanisms controlling villous vascularization are also unknown and although Asmussen (1982a, b) regards excessive villous vascularization, encountered in some placentas of diabetic patients, as a manifestation of diabetic microangiopathy this is a view to which few other pathologists would accede.

It is clear that in maternal diabetes mellitus the villous syncytiotrophoblast does suffer damage: it is also clear that this damage is efficiently repaired and that residual lesions within the syncytiotrophoblast are focal, few and detectable only on electron microscopy. The visible evidence of this repair mechanism is the proliferation of villous cytotrophoblast which is such a prominent feature of the diabetic's placenta. The cytotrophoblastic cells are the stem cells of the trophoblast, the syncytiotrophoblast being a postmitotic terminally differentiated tissue; these cytotrophoblastic stem cells form a "germinative zone" which is normally inconspicuous and relatively inactive in the third trimester but which can be provoked into a resurgence of mitotic activity if the need arises to replace damaged syncytiotrophoblast. Such a need does arise in maternal diabetes mellitus and the striking prominence and number of the villous cytotrophoblastic cells in these placentas bears eloquent witness to the adequacy and extent of the repair process. The trophoblastic basement membrane thickening seen in many of these placentas is an incidental by-product of the abnormal cytotrophoblastic cell proliferation: basement membrane protein is synthesized, in part at least, by these cells and excessive cytotrophoblastic cell division and growth will be associated with increased basement membrane substance production.

This still leaves undetermined the cause of the syncytial damage. It has often been suggested, either directly or by implication, that the trophoblast suffers hypoxic damage in maternal diabetes mellitus, either because of a reduced uteroplacental blood flow (Driscoll 1965; Emmrich et al. 1975) or because large, oedematous, immature villi encroach upon and narrow the intervillous space (Aladjem 1967; Jacomo et al. 1976). Studies of the maternal placental vasculature in uncomplicated diabetic pregnancies have, however, generally failed to reveal any significant arterial lesions (Pinkerton 1963; Magnin and Gabriel 1966) whilst it is now clear that, in the absence of superimposed pregnancy-induced hypertension, there is fully adequate and complete conversion of the spiral arteries of the placental bed into utero-placental vessels (Robertson 1979; Björk et al. 1984). It is therefore unlikely that utero-placental ischaemia plays any significant role in the pathogenesis of the syncytial damage in the diabetic patient's placenta and the concept of intervillous space reduction has been disposed of by Teasdale (1981) who showed that the volume of the intervillous space is either normal or increased in the diabetic's placenta. Further, the electron microscopic findings of unimpaired syncytial pinocytotic activity, increased syncytial secretory activity and lack of microvillous damage indicates a pattern quite unlike that found in hypoxic damage to the syncytiotrophoblast (Fox and Jones 1983).

Suggestions that the placental lesions in diabetic pregnancies may be immune-mediated (Galbraith 1979) have not been confirmed by immunopathological studies which have tended to show only that there is a degree of augmentation of the normal immune processes in the placenta in maternal diabetes but no specific immunopathological abnormalities. Electron microscopic studies have also failed to yield any evidence of immune-mediated damage.

Currently, therefore, the cause of the abnormalities in the placenta of the diabetic woman is unknown though it is generally assumed that "some component of the diabetic state" plays a pathogenetic role. Any attempt to attribute the placental abnormalities to maternal hyperglycaemia founders, however, on the evidence that the attainment of normal blood glucose levels both before and during pregnancy does not prevent the development of the placental lesions.

Functional Significance of Placental Changes in Diabetes Mellitus

Pregnancy in the diabetic woman is associated with a significant, though progressively diminishing, excess perinatal mortality and the temptation to ascribe this to placental damage has not always been resisted. It is true that the placenta does suffer a degree of damage in maternal diabetes mellitus but the vast bulk of the trophoblast is fully viable and syncytial injury is rapidly and efficiently repaired by an uninhibited cytotrophoblastic hyperplasia/repair reaction. Morphological indicators of trophoblastic functional activity also indicate that the trophoblast is functioning at a normal, or even enhanced, level. The dilatation of the syncytial rough endoplasmic reticulum and the increased number of secretory droplets could indicate either a failure of release of secretions and inhibited protein synthesis or, alternatively, increased secretory and synthetic activity. That the latter is the correct interpretation is clearly shown by the fact that pregnancy in the diabetic woman tends to be associated with raised maternal plasma levels of placental hormones and proteins (Gillmer and Beard 1975). The normal appearance of the trophoblastic microvilli, the enhanced number of microvilli, the increased number of syncytial pinocytotic vesicles and the greater surface area available for materno-fetal transfer all suggest that placental transfer activity is at least maintained and, indeed, almost certainly augmented.

There is thus no good reason for believing that placental functional capacity is in any way diminished in maternal diabetes.

Conclusions

The placenta suffers injury in maternal diabetes mellitus. The damaging factor does not appear to be hypoxia or immunological attack and it is assumed that a still unidentified factor in the diabetic woman is capable of producing trophoblastic lesions. This factor is independent, to a very significant extent, of the severity and duration of the diabetic state and is not eliminated by rigid control of blood sugar levels during the periconceptual period and throughout pregnancy.

The placental damage is rapidly and efficiently repaired and there is no evidence that the functional capacity of the placenta is impaired in the diabetic woman: indeed, the placenta appears to be functioning with greater than normal efficiency.

References

Aladjem S (1967) Morphologic aspects of the placenta in gestational diabetes. Am J Obstet Gynecol 99:341–349

Asmussen I (1982a) Ultrastructure of the villi and fetal capillaries of the placentas delivered by non-smoking diabetic women (White Group D). Acta Pathol Microbiol Immunol Scand [A] 90:95–101

Asmussen I (1982b) Vascular morphology in diabetic placentas. Contrib Gynecol Obstet 9:76–85

Björk O, Persson B (1982) Placental changes in relation to the degree of metabolic control in diabetes mellitus. Placenta 3:367–368

Björk O, Persson B, Strangenborg M, Baclavinkova V (1984) Spiral artery lesions in relation to metabolic control in diabetes mellitus. Acta Obstet Gynecol Scand 63:123–127

Desoye G (1988) The human placenta in gestational diabetes. In: Weiss PAM, Coustan DR (eds) Gestational diabetes. Springer, Vienna, pp 72–86

Driscoll SG (1965) The pathology of pregnancy complicated by diabetes mellitus. Med Clin North Am 49:1053–1067

Emmrich P, Birke R, Godëc E (1975) Beitrag zur Morphologie der myometrialen und dezidualen Arterien bei normalen Schwangerschaften, EPH-Gestosen und mütterlichen Diabetes mellitus. Pathologia et Microbiologia 43:38–61

Fox H (1969) Pathology of the placenta in maternal diabetes mellitus. Obstet Gynecol 34:792–798

Fox H (1978) Pathology of the placenta. Saunders, London Toronto Philadelphia

Fox H (1979) Placental changes in gestational diabetes. In: Sutherland HW, Stowers JM (eds) Carbohydrate metabolism in pregnancy and the newborn, 1978. Springer-Verlag, Berlin Heidelberg New York, pp 102–113

Fox H, Jones CJP (1983) Pathology of trophoblast. In: Luke YW, Whyte A (eds) Biology of trophoblast. Elsevier, Amsterdam New York Oxford, pp 137–185

Galbraith RM (1979) Immunological aspects of diabetes mellitus. CRC Press, Boca Raton

Galbraith RM, Faulk WP (1979) Immunologic considerations of the materno-fetal relationship in diabetes mellitus. In: Merkatz IR, Adams PAI (eds) The diabetic pregnancy: a perinatal perspective. Grune and Stratton, New York, pp 111–121

Galbraith GMP, Galbraith RM, Paulsen EP (1981) Placental immunopathology in gestational diabetes. Placenta [Suppl 3] 183–192

Galbraith RM, Sinha DP, Galbraith GMP, Faulk WP (1984) Immunohistological studies of placentae from insulin-dependent diabetic women. In: Sutherland HW, Stowers JM (eds) Carbohydrate metabolism in pregnancy and the newborn. Churchill Livingstone, Edinburgh London Melbourne New York, pp 23–33

Gillmer MDG, Beard RW (1975) Fetal and placental function tests in diabetic pregnancy. In: Sutherland HW, Stowers JH (eds) Carbohydrate metabolism in pregnancy and the newborn. Churchill Livingstone, Edinburgh, pp 168–194

Haust MD (1981) Maternal diabetes mellitus: effects on the fetus and newborn. In: Naeye RL, Kissane J (eds) Perinatal diseases. Williams and Wilkins, Baltimore, pp 201–285

Jacomo KH, Benedetti WL, Sala MA, Alvarez H (1976) Pathology of the trophoblast and fetal vessels of the placenta in maternal diabetes mellitus. Acta Diabetol Lat 13:216–235

Jones CJP, Fox H (1976a) An ultrastructural and ultra-histochemical study of the placenta of the diabetic woman. J Pathol 119:91–99

Jones CJP, Fox H (1976b) Placental changes in gestational diabetes: an ultrastructural study. Obstet Gynecol 48:274–280

Laurini RN, Visser GHA, van Ballegooie E, Schoots CJF (1987) Morphological findings in placentae of insulin-dependent diabetic patients treated with continuous subcutaneous insulin infusion (CS11). Placenta 8:153–165

Magnin P, Gabriel H (1966) Les scléroses vasculaires de la cadaque profonde. Gynécologie et Obstétrique 65:37–56

Nummi S (1972) Relative weight of the placenta and perinatal mortality: a retrospective clinical and statistical analysis. Acta Obstet Gynecol Scand [Suppl 17]

O'Herlihy C, O'Driscoll K (1987) Diseases associated with abnormal placenta. In: Lavery JP (ed) The human placenta – clinical perspectives. Aspen, Rockville, pp 237–256

Pinkerton JHM (1963) The placental bed arterioles in diabetes. Proc R Soc Med 56:1021–1022

Robertson WB (1979) Utero-placental blood supply in maternal diabetes. In: Sutherland HW, Stowers JM (ed) Carbohydrate metabolism in pregnancy and the newborn, 1978. Springer-Verlag, Berlin Heidelberg New York, pp 63–75

Rushton DI (1984) Placenta as a reflection of maternal disease. In: Perrin EVDK (ed) Pathology of the placenta. Churchill Livingstone, New York Edinburgh London Melbourne, pp 57–87

Singer DR, Liu CT, Widness JA, Ellis RA (1981) Placental morphometric studies in diabetic pregnancies. Placenta [Suppl] 3:193–202

Teasdale F (1981) Histomorphometry of the placenta of the diabetic woman: class A diabetes mellitus. Placenta 2:241–252

Teasdale F (1983) Histomorphometry of the human placenta in class B diabetes mellitus. Placenta 4:1–12

Teasdale F (1985) Histomorphometry of the human placenta in class C diabetes mellitus. Placenta 6:69–82

Teasdale F, Jean-Jacques G (1986) Morphometry of the microvillous membrane of the human placenta in maternal diabetes mellitus. Placenta 7:81–88

Thomson AM, Billewicz WZ, Hytten FE (1969) The weight of the placenta in relation to birthweight. J Obstet Gynaecol Br Commonwealth 76:865–872

12. Amniotic Fluid Levels of Insulin and C-Peptide in Pregnancies Complicated by Diabetes Mellitus

B. Persson, H. Pschera, U. Hanson and N. O. Lunell

Clinical and experimental evidence suggest that insulin plays a central role in the regulation of fetal growth, particularly during the last 10 weeks of gestation (Lin et al. 1981a; Persson 1981; Milner and Hill 1984).

An exaggerated insulin secretion is frequently recorded in offspring of diabetic mothers. The opposite, i.e. hyposecretion of insulin, is characteristic of infants who are small-for-gestational-age (SGA).

Newborn infants of insulin-dependent diabetic mothers (IDMs) used to be at risk of developing respiratory distress syndrome due to surfactant deficiency. The detection of surfactant in samples of amniotic fluid obtained by amniocentesis and the assessment of fetal lung maturation and the risk of developing respiratory distress syndrome was demonstrated by Gluck and co-workers in 1971 (Gluck et al. 1971). This important clinical contribution was confirmed by other investigators. Soon amniocentesis performed in the last trimester of pregnancy became a part of the routine management of pregnancies complicated by diabetes as well as of other high-risk pregnancies. The introduction of this diagnostic tool brought about the opportunity to analyse samples of amniotic fluid for other biochemical parameters such as hormones like insulin.

The object of this chapter is to summarize briefly some of these studies on amniotic fluid dealing with measures of fetal β-cell secretory function, especially in relation to fetal size and growth and to the concept of maternal hyperglycaemia–fetal hyperinsulinaemia–fetal hypoxia.

Levels of Insulin and C-Peptide in Amniotic Fluid

Extensive studies have suggested that the mammalian fetus possesses endocrine autonomy (Jost 1969). Differentiated β-cells capable of synthesizing and storing

Table 12.1. Insulin and C-peptide levels (mean±SEM) in amniotic fluid (AF) and their relation to fetal size

Gestational age at sampling (weeks)	Diagnosis	Numbers	Statistical method	Amniotic fluid		Relationship to birthweight (BW) or BW-percentile	References
				Insulin (nmol/l)	C-peptide (nmol/l)		
Around term	Controls	38	Values not given			Insulin vs BW: r=0.37, P<0.02	Spellacy et al. (1973)
35–40	IDDM	12		0.82±0.33		Insulin vs BW: positive correlation, r-value not given	Weiss (1979)
36–39	Controls	16		0.08±0.005		Not calculated	Ogata et al. (1980a)
36–40	GDM[1]	18		0.23±0.07			
	GDM[2]	15		0.13±0.03			
	IDDM	11		0.15±0.03			
	Controls	37	t-test:	0.05±0.007		P<0.01 (controls vs GDM, controls vs IDDM)	
≥36	IDDM	27/21		0.17±0.05	0.76±0.13	C-peptide vs BW: P<0.01; C-peptide vs BW-percentile: P<0.05; r-values not given	Tchobroutsky et al. (1980)
	Controls	15/14	Wilcoxon's test:	0.05±0.007	0.43±0.07	NS	
≥36	Controls SGA	11		P<0.01; 0.09±0.03	P<0.06; 0.34±0.07	Calculated on all values	Lin et al. (1981a)
	Controls AGA	75		0.09±0.01	0.51±0.03	C-peptide vs BW-percentile: r=0.43, P<0.001	
	Controls LGA	17	One-way analysis of variance:	0.10±0.01	0.88±0.09		
≥36	GDM+IDDM	33		NS; 0.16±0.03	P<0.001; 1.04±0.09	Not calculated	Lin et al. (1981b)
	Controls	126	t-test:	0.08±0.007; P<0.05	0.57±0.03; P<0.001		

		n	Test				Reference
34–35	IDDM	17			0.95±0.14	Calculated on all values C-peptide vs BW: $r=0.50$, $P<0.02$	Stangenberg et al. (1982)
	GDM	8	Mann-Whitney U-test:		1.92±1.09		
36–39	IDDM	43		0.08±0.02	NS 1.17±0.29	Insulin vs BW: $r=0.51$, $P<0.001$ Insulin vs BW-percentile: $r=0.45$, $P<0.01$ C-peptide vs BW: $r=0.38$, $P<0.01$ C-peptide vs BW: $r=0.54$, $P<0.05$	Persson et al. (1982)
	Controls	17	Mann-Whitney U-test: $P<0.001$	0.02±0.009	0.18±0.02		
36–39	GDM	6	Mann-Whitney U-test: $P<0.001$		$P<0.001$ 0.69±0.16	NS C-peptide vs BW-percentile: $r=0.63$, $P<0.05$	Persson et al. (1986)
	IDDM	12			0.54±0.07		
	Controls	18			0.38±0.02	NS	
	IUGR	10	Mann-Whitney U-test: $P<0.01$ (controls vs IUGR)		0.28±0.03	NS	

NS, not significant.
[a] Fasting plasma glucose <5.8 mmol/l.
[b] Fasting plasma glucose ≥5.8 mmol/l.

insulin and proinsulin are present at approximately 10–11 weeks of gestation. Insulin is present in the fetal circulation at around 12 weeks. From around the 17th week of gestation insulin is detectable at low concentrations in amniotic fluid (AF). There is no evidence of any significant transfer of insulin across the placenta from the mother to the fetus, or in the opposite direction. Infusions of pharmacological doses of either insulin, proinsulin or C-peptide into the maternal circulation of the pregnant rat have demonstrated clearly that the concentrations of these peptides in fetal blood and AF remain low regardless of the maternal concentrations achieved (Katz et al. 1975). The concept that AF C-peptide is entirely of fetal origin is further supported by the observation in diabetic pregnancies of significantly elevated AF C-peptide levels despite non-measurable levels of C-peptide in maternal blood (Stangenberg et al. 1982; Pschera et al. 1988b). Insulin of maternal origin, on the other hand, may in the presence of insulin-binding antibodies be transferred to the fetus. In a series of 38 insulin-dependent diabetic pregnancies insulin-binding antibodies of the IgG type were detected in 57% of the mothers (Persson et al. 1982). However, only around 15% of these antibody-positive subjects had insulin-binding antibodies in AF as well (Persson et al. 1982).

Insulin-binding antibodies may interfere with the radioimmunoassay of insulin and proinsulin but not with that of C-peptide. C-peptide therefore would seem to reflect fetal β-cell function more reliably. It is generally believed that the main route of hormones into the AF is by fetal urine. Theoretically, influx or efflux of hormones and metabolites into AF could also occur across the chorioamnion, or via the umbilical cord and the placenta. Fetal micturition and fetal swallowing seem to play a crucial role among the complex factors regulating AF volume during the later part of gestation (van Otterlo et al. 1977). Around term the infant swallows approximately 450 ml of amniotic fluid per day while there is a total water exchange in AF of 470 ml/h (Abramovich 1978). The volume of fetal urine formed is about equal to the volume of AF that is swallowed by the fetus.

In normal pregnancies the average AF insulin level increases from around 9 μU/ml in week 27 to about 15 μU/ml at term. Much higher AF concentrations of both insulin and C-peptide have been recorded in both insulin-dependent and gestational diabetic patients (Spellacy et al. 1973; Newman and Tutera 1976; Weiss et al. 1978; Ogata et al. 1980a; Tchobroutsky et al. 1980; Lin et al. 1981b; Persson et al. 1982; cf Table 12.1). Markedly elevated concentrations of insulin corresponding to those seen in amniotic fluid have also been reported in urine of the newborn IDMs (Weiss et al. 1978). These results clearly indicate an augmented β-cell activity in fetuses of diabetic mothers. The opposite observation, that of significantly decreased concentrations of AF C-peptide, has been found in pregnancies accompanied by fetal growth retardation (Lin et al. 1981a). These deviations from normal of AF C-peptide in pregnancies complicated by diabetes or intrauterine growth retardation become even more pronounced when considering the variation in AF volumes (Table 12.2) (Pschera et al. 1986). The AF volume usually does not exceed 1500 ml from 36 weeks of gestation (van Otterlo et al. 1977). The AF volumes determined by the p-amino hippuric acid (PAH) dilution technique were approximately 60% higher and 20% lower than normal in pregnancies complicated by diabetes and growth retardation, respectively (Pschera et al. 1986). In the absence of more precise turnover data of the β-cell peptides, comparative evaluation of results must be done with caution. The observation in diabetic pregnancies of significant correlations between C-peptide and both insulin and proinsulin in AF suggests that their concentrations reflect the secretory activity of the fetal β-cell (Persson et al. 1982).

Table 12.2. Amniotic fluid (AF) volumes and concentration and total amount of AF C-peptide in pregnant diabetic and non-diabetic women and women with intrauterine growth-retarded fetuses (IUGR) (mean values) (Pschera et al. 1986)

	Gestational diabetes ($n=10$)	Insulin-dependent diabetes ($n=16$)	Controls ($n=17$)	IUGR ($n=11$)
AF volume (ml)	864	1036*	614	486
C-peptide (nmol/l)	0.46	0.55*	0.38	0.31*
C-peptide × AF volume (nmol)	0.48	0.54**	0.23	0.15*

* $P<0.05$; ** $P<0.01$ (Mann–Whitney test, significant difference versus controls)

Amniotic Fluid C-Peptide/Insulin and Substrate Levels

The AF glucose concentration decreases with gestational age from around 2.5 mmol/l in early pregnancy (14–17 weeks) to around 1 mmol/l around term (Weiss et al. 1984). A weak positive correlation between glucose levels in maternal venous blood and AF has been recorded in non-diabetic pregnancies ($r = 0.18$, $P<0.05$) (Spellacy et al. 1973). Changes of maternal nutrition are reflected in the composition of AF. Prolonged fasting for 84–90 h by non-diabetic pregnant women during weeks 16–22 of gestation was accompanied by a parallel decrease of glucose in maternal blood and AF of around 40% (Kim and Felig 1972). Concurrently, the concentrations of acetoacetate and 3-hydroxybutyrate increased 10- and 30-fold, respectively. Levels of ketone bodies in maternal blood and in AF were highly significantly correlated as has also been found in diabetic pregnancies (Pschera et al. 1988b).

The AF glucose concentration in diabetic pregnancies on the other hand was statistically unrelated to the maternal pregnancy glucose level (Persson et al. 1982). Hourly measurements for 21 h of concentrations of glucose in maternal blood and AF in one White's class B patient showed, however, that changes in maternal blood glucose were reflected in AF with a time lag of around 3–4 h (Weiss et al. 1985). A significant interrelationship between glucose and C-peptide or insulin in AF has been described in some studies of insulin-dependent diabetic pregnancies (Tchobroutsky et al. 1980; Persson et al. 1982; Pschera et al. 1988a) but not in others (Lin et al. 1981b).

A significant impact of the quality of maternal diabetic control on fetal β-cell function has been recorded in some series of diabetic pregnancies. Based on several blood glucose determinations during the second half of pregnancy the degree of blood glucose control was arbitrarily defined as good, fair or poor (Lin et al. 1981b). The group with "good control", i.e. blood glucose values close to the physiological range, had AF C-peptide values equal to those seen in non-diabetic controls. In contrast, patients who had had hyperglycaemia, i.e. fair or poor control groups, had significantly elevated AF C-peptide values (Lin et al. 1981b). These observations and also the finding of a direct positive correlation between pregnancy glucose value and AF C-peptide (Persson et al. 1986) support the concept of maternal hyperglycaemia–fetal hyperinsulinism. Further evidence of this hypothesis is the finding in gestational diabetic pregnancies of a significant association between the degree of glucose intolerance (area under the blood glucose curve) and the concentration of C-peptide both in AF ($r = 0.40$, $P<0.03$; Persson, unpublished) and in urine of the newborn infant collected during the first 12 h after birth ($r = 0.60$, $P<0.01$; Lunell et al. 1988).

Amino acids have also been ascribed an important role in the regulation of fetal β-cell replication as well as insulin production (de Gasparo et al. 1978; Freinkel and Metzger 1979; Milner 1979). The finding of a significant interrelationship between maternal branched-chain amino acids in plasma and AF C-peptide in insulin-dependent diabetic pregnancies ($r = 0.63$, $P<0.05$) lends support to this expanded theory of Pedersen (Persson et al. 1986).

Amniotic Fluid C-Peptide/Insulin and Fetal Size

The concept that insulin is an important fetal growth factor is supported by significant correlations between C-peptide or insulin in AF and the size at birth of the offspring of both diabetic and non-diabetic mothers (Spellacy et al. 1973; Tchobroutsky et al. 1980; Lin et al. 1981a; Stangenberg et al. 1982; Persson et al. 1982, 1986; Table 12.2). Fetal C-peptide values could at best explain around 40% of the variation in birthweight in IDMs and around 30% in controls. In this context, it is of interest to note that Lin and co-workers reported that a group of 13 large-for-gestational-age (LGA) infants (birthweight >90th percentile) of non-diabetic mothers had AF C-peptide values that were significantly above normal, but not different from those of nine LGA infants of insulin-dependent diabetic mothers. These authors therefore suggested that the basic mechanism of fetal macrosomia due to other causes is not different from the mechanism underlying diabetogenic macrosomia (Lin et al. 1981b). The criteria for the "non-diabetic" assessment are not clearly stated. Therefore, one cannot exclude the possibility that some of these LGA infants were born to mothers with undiagnosed gestational diabetes.

Fetal growth acceleration seems to be particularly prominent in mothers with a short duration of diabetes. This may be illustrated by the following case history. A 17-year-old woman developed insulin-requiring diabetes at 28 weeks of gestation. She was kept normoglycaemic and 4 weeks later an infant girl weighing 5100 g and with a length of 56 cm was born. Amniotic fluid C-peptide (prior to insulin treatment) was 12 nmol/l, the highest value that we have ever recorded. It should also be recalled that maternal duration of diabetes, degree of diabetic angiopathy and hypertension are other important variables determining fetal growth as they may influence utero-placental blood perfusion and, hence, the fetal supply line (Nylund et al. 1983; Semmler et al. 1985).

Serial ultrasonic measurements of fetal dimensions such as abdominal circumference have been used to illustrate the accelerated somatic growth in pregnancies complicated by insulin-dependent diabetes (Ogata et al. 1980b). In a series of gestational diabetic pregnancies we related AF C-peptide to a measure of growth velocity, based on serial ultrasonic measurements of an abdominal transverse section, expressed as mm/d. In six patients, where AF C-peptide was sampled at the time of delivery, a positive interrelationship between these two variables ($r = 0.82$, $P<0.05$) was found.

Amniotic Fluid C-Peptide and other Hormones in Amniotic Fluid

The possibility that the fetus of the diabetic mother may suffer chronic hypoxia was suggested as early as 1954 (Berglund and Zetterström 1954). Experimentally induced hyperinsulinaemia and hyperglycaemia in the fetal lamb have been shown to be associated with increased fetal glucose utilization and oxygen consumption, a decrease of arterial oxygen content and elevation of plasma erythropoietin (Simmons et al. 1978; Philipps et al. 1982; Milley et al. 1984). It has been speculated that erythrocytosis, increased extramedullary erythropoiesis and increased plasma concentrations of erythropoietin in newborn IDMs (Widness et al. 1981) represent the response to hypoxia induced by chronic elevations of fetal insulin and glucose.

Fetal hypoxia is known to activate the fetal sympatho-adrenal system. Elevated AF concentrations of catecholamine metabolites in pregnancies with growth-retarded fetuses have been suggested to indicate a state of intrauterine stress (Lagercrantz et al. 1980). However, in both gestational and insulin-dependent diabetic pregnancies AF concentrations of noradrenaline and adrenaline were not significantly different from those of controls despite significantly higher concentrations of AF C-peptide (Pschera et al. 1988a). The concentration of AF C-peptide, however, was positively correlated with the concentration of noradrenaline, perhaps reflecting maturation of these two hormonal systems in parallel. These data did not suggest that there were any major differences in fetal sympathetic nervous activity between offspring of diabetic women and of controls. This interpretation is also in accordance with the finding of similar plasma concentrations of catecholamines at birth in IDMs and offspring of controls (Broberger et al. 1984). Similarly, no significant difference has been found in AF cortisol levels between diabetic and non-diabetic pregnancies (Pschera et al. 1986). In insulin-dependent diabetic pregnancies the C-peptide/cortisol ratio in amniotic fluid was increased favouring a state of functional hyperinsulinism whereas the opposite, i.e. a significantly lower ratio between these two components, was present in pregnancies with fetal growth retardation. It is tempting to speculate that a decreased C-peptide/cortisol ratio could indicate a reduced insulin effectiveness similar to that recorded in malnourished children and rats where a close association was found between the insulin/cortisol ratio and growth velocity (Lunn et al. 1979).

Evidence supporting the view that chronic maternal hyperglycaemia leads to fetal hypoxaemia was recently presented by Teramo et al. (1987a, b). These authors found a significant correlation between concentrations of erythropoietin in umbilical venous plasma and in AF ($r = 0.87$) and also that the values were significantly elevated above normal. Multiple regression analysis showed that maternal HbA_{1c} was the most important variable accounting for around 30% of the variance in erythropoietin levels in umbilical venous plasma and AF, supporting the impact of maternal hyperglycaemia on fetal oxygen metabolism (Teramo et al. 1987a, b).

Amniotic Fluid C-Peptide/Insulin and Perinatal Outcome

It has been claimed that the concentration of insulin or C-peptide in AF could be used as a prognostic variable in predicting perinatal outcome in diabetic pregnancy. Newman and Tutera (1976) determined the glucose/insulin ratio in 29 insulin-dependent diabetic patients and 349 non-diabetic controls. These authors found markedly elevated insulin values in three of the diabetic patients. Two of these were associated with intrauterine death of the fetus and in the third case, the newborn baby experienced considerable difficulty with marked hypoglycaemia after delivery (Newman and Tutera 1976). Other investigators have proposed that serial determinations of either insulin or C-peptide in AF could be used to monitor the impact of maternal diabetes on the fetus (Weiss et al. 1978; Lin et al. 1981b). Thus, significantly elevated AF insulin was associated with neonatal morbidity (Weiss et al. 1978) and elevation of AF C-peptide was associated with an increased risk of macrosomia (Lin et al. 1981b).

On the basis of a very extensive experience with amniocentesis, with practically no complications, Weiss and co-workers concluded that monitoring of AF insulin every second week during the last trimester gives important information of value in the clinical management (Weiss et al. 1978). This suggestion is difficult to evaluate as this study provided no information about the quality of maternal metabolic control. Another study using more precise definitions of neonatal morbidity than are given by Weiss et al. (1978) disclosed significantly elevated AF concentrations of both insulin and C-peptide in diabetic pregnancies associated with neonatal morbidity, supporting the concept that neonatal complications such as hyperglycaemia, polycythaemia and transient tachypnoea are related to fetal and, subsequently, neonatal hyperinsulinism (Persson et al. 1982). There was, however, a wide individual variation and overlap in AF C-peptide values among patients with and without neonatal morbidity. It was therefore concluded that AF C-peptide could not be used in the individual case as a prognostic variable to predict neonatal morbidity.

Today, amniocentesis on clinical grounds for assessment of fetal lung maturation or for determination of insulin or C-peptide as a prognostic variable seems unnecessary in the majority of cases. Management of the pregnant diabetic has improved markedly following the introduction of self-control of blood glucose and the aim of trying to maintain maternal blood glucose close to or within the physiological range and to avoid premature delivery.

Acknowledgement. Supported by the Swedish Medical Research Council, Thielman's Fund for Pediatric Research, Allmänna BB Minnesfond and The Samariten Fund for Pediatric Research.

References

Abramovich DR (1978) The volume of amniotic fluid and its regulating factors. In: Fairweather DVI, Eskes TKAB (eds) Amniotic fluid – research and clinical application. Excerpta Medica, Amsterdam, pp 31–49

Berglund G, Zetterström R (1954) Infants of diabetic mothers. I. Foetal hypoxia in maternal diabetes. Acta Paediatr Scand 43:368–373

Broberger U, Hanson U, Lagercrantz H, Persson B (1984) Sympatho-adrenal activity and metabolic adjustment during the first 12 hours after birth in infants of diabetic mothers. Acta Paediatr Scand 73:602–609

de Gasparo M, Milner GR, Norris PD, Milner RDG (1978) Effect of glucose and amino acids on foetal rat pancreatic growth and insulin secretion in vitro. J Endocrinol 77:241–248

Freinkel N, Metzger BE (1979) Pregnancy as a tissue culture experience: the critical implications of maternal metabolism for fetal development. In: Pregnancy, metabolism, diabetes and the fetus. Ciba Foundation Symposium 63. Excerpta Medica, Amsterdam, pp 3–23

Gluck L, Kulovich MV, Borer RC, Brenner PH, Anderson GG, Spellacy WN (1971) Diagnosis of the respiratory distress syndrome by amniocentesis. Am J Obstet Gynecol 109:440–445

Jost A (1969) The extent of foetal endocrine autonomy. In: Wolstenholme GEW, O'Connor M (eds) Foetal autonomy. Churchill, London, pp 79–89

Katz AI, Lindheimer MD, Mako ME, Rubenstein AH (1975) Peripheral metabolism of insulin, proinsulin, and C-peptide in the pregnant rat. J Clin Invest 56:1608–1614

Kim YJ, Felig P (1972) Maternal and amniotic fluid substrate levels during caloric deprivation in human pregnancy. Metabolism 21:507–512

Lagercrantz H, Sjöqvist B, Bremme K, Lunell N-O, Somell C (1980) Catecholamine metabolites in amniotic fluid as indicators of intrauterine stress. Am J Obstet Gynecol 136:1067–1070

Lin C-C, Moawad AH, River P, Blix P, Abraham M, Rubenstein AH (1981a) Amniotic fluid C-peptide as an index for intrauterine fetal growth. Am J Obstet Gynecol 139:390–396

Lin C-C, River P, Moawad AH et al. (1981b) Prenatal assessment of fetal outcome by amniotic fluid C-peptide levels in pregnant diabetic women. Am J Obstet Gynecol 141:671–676

Lunell N-O, Persson B, Devarajan LV, Hassan S et al. (1988) Urinary C-peptide in the neonate correlates both to maternal glucose tolerance and to fetal size at birth. Am J Perinatol 5:144–145

Lunn PG, Whitehead RG, Cole TJ, Austin A (1979) The relationship between hormonal balance and growth in malnourished children and rats. Br J Nutr 41:73–84

Milley JR, Rosenberg AA, Philipps AF, Molteni RA, Jones DM Jr, Simmons MA (1984) The effect of insulin on ovine fetal oxygen extraction. Am J Obstet Gynecol 149:673–678

Milner RDG (1979) Amino acids and beta cell growth in structure and function. In: Merkatz IR, Adam PAJ (eds) The diabetic pregnancy. A perinatal perspective. Grune and Stratton, New York, pp 145–153

Milner RD, Hill DJ (1984) Fetal growth control: the role of insulin and related peptides. Clin Endocrinol 21:415–433

Newman RL, Tutera G (1976) The glucose–insulin ratio in amniotic fluid. Obstet Gynecol 47:599–601

Nylund L, Lunell NO, Lewander R, Persson B, Sarby B (1983) Utero-placental blood flow in diabetic pregnancy – measurements with indium 113 m and a computer-linked gamma camera. Am J Obstet Gynecol 144:298–302

Ogata ES, Freinkel N, Metzger BE et al. (1980a) Perinatal islet function in gestational diabetes: assessment by cord plasma C-peptide and amniotic fluid insulin. Diabetes Care 3:425–429

Ogata ES, Sabbagha R, Metzger BE, Phelps RL, Depp R, Freinkel N (1980b) Serial ultrasonography to assess evolving fetal macrosomia. J Am Med Assoc 243:2405–2408

Persson B (1981) Insulin as a growth factor in the fetus. In: Ritzén M, Aperia A, Hall K, Larsson A, Zetterberg A, Zetterström R (eds) The biology of normal human growth. Raven Press, New York, pp 213–221

Persson B, Heding LG, Lunell NO, Pschera H, Stangenberg M, Wager J (1982) Fetal beta cell function in diabetic pregnancy. Amniotic fluid concentrations of proinsulin, insulin, and C-peptide during the last trimester of pregnancy. Am J Obstet Gynecol 144:455–459

Persson B, Pschera H, Lunell N-O, Barley J, Gumaa KA (1986) Amino acid concentrations in maternal plasma and amniotic fluid in relation to fetal insulin secretion during the last trimester of pregnancy in gestational and type I diabetic women and women with small-for-date-gestational-age infants. Am J Perinatol 3:98–103

Philipps AF, Widness JA, Garcia JF, Raye JR, Schwartz R (1982) Erythropoietin elevation in the chronically hyperglycemic fetal lamb. Proc Soc Exp Biol Med 170:42–47

Pschera H, Persson B, Lunell NO (1986) Amniotic fluid C-peptide and cortisol in normal and diabetic pregnancies and pregnancies accompanied by fetal growth retardation. Am J Perinatol 3:16–21

Pschera H, Persson B, Lunell N-O (1988a) Interrelationship between amniotic fluid C-peptide and catecholamines in the last trimester of diabetic pregnancy. Am J Obstet Gynecol 154:48–52

Pschera H, Persson B, Lunell NO (1988b) Interrelation between glucose, insulin, C-peptide and 3-hydroxybutyrate in plasma and amniotic fluid in last trimester diabetic women without residual beta cell function. Horm Metab Res (in press)

Semmler K, Kirsch G, Zöllner P, Fuhrmann K, Jutzi E (1985) Die Messung der uteroplazentaren Durchblutung mit [113]m In in der diabetischen Schwangerschaft. Zentralbl Gynäkol 107:793–802

Simmons MA, Jones MD Jr, Battaglia FC, Meschia G (1978) Insulin effect on fetal glucose utilization. Pediatr Res 19:90–92

Spellacy WN, Buhi WC, Bradley B, Holsinger KK (1973) Maternal, fetal and amniotic fluid levels of glucose, insulin and growth hormone. Obstet Gynecol 41:323–331

Stangenberg M, Persson B, Vaclavinkova V (1982) Amniotic fluid volumes and concentrations of C-peptide in diabetic pregnancies. Br J Obstet Gynaecol 89:536–542

Tchobroutsky G, Heard I, Tchobroutsky C, Eschwege E (1980) Amniotic fluid C-peptide in normal and insulin-dependent diabetic pregnancies. Diabetologia 18:289–292

Teramo KA, Widness JA, Clemons GK, Voutilainen P, McKinlay S, Schwartz R (1987a) Amniotic fluid erythropoietin correlates with umbilical plasma erythropoietin in normal and abnormal pregnancy. Obstet Gynecol 69:710–716

Teramo KA, Widness JA, Clemons GK, Voutilainen P, McKinley SM, Schwartz R (1987b) Direct association of maternal glycemic control (HbAI$_c$) with fetal erythropoietin (Ep) in diabetic pregnancy. Abstract. Diabetes and pregnancy study group of the European Association for the Study of Diabetes. XVIII Annual meeting. Berlin, GDR, 13–15 September

van Otterlo LC, Wladimiroff JW, Wallenburg HCS (1977) Relationship between fetal urine production and amniotic fluid volume in normal pregnancy and pregnancy complicated by diabetes. Br J Obstet Gynaecol 84:205–209

Weiss PAM (1979) Die Ueberwachung des Ungeborenen bei Diabetes mellitus an Hand von Fruchtwasserinsulinwerten. Wien Klin Wochenschr 91:293–304

Weiss PAM, Lichtenegger W, Winter R, Pürstner P (1978) Insulin levels in amniotic fluid. Management of pregnancy in diabetes. Obstet Gynecol 51:393–398

Weiss PAM, Pürstner P, Winter R, Lichtenegger W (1984) Insulin levels in amniotic fluid of normal and abnormal pregnancies. Obstet Gynecol 63:371–375

Weiss PAM, Hofmann H, Winter R, Pürstner P, Lichtenegger W (1985) Amniotic fluid glucose values in normal and abnormal pregnancies. Obstet Gynecol 65:333–339

Widness JA, Susa JB, Garcia JF et al. (1981) Increased erythropoiesis and elevated erythropoietin in infants born to diabetic mothers and in hyperinsulinemic rhesus fetuses. J Clin Invest 67:637–642

13. Prepregnancy Preparation

Judith M. Steel, F. D. Johnstone and A. F. Smith

It is now widely accepted that prepregnancy clinics for insulin-dependent diabetics are both logical and desirable (Hadden 1986). Many centres around the world are using this approach to the management of diabetic pregnancy.

We feel that the aims which we first suggested in 1980 (Steel et al.) and expanded in 1982 (Steel et al.) remain important. Of these the purpose which has attracted the most attention, because of its obvious clinical impact, is the attempt to reduce the incidence of congenital abnormalities by improving diabetic control during the early weeks after conception.

Congenital Abnormalities

Relevance of Hyperglycaemia

Mølsted-Pedersen et al. (1964) first described a high incidence of congenital malformations in the infants of diabetic mothers. Others have since confirmed their observations (Soler et al. 1976; Glasgow et al. 1979). There was a report in 1945 (Landauer) of abnormalities produced in chick embryos by injection of insulin. It was thought that this was unlikely to be relevant to human pregnancy and there was no clinical evidence to support a theory that hypoglycaemia in early pregnancy might be related to congenital malformation. On the contrary Pedersen (1977) states in his now-classic book *The Pregnant Diabetic and her Newborn* that "There is at least a strong negative tendency between insulin reaction including insulin coma in the first trimester and the incidence of malformations pointing to a rather high maternal blood glucose level in this period in diabetics with malformed fetuses'.

Over the following years there were several studies which showed that hyperglycaemia in early pregnancy in the rat is associated with a high rate of abnormal development in the fetus (Deuchar 1978; Baker et al. 1981). Experiments incubating rat embryos in vitro with increasing concentrations of glucose showed that high levels of glucose increased the incidence of developmental abnormalities. These studies are comprehensively reviewed by Sadler et al. (1986). Several studies looking at control over the period of organogenesis by measuring HbA$_1$ in early pregnancy have suggested an association between high blood glucose levels and congenital abnormalities (Leslie et al. 1978; Miller et al. 1981; Ylinen et al. 1981; Stubbs et al. 1987). The recent large multi-centre study of the National Institute of Child Health and Human Development (Mills et al. 1988) throws some doubt on the subject but their failure to show a relationship between congenital malformations and glycaemic control is probably because they only studied a highly selected, well-controlled group.

Large numbers of patients must be studied before one can expect to be able to demonstrate a statistically significant difference in the frequency of congenital abnormalities between patients attending and those not attending a prepregnancy clinic. Fuhrmann's department in Karlsburg, East Germany has the greatest experience in caring for large numbers of patients and they have been able to show a significant reduction in congenital abnormalities (Fuhrmann et al. 1983; Fuhrmann et al. 1984). They started prepregnancy counselling in 1977 and report separately their experience from 1977 to 1981 and from 1981 to 1983. Over the whole 7-year period they have seen only two congenital malformations in 185 insulin-dependent diabetics attending their prepregnancy clinic (1.1%) and 31 malformations in 473 patients not attending the prepregnancy clinic (6.6%). The two groups were comparable in terms of severity of diabetes, as measured by White's classification. Blood glucose control as measured by mean daily measurements during hospitalization at 5–7 weeks in those attending the clinic, and at 8–14 weeks in those not attending, was clearly better in the group attending the prepregnancy clinic. HbA$_1$ results are not reported nor are the details of blood glucose control in those who did have offspring with abnormalities except a comment that one of the abnormalities in the prepregnancy group was in the infant of a patient with unstable diabetes.

This achievement of the East German group is most impressive but it would be difficult in many centres to follow this successful form of management. The prepregnancy patients were hospitalized every 3 months up to conception and had nine blood glucose determinations daily. They were then hospitalized as soon as the basal body temperature had been elevated for more than 16 d. All pregnant patients were seen twice weekly as out-patients and had five to seven periods of hospitalization during pregnancy.

Our own experience, which now extends over 12 years, is based largely on out-patient management. We described our prepregnancy clinic at the International Colloquium in Aberdeen in 1983 (Steel et al. 1984). The majority of our patients are hospitalized just before delivery although a few are admitted because of unsatisfactory diabetic control, vomiting or obstetric complications. From 1976 to 1987, 189 couples have been seen at our prepregnancy clinic. One hundred and ten of these patients have had pregnancies continuing beyond 28 weeks. Over the same period we have had 84 pregnancies continuing beyond 28 weeks in patients not attending the prepregnancy clinic.

The HbA$_1$ results of the 155 patients seen since the assay became available to us are shown in Table 13.1. Stratification by White's class is shown in Table 13.2. To the end of 1987 we have had 10 major congenital abnormalities, two in those attending the clinic (1.8%) and eight in those not attending (9.5%). The proportion of infants with congenital abnormalities born to mothers who did not attend the clinic is significantly greater ($P<0.05$) than the proportion born to

Table 13.1. HbA$_1$ in 155 pregnancies

	Prepregnancy clinic				Others				P
	n	Mean HbA$_1$	SE	% below 8%[a]	n	Mean HbA$_1$	SE	% below 8%	
First attended	86	11.67	0.23	0					
Booking	100	8.96	0.16	26	55	10.94	0.28	8	0.00001
1st trimester	100	8.65	0.13	30	39	10.06	0.29	15	0.00001
2nd trimester	100	8.0	0.09	59	53	8.72	0.22	45	0.0005
3rd trimester	100	7.63	0.09	70	55	8.03	0.14	59	0.01

[a] Normal range 5%–8%.

Table 13.2. Pregnancies over 28 weeks, 1976–1987 (stratification by White's class)

White's class	Prepregnancy clinic (n=110)	Others (n=84)	Total (n=94)	% of total
B	21	20	41	21
C	28	21	49	25
D	48	30	78	40
F/R	13	13	26	13

mothers who did attend the clinic. In early 1988 we have had a further major abnormality in the group not attending the prepregnancy clinic, now making 2/114 (1.8%) in the group attending prepregnancy clinic and 9/86 (10.5%) in the group not attending prepregnancy clinic ($P<0.01$). Details are shown in Table 13.3. Among the nine "non-clinic" patients with affected babies, one abnormality occurred before the HbA$_1$ assay became available and three came too late to have HbA$_1$ measured in early pregnancy. This is an inevitable problem of this type of study as poorly motivated, poorly controlled patients tend to present late, but we do have circumstantial evidence that these three patients were poorly controlled, two of them to the extent of completely omitting their insulin injections on several occasions. The five non-clinic patients who presented early did have high HbA$_1$ levels. Of the two patients who had attended the prepregnancy clinic, but who nevertheless gave birth to infants with congenital abnormalities, one had an HbA$_1$ of 9.5% which we had accepted as satisfactory. In the other, the HbA$_1$ level was 8.1% at 7 weeks. She then suffered a viral illness and vomiting of pregnancy and the HbA$_1$ rose to 11.3% at 10 weeks.

Our experience continues to emphasize the importance of long follow-up on these babies in order to identify abnormalities. The baby who died of a transposition of the great vessels was not diagnosed until the age of 6 weeks, one with kyphoscoliosis was diagnosed at 3 months and the other at 15 months. The baby with sacral hypoplasia was not diagnosed until the age of 3 years, mainly because she was not brought back to a follow-up clinic. These four abnormalities would all have been missed using Mølsted-Pedersen's criterion (1964) of malformation recognized before the 10th day of life.

Table 13.3. Major congenital abnormalities, 1976–February 1988

Case no.	Prepregnancy clinic	White's class	HbA$_1$, first trimester	Defect	Outcome
1	No	R	Before assay	Encephalocele	Surgically removed, survived retarded
2	No	C	Too late, omitted insulin	Anencephaly	Induced abortion
3	No	R/F	Too late, omitted insulin	Sacral hypoplasia	Diagnosed 3 years, urinary incontinence
4	No	C	Too late	Microcephaly	Survived severely handicapped
5	No	C	13.4%	Sirenomelia	Died 3 h
6	No	D	11.6%	Vertebral abnormalities, kyphoscoliosis	Diagnosed 6 months, spinal fusion, survived
7	No	C	11.4%	Monomelia	Died 4 h
8	No	C	13.8%	Vertebral abnormalities, kyphoscoliosis	Diagnosed 15 months, spinal fusion, survived
9	No	B	13.9%	Single ventricle, mitral atresia, aortic arch hypoplasia	Died 2 d
10	Yes	D	9.5%	Transposition great vessels	Died 8 weeks
11	Yes	D	8.1% (7 weeks) 11.3% (11 weeks)	Anencephaly	Aborted induced abortion

The proportion who did not attend the prepregnancy clinic is significantly greater ($P<0.01$) than those who did attend.

Possible Relevance of Hypoglycaemia

In the last few years Freinkel has drawn our attention to the possible relevance of studies in rats showing that interference with glycolytic processes at the time of organogenesis can result in growth retardation and congenital abnormalities (Buchanan et al. 1986). In 1983 Freinkel et al. described the "honey-bee syndrome" where they showed that D-mannose will cause growth retardation and faulty neural tube closure associated with the inhibition of glycolysis in rats. His group then reported (Buchanan et al. 1986) that the fetuses of pregnant rats made hypoglycaemic at day 9.5 (when the neural plate is established) and at day 9.75 (when somites are forming and the neural folds are beginning to oppose) were growth retarded and displayed a small but significantly raised incidence of gross developmental anomalies compared with embryos from insulin-infused euglycaemic mothers. This was not a direct effect of insulin.

These observations have been extended studying rat embryos grown in vitro and it has been shown that if these are exposed to hypoglycaemia on days 9.5–11.5 they show marked growth retardation and 42.7% had neural lesions versus 0% in the euglycaemic group (Akazawa et al. 1987). Ellington (1987) showed that at glucose concentrations <2.5 mmol the rate of glucose uptake by the rat embryos progressively decreased. Embryonic growth and differentiation became increasingly retarded and many of the embryos developed severe dysmorphic lesions. It is not known if analogous glycolytic dependence occurs in human embryos at a comparable developmental period which would be between day 18 and day 26. To those of us attempting to tighten diabetic control in early pregnancy these studies are very worrying indeed. Hypoglycaemia is very common in pregnancy. Defining severe hypoglycaemia as altered consciousness to the extent that self-treatment is impossible, Rayburn et al. (1986) found an incidence of 33% (19 out of 57) in insulin-dependent diabetic (IDD) pregnant patients and a similar percentage (30%) was reported by Tymms in 46 IDD pregnancies (Tymms et al. 1987). Neither of these authors comment on a relationship (if any) with congenital abnormalities but Bergman et al. (1986), looking at blood glucose determinations in eight insulin-dependent diabetics, found that 19% of values were below 60 mg/dl. None of their patients had infants with abnormalities but it is possible that damage could be caused at a critical stage of development and they advocated caution in treating these patients (Bergman et al. 1986; Bergman and Newman 1987).

In a retrospective study of 143 insulin-dependent diabetics delivered between 1980 and 1987 we found that 63 (44%) had had at least one (and in most cases several) episode of hypoglycaemia, so severe that self-treatment was impossible. It is clear that hypoglycaemia is not simply due to tightening diabetic control as we do this at our prepregnancy clinic and in some cases we can diagnose pregnancy before we receive a positive pregnancy test because our patient develops severe hypoglycaemia, often accompanied by unawareness. We agree with Rayburn et al. (1986) that defective recovery from hypoglycaemic occurs temporarily during pregnancy in some patients. In a retrospective study it is not easy to be sure of the exact timing of all the severe episodes but it is particulary worrying that the susceptible time in the rat embryos, equivalent to 18–22 d in human pregnancy, is a time when some of our patients first experience severe hypoglycaemia. Of our 11 patients who delivered infants with major congenital malformations only two had severe hypoglycaemia at any stage during pregnancy and only one before the ninth week. This is a relatively low incidence (18% compared to 44% in the whole group) of severe hypoglycaemia during pregnancy and only 1 (9%), compared with 26 (18%) for the whole group, had severe hypoglycaemia before the ninth week.

Our findings are therefore moderately reassuring in that they indicate a negative correlation between hypoglycaemia during pregnancy and congenital malformation. A prospective study has recently been published (Mills et al. 1988) looking at 347 insulin-dependent diabetic women over the period of organogenesis and no relationship was seen between the incidence of congenital malformations and the frequency of hypoglycaemia in the mothers. While there is as yet no clinical evidence to implicate hypoglycaemia in the aetiology of congenital malformations in humans, we are very concerned about the danger to our mothers. We have had numerous episodes of grand mal seizures and five episodes of transient hemiplegia; two patients have "written-off" their cars, two have had severe cerebral oedema and been unconscious for more than 24 h and one fractured her tibia and fibula during a convulsion. Our most severely affected patient used 68 vials of glucagon in her first pregnancy and 72 vials in her second. Throughout the other 20 years of her diabetic life she has not used more than six vials.

It is not clear to us why some patients should have so much trouble with hypoglycaemia while others have little or none. We see very well-controlled diabetics with HBA_1 levels in the normal range in both groups. There is, as one would expect, some relationship with White's classification. When our 63 patients with severe hypoglycaemia are compared with the total clinic population, they comprised 7/27 (26%) of White's class B, 20/41 (49%) of White's class C and 35/75 (48%) of White's class D. This correlation is not very impressive and we have no way of predicting which individuals will have problems. It is our practice to teach all our patients' partners and sometimes other friends or relatives how to use glucagon. We warn our patients of the dangers of falling asleep during the day and advise them not to be alone for more than short periods of time during the day and never at night. We advise them not to drive while pregnant and in some cases we use "sleep sentry" devices (Landon and Gabbe 1985). None of our patients has suffered permanent injury and none has died but the possibility cannot be disregarded (Tunbridge 1981).

Complications of Diabetes

We advised 18 of the 189 clinic patients against pregnancy, mainly because of severe renal disease and hypertension or ischaemic heart disease. In only one patient was the advice given chiefly because of severe proliferative retinopathy. That was in 1976 when our clinic had just started. With advances in management of retinopathy this would not be a major contraindication to pregnancy nowadays.

Retinopathy

There is no doubt that deterioration of retinopathy can occur in pregnancy (Beetham 1950; Maloney and Drury 1982) and until the mid-1970s proliferative retinopathy was often considered to be a contraindication to pregnancy (White 1971). It is now clear that if retinopathy has been successfully treated by panretinal photocoagulation it rarely deteriorates during pregnancy (Dibble et al. 1982).

Since 1976 at the prepregnancy and pregnancy clinic we have seen a total of 18 pregnancies in patients with proliferative retinopathy. Of the eight treated with laser therapy during pregnancy four were seen in the year in which we were just starting the prepregnancy clinic, three were referred to us already pregnant because they had proliferative retinopathy which was treated subsequently during the second or third trimester and one patient had not attended our prepregnancy clinic. She was poorly controlled and presented with rapidly progressive proliferative retinopathy in the first trimester of pregnancy. The prognosis for vision is often poor in this situation and some authorities have recommended termination of pregnancy (Sinclair et al. 1975). She refused to consider this option and her new vessels regressed after laser treatment. All these eight patients responded well to laser treatment; none had any deterioration of vision and all had good visual acuity. All mothers delivered live infants; one had sacral hypoplasia and the others were normal.

Nine patients with proliferative retinopathy and four with preproliferative retinopathy were diagnosed at our prepregnancy clinic and were treated with laser therapy before conception. All patients responded; all maintained excellent visual acuity during pregnancy; and none showed any deterioration in the appearance of their fundi and therefore did not require further treatment during pregnancy. All delivered live, healthy infants.

The remaining patient with proliferative retinopathy was referred to us from another centre, poorly controlled in early pregnancy. She had a spontaneous abortion. She then had extensive laster treatment, conceived again against medical advice and had a second spontaneous abortion. Despite treatment she had dense bilateral vitreous haemorrhages and became blind. She was then persuaded to improve her diabetic control and to use contraception. One vitreous haemorrhage gradually cleared spontaneously. The other did not and she had a successful vitrectomy in that eye (Michels et al. 1983; Young et al. 1987). She was determined to embark on another pregnancy and in fact has since had two successful pregnancies with no deterioration in her retinopathy. She maintains vision of 6/6 in the eye treated by vitrectomy and 6/9 in the other eye.

We recommend that all patients attending a prepregnancy clinic should have their eyes examined and treated, if this is indicated, before conception.

Nephropathy

Pregnancy in patients with severe renal disease may have a poor outcome and the mother's life expectancy may be very limited (Bear 1976; Grenfell et al. 1986). Pregnancies in those with nephropathy who have good renal function are usually successful (Grenfell et al. 1986). The outcome of pregnancy is related to the creatinine clearance, the degree of proteinuria and the degree of hypertension (Main et al. 1984). In patients with good renal function or extremely poor renal function a decision is easy to make but there are others where it may be quite difficult. Kitzmiller et al. (1981) described successful pregnancies in a few very high-risk patients.

We have assessed renal function, proteinuria and blood pressure in patients attending our prepregnancy clinic. Ten have been advised against pregnancy mainly because of nephropathy. Five of these have since died, two are now on dialysis and one will soon receive dialysis. The other two patients are of some interest. One, diabetic since the age of 3 years, developed very rapidly progressive nephropathy and retinopathy at the age of 19 years a few months after starting the combined oral contraceptive pill. A renal biopsy was carried out because of a rapid increase in proteinuria and a fall in creatinine clearance from 90 ml/min to 40 ml/min over 6 months. It showed classical changes of diabetic nephropathy complicated by a disproportionate tendency to fibrin deposition. She stopped the pill and was sterilized on the recommendation of the pathologist who felt very strongly that pregnancy would precipitate further fibria deposition in her kidneys. Ten years later she is blind in one eye and requires anti-hypertensive therapy but her creatinine clearance remains around 40 ml/min and she is well. We shall never know if we gave the correct advice in her case. The remaining patient has not deteriorated as fast as we had anticipated. She has maintained a creatinine clearance of around 20 ml/min and her hypertension is reasonably controlled. She was told she would be able to become pregnant after she received a transplant from her mother who is a willing and compatible donor. Both she and her mother would like this to be done but naturally the renal physicians will not consider such treatment until it is necessary for the patient. This is now likely to be when she is too old to conceive.

We have had 17 pregnancies in patients with nephropathy as defined by albustrix +ve on more than three consecutive occasions in the absence of infection. All these patients had a creatinine clearance greater than 40 ml/min. Three of them had significant hypertension which was treated before conception. None of them had significant deterioration in their renal function during pregnancy. All delivered live babies, one with a congenital abnormality.

We recommend that renal function should be assessed and hypertension treated (if present) before conception.

Attendance at Prepregnancy Clinic

In any type of preventive medicine such as the running of a prepregnancy clinic, there are inevitably problems in persuading patients to attend. There is a tendency for those who most need to attend not to do so.

It is very difficult to run a prepregnancy clinic in centres where pregnant patients are referred in largely from other clinics. We are fortunate in that this applies to only about 15% of our pregnancies. Excluding the first 2 years, when the clinic was starting, 65% of insulin-dependent pregnant diabetics seen in our department have attended the prepregnancy clinic. The corresponding figure for Fuhrmann et al. (1984) was 33%, for Goldman et al. (1986) 59%, for Pearson (personal communication) 43% and, in smaller series, Rowe et al. (1987) reported 14 out of 21 (67%) and Tindall et al. (1986) 8 out of 16 (50%).

Fuhrmann, Tindall and Pearson discuss the motivation of their separate groups of patients. In Fuhrmann's experience, previous perinatal loss appeared to be important in motivating patients to come to the prepregnancy clinic. Of those attending his prepregnancy clinic, 31.7% had had a previous perinatal loss and 13.3% an infant with a congenital malformation. This was compared with a previous perinatal loss rate of 13.9% and previous congenital malformation rate of 5.6% in his group not attending the prepregnancy clinic. Tindall asked the eight patients not coming to her prepregnancy clinic why they had not attended. Three had unplanned pregnancies, one did not know about the clinic, the other four had known but not attended, one stating that she was "far too busy". Pearson (personal communication), looking at 66 sequential pregnancies, saw 26 (43%) for prepregnancy counselling. He found that those attending for prepregnancy counselling were slightly more likely to be primigravida, 46% versus 38% (62% of the latter unmarried). City dwellers were more likely to attend than country dwellers, 38% versus 28%.

For the last 7 years we have asked those not coming through the clinic why they have not attended. Over that period we have had 126 pregnancies. Seventy-nine patients (63%) have attended the prepregnancy clinic. If we exclude the 19 patients referred to us from other centres, already pregnant, 74% attended the prepregnancy clinic (79/107). In the whole series five patients (4.0%) had had previous perinatal losses. Those were three (one due to congenital malformation) in the prepregnancy group (3.8%) and two, both due to congenital malformation (7%), in those not attending. Previous pregnancy loss therefore does not appear to have been a major motivating factor for coming to the clinic. Unlike Pearson we found that those attending the prepregnancy clinic were slightly less likely to be primigravida (50% compared with 62%) but like him we found a higher proportion of unmarried mothers among those not attending (37% compared with only 4% in the group attending for prepregnancy counselling).

I have found it very interesting and encouraging over the years that many of my rather rebellious girls, who have not attended the prepregnancy clinic, have been booking very early in pregnancy and coming in with a carefully compiled record of blood tests, when previously they have been rather poorly controlled. In many of these patients the haemoglobin A_1 at the booking clinic was far better than previous levels.

I asked the 28 patients attending our diabetic clinic, but not attending the prepregnancy clinic, if they had known about the clinic and, if they did know why did they not attend. Twenty of these patients had known about the clinic. Three had not attended because they had attended before with a previous pregnancy and had improved their control themselves. Two thought that the only purpose of the clinic was to achieve good control and judged themselves to be already well controlled. There were six who planned a pregnancy, but for a variety of reasons did not want us to know (and in four cases did not want their partner to know) and there were another eight who knew they ought to come but had not arranged to do so. All these patients did improve their control themselves and they booked early. These apparently "unplanned" pregnancies were in fact quite carefully planned. We only had one patient with a genuinely unplanned pregnancy and she was poorly controlled. The control was significantly better ($P<0.0005$) in the group who had known about the clinic, mean HbA_1 10.0% (SE 0.337), compared with the nine patients who had not known about the clinic, HbA_1 13.5% (SE 0.713). The eight patients who did not know about the clinic included two who had recently moved into our area, one who had just been diagnosed, three chronic defaulters and two whom somehow we had failed to inform. We are working hard to try to reduce the size of this group.

Infertility

The number of couples investigated for infertility is still rather high; 32 of our 165 couples (i.e. 189 attending the prepregnancy clinic but excluding 18 couples advised against pregnancy and six couples who decided against pregnancy). The findings, treatment and pregnancy rate in this group are shown in Table 13.4. The

Table 13.4. Findings in 32 infertile couples, 1976–1987

Diagnosis	No.	% total	Treatment	No.	Pregnancies
Ovulatory	5	16	Ovulation induction	4	3 (1 × 2)
Tubal	4	13	Salpingolysis	2	1 × 2
Male	7	22	AIH	2	1
			AID	1	1 × 2
			None	4	1
Unexplained	16	50	None	15	5
			GIFT	1	1

incidence of infertility may appear falsely high as we start to investigate couples after just over a year of infertility, but the frequent delays in conception are a problem when running a prepregnancy clinic (Steel 1984). Knowing that the risks of pregnancy are related to the duration of diabetes and the presence of complications, we feel it is important not to delay too long. With new methods of treatment of infertility becoming available and an almost negligible chance of a diabetic patient being able to adopt a young baby in Britain, we feel it is very important to take an active interest in this problem.

Conclusion

We continue to feel that running a prepregnancy clinic contributes to closer cooperation between patient, partner, physician and obstetrician in the management of diabetic pregnancy. It is encouraging that we now see a significant difference between the major congenital abnormality rate in patients coming through our prepregnancy clinic compared with those who have not. Increasing the proportion of patients coming through our clinic remains a challenging problem but with growing evidence of tangible benefits, we are able to publicize and promote the service with renewed vigour.

References

Akazawa S, Akazawa M, Hashimoto M et al. (1987) Effects of hypoglycaemia on early embryogenesis in rat embryo organ culture. Diabetologia 30:791–796

Baker L, Egler J, Kein S, Goldman AS (1981) Meticulous control of diabetes during organogenesis prevents congenital lumbo-sacral defects in rats. Diabetes 30:955–959

Bear RA (1976) Pregnancy in patients with renal disease. Obstet Gynecol 48:13–18

Beetham WP (1950) Diabetic retinopathy in pregnancy. Trans Am Ophthalmol Soc 48:205–219

Bergman M, Newman S (1987) Hypoglycaemia in pregnancy, unknown risks. Diabetes Care 10:180

Bergman M, Seaton TB, Auerhahn CC, Aaron-Young C, Glasser M, Shapiro L (1986) The incidence of gestational hypoglycaemia in insulin-dependent and non-insulin dependent diabetic women. New York State J Med 86:174–177

Buchanan TA, Schemmer JK, Freinkel N (1986) Embryotoxic effects of brief maternal insulin-hypoglycaemia during organogenesis in the rat. J Clin Invest 78:643–649

Deuchar E (1978) Experimental evidence relating fetal anomalies to diabetes. In: Sutherland HW, Stowers JM (eds) Carbohydrate metabolism in pregnancy and the newborn. Springer-Verlag, Berlin Heidelberg New York, pp 247–263

Dibble CM, Kochenour NK, Worley RJ, Tyler FH, Swartz M (1982) Effect of pregnancy on diabetic retinopathy. Obstet Gynecol 59:699–702

Ellington SKL (1987) Development of rat embryos cultured on glucose-deficient media. Diabetes 36:1372–1378

Freinkel N, Lewis S, Akazawa S, Gorman L, Potaczek M (1983) The honey bee syndrome, teratogenic effects of mannose during organogenesis in rat embryo culture. Trans Assoc Am Physicians 96:44–55

Fuhrmann K, Reiher H, Semmler K, Fischer F, Fischer M, Glockner E (1983) Prevention of congenital malformation in infants of insulin dependent diabetic mothers. Diabetes Care 6:219–223

Fuhrmann K, Reiher H, Semmler K, Glockner E (1984) The effect of intensified conventional insulin therapy before and during pregnancy on the malformation rate in offspring of diabetic mothers. Exp Clin Endocrinol 83:173–177

Glasgow ACA, Harley JMG, Montgomery DAD (1979) Congenital malformations in infants of diabetic mothers. Ulster Med J 48:109–117

Goldman JA, Dicker D, Feldberg D, Yeshaya A, Samuel N, Karp M (1986) Pregnancy outcome in patients with insulin-dependent diabetes mellitus with pre-conceptual diabetic control. A comparative study. Am J Obstet Gynecol 155:292–297

Grenfell A, Brudenell JM, Doddridge MC, Watkins PJ (1986) Pregnancy in diabetic women who have proteinuria. Q J Med 228:379–386

Hadden DR (1986) Diabetes in pregnancy 1985. Diabetologia 29:1–9

Kitzmiller JL, Brown ER, Phillippe M et al. (1981) Diabetic nephropathy and perinatal outcome. J Obstet Gynecol 141:741–751

Landauer W (1945) Rumplesness of chicken embryos produced by injections of insulin and other chemicals. J Exp Zool 98:65–77

Landon MB, Gabbe SG (1985) Glucose monitoring and insulin administration in the pregnant diabetic patient. Clin Obstet Gynaecol 28:496–506

Leslie RDG, John PN, Pyke DA, White JM (1978) Haemoglobin A$_1$ in diabetic pregnancy. Lancet II:958–959

Main EK, Main DM, Gabbe SG (1984) Factors predicting perinatal outcome in pregnancies complicated by diabetic nephropathy. Diabetes [Suppl 1] 33:201A

Maloney JM, Drury MI (1982) The effect of pregnancy on the natural course of diabetic nephropathy. Am J Ophthalmol 93:745–756

Michels RG, Rice TA, Rice EF (1983) Vitrectomy for vitreous haemorrhage. Am J Ophthalmol 95:12–21

Miller E, Hare JW, Cloherty JP (1981) Elevated maternal haemoglobin A$_1$ in early pregnancy and major congenital anomalies in infants of diabetic mothers. N Engl J Med 304:1331–1334

Mills JL, Knopp RH, Simpson JL et al. (1988) Lack of relation of increased malformation rates in infants of diabetic mothers to glycemic control during organogenesis. N Engl J Med 318:671–676

Mølsted-Pedersen L, Tygstrup I, Pedersen J (1964) Congenital malformations in new born infants of diabetic women. Lancet I:1124–1126

Pedersen J (1977) Congenital malformations. In: The pregnant diabetic and her newborn, 2nd edn. Munksgaard, Copenhagen, pp 191–196

Rayburn W, Piehl E, Jacober S, Schork A, Ploughman L (1986) Severe hypoglycaemia during pregnancy, its frequency and predisposing factors in diabetic women. Int J Gynaecol Obstet 24:263–268

Rowe BR, Rowbotham CJF, Barnett AH (1987) Pre-conception counselling, birth weight and congenital abnormalities in established and gestational diabetic pregnancy. Diabetes Res 6:33–35

Sadler TW, Horton WE, Hunter ES (1986) Mechanisms of diabetes-induced congenital malformations as studied in mammalian embryo culture. In: Jovanovic L, Peterson CM, Fuhrmann K (eds) Diabetes and pregnancy, teratology, toxicity and treatment. Praeger, New York, pp 51–71

Sinclair SH, Nesler CL, Schwartz SS (1975) Retinopathy in the pregnant diabetic. Clin Obstet Gynecol 28:536–552

Soler NG, Walsh CH, Malins JM (1976) Congenital malformations in infants of diabetic mothers. Q J Med 45:303–313

Steel JM, Parboosingh J, Cole RA, Duncan LJP (1980) Pre-pregnancy counselling, a logical prelude to the management of the pregnant diabetic. Diabetes Care 3:371–373

Steel JM, Johnstone FD, Smith AF, Duncan LJP (1982) Five years experience of a pre-pregnancy clinic for insulin-dependent diabetics. Br Med J 285:353–356

Steel JM, Johnstone FD, Smith AF, Duncan LJP (1984) The pre-pregnancy clinic approach. In: Sutherland HW, Stowers JM (eds) Carbohydrate metabolism in pregnancy and the newborn. Springer-Verlag, Berlin Heidelberg New York, pp 75–86

Stubbs SM, Doddridge MC, John PN, Steel JM, Wright AD (1987) Haemoglobin A$_1$ and congenital malformation. Diabetic Medicine 4:156–159

Tindall H, Vinall PS, Stickland M, Wales JK (1986) Improved results for diabetic pregnancies after pre-pregnancy counselling. Practical Diabetes 3:250–252

Tunbridge WHG (1981) Factors contributing to deaths in diabetics under fifty years of age. Lancet II:569–572

Tymms DJ, Callaway PL, Leatherdale BA, Wheeler T (1987) Audit of out-patient management of 99 pregnancies in patients with diabetes. Diabetic Medicine 4:578A

White P (1971) Pregnancy and diabetes. In: Marble A, White P, Bradley R, Krall L (eds) Joslins diabetes mellitus. Lea and Febiger, Philadelphia, pp 595–597

Ylinen K, Rawo K, Teramo K (1981) Haemoglobin A$_1$c predicts the perinatal outcome in insulin-dependent diabetic pregnancies. Br J Obstet Gynaecol 88:961–967

Young LB, Steel JM, West CP, Chawla H (1987) Pregnancy after vitrectomy for proliferative diabetic retinopathy. Diabetic Medicine 4:77–78

14. Management of the Insulin-Dependent Diabetic Woman: Problems with Pregnancy

D. W. M. Pearson and H. W. Sutherland

Introduction and Historical Perspective

Although the earliest description in the English language of diabetic pregnancy was provided in the nineteenth century (Duncan 1833), management of diabetic pregnancy was infrequently mentioned in the literature until the discovery of the clinical use of insulin which returned fertility to young women with diabetes. Almost 200 years ago, when the condition was discussed by the local Medico-Chirurgical Society in Aberdeen, the minutes report "the pathology and method of cure of this disease is wrapped up in obscurity, very little being said upon it". The link between diabetes and the pancreas was first suggested around that time when Thomas Cawley reported a case of diabetes with marked pancreatic damage to the *London Medical Journal*, but 100 years passed before Von Mering and Minkowski confirmed the central role of the pancreas in the development of diabetes and the search intensified for a pancreatic factor which controlled blood glucose.

Many groups were investigating this actively and two Aberdonians, a zoologist, Dr. John Rennie, and a physician, Dr. Thomas Fraser, reported in 1905 that in the fish species *Lophius piscatorius* the islets of Langerhans were separate from the remainder of the pancreas (Rennie and Fraser 1906/7). The anatomically distinct islets were dissected and saline extracts given orally and by injection to animals and people with diabetes mellitus. However, no significant glucose-lowering effect was demonstrated and experiments had to be discontinued due to the lack of supply of suitable fish! Sixteen years later insulin became available following Banting and Best's isolation and purification of it in the laboratory of J. J. R. MacLeod, Professor of Physiology in Toronto, who was an Aberdeen graduate and who returned to Aberdeen in 1928 as Professor of Physiology. Fertility was restored by the therapeutic administration of insulin to women who so recently had been barren due to diabetes. The most obvious effect was that maternal mortality associated with diabetic pregnancy almost disappeared and morbidity was reduced, but the perinatal mortality rate remained very high during the 1920s, 1930s and 1940s. In 1946, 25 years after the discovery of insulin, Sir Derek Dunlop quoted a perinatal mortality rate of between 50% and 70% in women with diabetes mellitus, although he stated that in women with carefully controlled diabetes it could be reduced to 25%.

Over the last 40 years increasing emphasis has been placed on optimizing metabolic control. It has also become apparent, however, that with increasing duration of diabetes, microvascular complications produce functional and anatomical abnormalities in the retina, kidneys and cardiovascular system. When Leonard Thomson, the first person treated with insulin, died from pneumonia in 1935 he had evidence already of atherosclerosis, although aged only 27 (Burrow et al. 1982). In 1949 Priscilla White reviewed her extensive experience of diabetic pregnancy and produced for pregnant diabetic women a classification which, although it has been modified (Hare and White 1980), continues to find favour in many centres (Table 14.1). Similarly, the prognostically bad signs during pregnancy described by Jorgen Pedersen and Lars Mølsted-Pedersen in 1965 (Pedersen and Mølsted-Pedersen 1965) are still relevant to clinical practice in the 1980s (Table 14.2). In 1987 Diamond et al. (1987) reassessed White's classification and Pedersen's prognostically bad signs during pregnancy in the light of modern management, and they found both continued to be appropriate and useful.

Table 14.1. Diabetic pregnancy: classification of Priscilla White

Gestational diabetes	Abnormal GTT, but euglycaemia maintained by diet alone
	Diet alone insufficient, insulin required
Class A	Diet alone, any duration or onset age
Class B	Onset age 20 or older and duration less than 10 years
Class C	Onset age 10–19 or duration 10–19 years
Class D	Onset age under 10 or duration of over 20 years or background retinopathy or hypertension
Class R	Proliferative retinopathy or vitreous haemorrhage
Class F	Nephropathy with over 500 mg/d proteinuria
Class RF	Criteria for both classes F and R
Class H	Atherosclerotic heart disease
Class T	Prior renal transplantation

Table 14.2. Prognostically bad signs during diabetic pregnancy

1. Hyperpyretic pyelitis
2. Pre-coma or severe acidosis
3. Toxaemia
4. "Neglectors"

Since the discovery of insulin, knowledge about diabetes mellitus has advanced considerably and outwith pregnancy a new classification has developed which clearly delineates two major types of diabetes (National Diabetes Data Group 1979). During reproductive life, most women with established diabetes mellitus will have type I or insulin-dependent diabetes mellitus (IDDM). They will have presented classically in childhood or adolescence with a fairly rapid onset of thirst, frequency of micturition and weight loss. Ketonuria and a predisposition to ketoacidosis result from insulin deficiency due to a progressive destruction of the beta cells in the islets of Langerhans. Although the symptoms may have been present for only a short time at diagnosis, it is known that immunological abnormalities, such as islet cell antibodies, may have been present for many months or years prior to the clinical diagnosis. The predisposition to IDDM is associated with certain HLA tissue types, e.g. DR3 or DR4, and current evidence suggests that an insult by a virus, chemical agent or both initiates an immunological response in a susceptible individual producing insulinitis and eventual beta cell failure leading to clinical diabetes mellitus. The other common type of diabetes is type II or non-insulin-dependent diabetes mellitus (NIDDM) which appears classically in middle aged or elderly subjects who are overweight, but it can appear in younger women. The condition is characterized by a relative but not absolute deficiency of insulin, resistance to the metabolic action of insulin with regard to carbohydrate metabolism and no ketonuria. If a woman with NIDDM is still in her reproductive years, she requires advice about careful monitoring prior to and during pregnancy, similar to that given to a woman with pre-existing IDDM. Women with NIDDM will often be older and may have macrovascular disease.

As information about the importance of prepregnancy control and methods of early detection of diabetic complications, such as measurement of microalbuminuria, become available, a new classification to distinguish high-risk pregnancy may evolve but the present systems remain useful since they allow comparison of data from different centres. In the numerous series of diabetic pregnancies which have been reported during this decade (Murphy et al. 1984; Drury 1986; Mølsted-Pedersen and Kuhl 1986; Martin et al. 1987), the perinatal mortality has been approaching that of the background population. However, diabetic pregnancy remains a high-risk situation and it is important to consider in detail the particular problems associated with the condition.

The Problem of Increasing Numbers: Epidemiology of Diabetes and Diabetic Pregnancy

The organization of care during diabetic pregnancies in many countries will need to cope in future with increasing numbers of patients. During reproductive life, IDDM is more common than NIDDM and the incidence of IDDM is increasing in many countries (Diabetes Epidemiology Research International 1987). One of the most striking characteristics of IDDM is its great geographical variability with a high incidence in northern European countries such as Finland, Sweden and Scotland, and a relatively low incidence in countries such as Japan and France. In several populations there have been quite rapid changes in incidence over a relatively short time period. In Poland a rapid increase between 1970 and 1982 has been reported (Rewers et al. 1987) and a similar increase has been reported between 1968 and 1976 in Scotland (Stewart-Brown et al. 1983). In the North-East of Scotland the increasing incidence over the last 60 years is reflected in the number of new cases reported to the Royal Aberdeen Children's Hospital, particularly since the Second World War, and also by the increasing number of diabetic pregnancies seen each year which has risen from around 10 in the late 1970s to around 30 in 1987.

Partly as a consequence of this increasing incidence, many fertile women have longstanding complicated diabetes, but these women are strongly motivated for successful procreation and increasing resources will need to be allocated to services providing care for children, teenagers and mothers with type I diabetes mellitus. A report of the accounts of our hospital in 1926 expressed concern that 20% of the total pharmacy budget was being spent on the new treatment of insulin; in the 1990s increasing resources will be required to maintain present standards in the management of the increasing numbers of people with diabetes. The requirement for resources will increase further as more effective treatment becomes available. Complications of diabetes may already be present during childhood and adolescence (Dahlquist and Rudberg 1987) and the outcome of diabetic pregnancy may be determined largely by the attitudes developed and degree of control achieved during the childhood and teenage years.

Organization of Diabetic Care: The Combined Clinic Approach

Many of the problems associated with diabetic pregnancy can be reduced significantly by organizing a centralized multidisciplinary team who will provide experienced care to tackle the unique metabolic and pathophysiological problems precipitated by the combination of the metabolic disorder of diabetes mellitus and the metabolic re-adjustments of pregnancy. The combined obstetrician and diabetologist approach can be extended to include many other health care professionals, thereby ensuring appropriate education and care for diabetic women during pregnancy. Different countries have evolved different approaches to suit their particular health care systems. In the Grampian Region, which is an area in the North-East of Scotland with a population of around 500000, pregnancy care is centralized at the combined Obstetric/Diabetic Clinic, established in 1962 at Aberdeen Maternity Hospital. The Clinic provides combined obstetric, metabolic and diabetic care for women from the peripheral islands of Orkney and Shetland, in addition to those from rural areas in the North-East of Scotland and from the City of Aberdeen. Patients are reviewed frequently at the combined clinic by an obstetrician and diabetologist simultaneously (see Fig. 14.3). Excellent support is provided by interested and enthusiastic midwifery, laboratory and dietetic staff. A structured programme is followed to ensure comprehensive care, but flexibility is required to accommodate the needs of individual women and their families.

The importance of prepregnancy assessment has been discussed in the previous chapter. Women are encouraged to attend the combined clinic as soon as they suspect pregnancy. When pregnancy is confirmed a short hospital admission is often arranged to optimize blood glucose control and to establish effective communication and good relationships with the care team. Reinforcement of educational messages which may or may not have been given some time previously is essential. At the monthly out-patient visits until 28 weeks, women have routine assessments of weight, blood pressure, urine (for glucose, ketones and protein) and haemoglobin A_{1C}, as well as laboratory blood glucose estimation and review of home blood glucose monitoring results. If control and progress are satisfactory women are seen at fortnightly intervals until 36 weeks and then weekly until delivery. Regular assessments of fetal growth by ultrasonography and of maternal metabolism and physiology by measurement of creatinine, haemoglobin and free thyroxine and by clinical examination of the retinae are performed. Occult urine infection is sought at first presentation, and at 28 and 36 weeks. Alpha-fetoprotein and C-peptide are measured at 16 weeks (see Fig. 14.1).

A review of 103 sequential deliveries between 1979 and 1986 in 94 women with pre-existing type I diabetes mellitus is summarized in Fig. 14.2. In this series there was one twin pregnancy and 17 women had two babies. The distribution of White classes was similar to that seen in other series. Just under 70% of the babies were delivered between 38 and 41 weeks with a total Caesarean section rate of 43%;

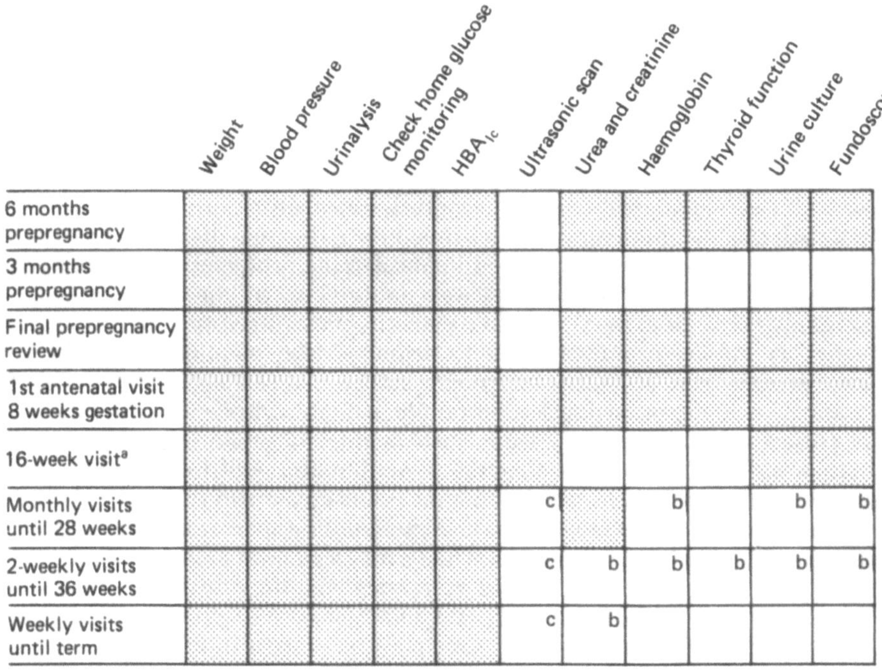

	Weight	Blood pressure	Urinalysis	Check home glucose monitoring	HBA$_{1c}$	Ultrasonic scan	Urea and creatinine	Haemoglobin	Thyroid function	Urine culture	Fundoscopy
6 months prepregnancy											
3 months prepregnancy											
Final prepregnancy review											
1st antenatal visit 8 weeks gestation											
16-week visit[a]											
Monthly visits until 28 weeks						c		b		b	b
2-weekly visits until 36 weeks						c	b	b	b	b	b
Weekly visits until term						c	b				

[a] Also measure C-peptide and α-fetoprotein.
[b] Required at one of these visits only.
[c] See text.

Fig. 14.1.   Aberdeen Combined Antenatal/Diabetic Clinic.

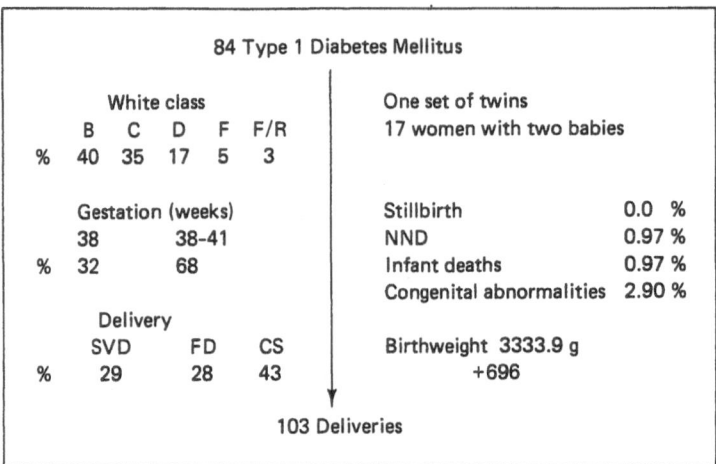

Fig. 14.2.   Outcome of diabetic pregnancies, Grampian Region (1 January 1979 to 1 April 1986).

this rate is significantly higher than that of the background population. There were no stillbirths during this period in women with insulin-dependent diabetes mellitus. One neonatal death at 33 weeks gestation was associated with severe central nervous system congenital malformation and one infant death at 29 d followed severe asphyxia due to a placental abruption at term. The abruption happened without warning while the patient was in the Ultrasound Department and an emergency Caesarean section was unsuccessful in preventing severe foetal asphyxia. The mean birthweight for the group as a whole was approximately 200 g above that of the background population.

Could all the problems of diabetic pregnancy therefore be solved if efficient organization provided good metabolic control, especially prior to pregnancy? A more detailed study of the reproductive outcome in the total diabetic population during 1979–1986 reveals there are still considerable problems associated with diabetes mellitus. A careful review was undertaken of the gynaecological, prepregnancy and combined obstetric diabetic clinic services. The same 103 deliveries in insulin-dependent diabetic women were identified (Fig. 14.3). Sixteen women who attended for prepregnancy counselling in the hope of commencing a family or having further family had not conceived by the time the study period was complete. Reasons such as infertility and complications of diabetes are discussed in other chapters. One hundred and twenty-six conceptions were confirmed but the problem of first-trimester abortion reduced the total number of fetuses surviving to 14 weeks. Hyperemesis gravidarum posed a major problem for three women, one of whom had a miscarriage at 22 weeks. The other two women had persistent nausea and occasional vomiting for the remainder of pregnancy. Neither had a history of peptic ulcer disease or previous symptoms suggestive of autonomic neuropathy. One gave a family history of hyperemesis gravidarum in non-diabetic relatives. Both lost weight during pregnancy and required frequent admissions for treatment with intravenous fluids, feeding and vitamin supplements. Mild ketosis produced an exacerbation of symptoms. Both women gave birth to healthy infants and nausea resolved after delivery. One has subsequently developed cardiological evidence of autonomic neuropathy. Both

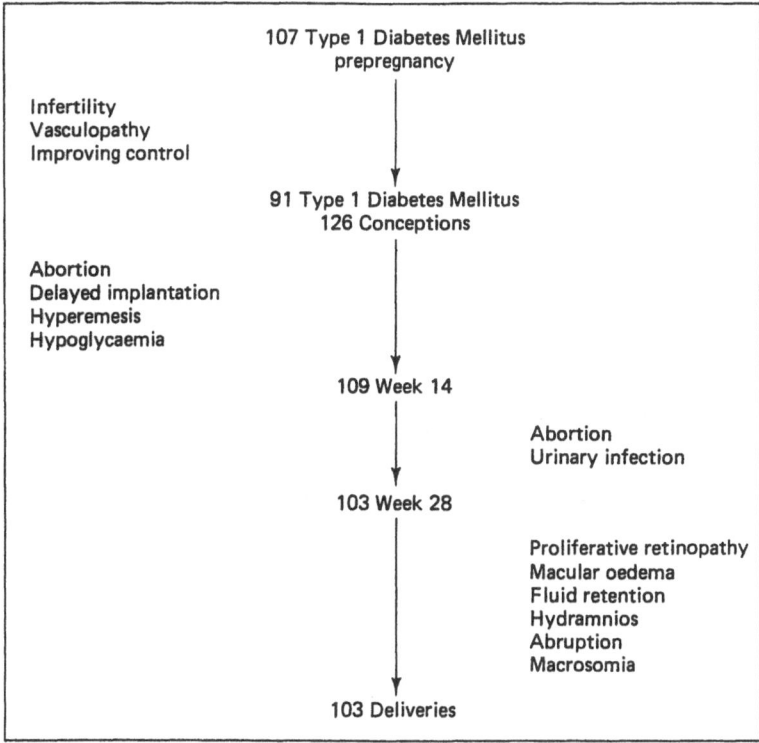

Fig. 14.3. Reproductive outcome in diabetes mellitus. Grampian Region (1 January 1979 to 1 April 1986).

decided after pregnancy that they did not wish further pregnancies and their husbands have undergone vasectomies.

Urinary infection was reduced by prepregnancy screening but even in the group who were seen before pregnancy, urinary infection was more common than in the background population. After a woman was stabilized on an effective insulin regimen, infection was the commonest reason for loss of control. Many of the problems in later pregnancy relating to the complications of diabetes are discussed in other chapters.

In addition to this experience in insulin-dependent diabetic women five women with non-insulin dependent diabetes mellitus attended the clinic during this period. A total of nine pregnancies were confirmed, two of which resulted in first-trimester abortion and two in stillbirth. These older, generally obese, women represent a high-risk category.

Problems with Metabolic Control

In diabetic pregnancy the main aims are to achieve normal metabolism at conception, throughout pregnancy and during delivery with a view to a healthy baby being delivered vaginally at term. Modern management strives to achieve these aims but, in the absence of appropriate levels of endogenous insulin secretion, they are not always possible, since insulin is delivered by a non-physiological route and the amount injected is adjusted by monitoring a single substrate, namely glucose. Notwithstanding, in practical terms blood glucose relates to many of the problems of diabetic pregnancy and control of glycaemia is the cornerstone of management. Blood glucose levels should be maintained within a narrow range and the subtle changes of carbohydrate metabolism in pregnancy should be mimicked as far as is possible. Blood glucose is the simplest and most practical substrate to measure, but amino acids, free fatty acids, ketones and glycerol are all available to the fetus as energy substrates. Monitoring circulating levels of all of these substrates during routine pregnancy care to assess the degree to which the intact fetal islets of Langerhans are exposed to each is currently impossible. Nevertheless an awareness of subtle derangements in handling these metabolites may yet provide an explanation for macrosomia or other problems in apparently "well-controlled" diabetic pregnancies.

The major determinants of glycaemic control are motivation, understanding of management principles, appropriate advice, a planned education programme and facilities for the woman and her care team to assess the degree of control and progress of fetal development during pregnancy.

Social and Psychological Aspects of Management

While a highly organized, centralized, combined system may be acceptable to most women, geographical, domestic or other constraints may mitigate against the usual programme. If women live far from the centralized clinic, a degree of supervision can be shared with primary care physicians or colleagues in peripheral clinics, provided excellent lines of communication exist. Brief admissions to the centralized unit can be utilized to assess metabolic control and pregnancy progress. We follow such a regimen for women living on the distant Orkney and Shetland islands with good results, although such women need to be admitted around 3 weeks prior to delivery.

Major problems in pregnancy are met by the group of women designated by Jorgen Pedersen as "neglectors". The reasons for non-compliance must be analysed critically and the system modified to optimize care in differing situations. The diabetic liaison health visitor or domiciliary midwife, with support from the primary care physician, can follow the guidance of the centralized care team. Paediatricians and adult physicians with an interest in the management of childhood or adolescent diabetes have been encouraging the development of self-help groups for adolescents with diabetes to promote positive attitudes in teenagers affected by diabetes. Much research needs to be done on the psychological impact of diabetes in the teenage years. Relationships should be fostered carefully with teenagers and younger mothers, either by group or individual counselling. The prepregnancy and pregnancy clinics should be seen as a continuum of the local diabetic service providing optimal care for diabetic women throughout life.

Newly Diagnosed Insulin-Dependent Diabetes Mellitus (IDDM) in Pregnancy

If IDDM develops during pregnancy, insulin is essential to maintain normogly-caemia. Urgent admission is arranged to stabilize metabolism, initially with intravenous fluids and insulin. The daily dosage of subcutaneous insulin may be less than the usual 0.7–1.0 unit/kg. Intermediate- and short-acting human insulin should be given using the regimen described below for established diabetic women. Newly diagnosed patients should not be discharged until normoglycae-mia has been achieved and they are competent in the practical aspects of insulin therapy, dietary management and home blood glucose measurement. The symptoms and management of hypoglycaemia must be explained and family education about diabetes should be initiated. Domestic support by the liaison diabetic health visitor helps to maintain good control, and frequent out-patient review is necessary initially. While diabetes may temporarily remit after delivery, careful follow-up is required, since most women will develop insulin-dependent diabetes mellitus in due course.

Management of Established Diabetes Mellitus in Pregnancy

Residual beta cell function may make glycaemic control easier (Pistaiato et al. 1987). This can be estimated by measurement of plasma C-peptide, but at present this is an expensive assay which cannot be regarded as an essential clinical tool, although it provides interesting information.

Insulin Therapy

The insulin regimen needs to be tailored to individual requirements with the aim of ideally producing normal fasting and postprandial glycaemia. The dosage of insulin required to maintain normal blood glucose will be influenced by gestation, body weight, diet, activity and residual beta cell function. There may be a slight fall in insulin requirements in the first trimester with a subsequent increase, and on average the dosage required will double by the time of delivery due to insulin resistance (Ryan et al. 1985). The insulin regimen must be flexible to allow for such increased requirements. There is usually a need to change from twice-daily premixed insulin to multiple insulin injections. Soluble and Isophane insulins before breakfast will usually provide satisfactory control by day, but often it is necessary to separate the evening insulins and give Soluble (fast-acting insulin) before the main evening meal and Isophane (intermediate-acting insulin) before bedtime. Additional insulin may also be required before lunch to avoid late afternoon hyperglycaemia.

The use of human insulins or highly purified porcine insulins is recommended during pregnancy, since such insulins are less immunogenic and thus less likely to stimulate production of anti-insulin antibodies which could cross the placenta (Mylvaganam et al. 1983). In our experience the change from highly purified porcine insulin to biosynthetic human insulin does not lead to a significant change in insulin antibody levels. It is particularly important during pregnancy that women should avoid injecting into fibrotic areas, which may lead to irregular absorption of insulin. This is particularly liable to happen in women with longstanding diabetes mellitus and injection sites should be carefully inspected at the first visit. Rotation of injection sites should be emphasized, but the rate of absorption of subcutaneous insulin varies according to the site of injection and patients should be aware that abdominal, as opposed to lower limb, injection of insulin leads to slightly faster absorption. Newer and more intensive methods of insulin treatment are described in the next chapter.

Poor Glycaemic Control

Poor glycaemic control is the commonest reason for hospital admission in our patients and is frequently signalled by the development of excessive liquor amnii found clinically or by ultrasound. Inadequate insulin dosage is the usual explanation for persistent non-ketonuric hyperglycaemia and while adequate education should decrease this problem, some women lack the confidence to increase insulin dosage. Ideally, in the matter of increasing insulin dosage, the care team should be proactive rather than reactive. Patients, after proper instruction and depending on their understanding, should be encouraged to take the appropriate measures throughout pregnancy. Rebound hyperglycaemia may occur in response to an episode of nocturnal hypoglycaemia and measurement of blood glucose overnight may confirm a need to reduce rather than increase the before-tea or bedtime insulin dosage. After a period of metabolic stability on an effective insulin regimen, extreme variability of diabetic control is usually due to infection, particularly in the urinary tract, but occasionally in the respiratory tract and it is important to remember that dental root abscess may be the cause of variable glycaemic control. A short hospital admission to identify and treat aggressively such infection may avoid decompensation to diabetic ketoacidosis. On the other hand, vaginal candidiasis may be severe without metabolic upset.

We have seen one young pregnant diabetic recently who was a "neglector" and who had previously had sterile urine, but who developed a urinary tract infection at home. She was seen by two primary care physicians who did not appreciate that her dyspnoea was due to diabetic ketoacidosis and by the time of hospital admission the fetus had died in utero. Diabetic ketoacidosis is a rare but very serious development in diabetic pregnancy (Brumfield and Huddlestone 1984) and patients must be aware of the importance of making contact with the hospital if they develop persistent non-fasting ketonuria. We have modified our home monitoring sheets to include advice about testing for ketonuria and a contact telephone number to use if ketonuria develops. A potential disadvantage of a very centralized care system is that other practitioners may not appreciate the speed and severity with which diabetic ketoacidosis can develop during pregnancy. Fetal survival has been reported following the presentation of diabetes in pregnancy with diabetic ketoacidosis (Robertson et al. 1986) and pre-existing metabolic control appears to be important. The most important consideration, however, is the early recognition of developing ketosis to ensure effective management.

Problems with Diet

Regular dietetic review during pregnancy is essential and the dietitian is an integral member of the diabetic pregnancy combined care team. Our patients are routinely reviewed by the dietitian at the first visit, at 20 weeks and at 30 weeks, but are encouraged to discuss uncertainties as frequently as is required. Dietary advice for diabetic pregnant women aims to promote a diet high in fibre and unrefined carbohydrate and low in fat. This type of regimen has been shown to improve short-term metabolic control in non-pregnant diabetic women and in women with gestational diabetes mellitus. The increased bulk of such meals may pose a problem for women during the later stages of pregnancy and they should be given careful advice about eating small or regular meals. This approach may also be advantageous in tackling the problem of mid-morning hypoglycaemia. It is also worthwhile remembering that the fine tuning of maternal metabolic control may be as readily achieved by dietary manipulation as by adjusting insulin dose.

Hypoglycaemia

First-trimester hypoglycaemia is a well-recognized feature of diabetic pregnancy and may indeed be the presenting symptom of pregnancy. In our series 40% of women had been seen at the prepregnancy clinic and for those who were not, the majority were seen prior to the 14th week of gestation. Many reported mild hypoglycaemia at routine clinic visits and at some stage in pregnancy almost all women revealed self-monitored blood glucose results lower than the physiological range. This may be expected, since the target set for home blood glucose values is between 4 and 6 mmol/l. Careful history will usually identify if diet, exercise, alcohol or inappropriate insulin dosage or type is the reason for hypoglycaemia (Rayburn et al. 1986).

A change from beef to human or purified porcine insulin prepregnancy may produce a sudden or gradual fall in antibody levels with a concomitant reduction in insulin requirement. This should be anticipated and more frequent blood glucose measurements should be taken during any changeover period. If the changeover occurs after conception it is prudent to carry this out under in-patient conditions to avoid loss of control. Hypoglycaemia occurs commonly in the mid-morning or overnight; mid-morning episodes can be alleviated by having an extra snack in the late morning or by reducing the before-breakfast soluble insulin. The most important factor in the avoidance of hypoglycaemia appears to be a mother's understanding of the interaction between her insulin, food and energy expenditure and her understanding of the duration of action of individual insulins. Most women with diabetes will recognize mild hypoglycaemia and a simple list of foods to relieve such symptoms should be available. Some women, however, do not, and husbands/partners must have instruction on the recognition and management of hypoglycaemia and should be shown how to use glucagon

(Rayburn et al. 1987). A neighbour or relative may need education in the management of hypoglycaemia if the husband is working away from home.

Morning sickness and anorexia are particular problems if associated with diabetes. Often there is an underlying urinary tract infection and this should be identified and treated.

Problems in Monitoring Control

Poor metabolic control can be identified in the absence of symptoms by home blood glucose monitoring profiles (Stubbs et al. 1980) (see Fig. 14.4), glycosylated haemoglobin (Kennedy and Baynes 1984) or other glycosylated protein estimation (Baker et al. 1983). Poor control may also be suspected clinically in the event of development of polyhydramnios from mid-pregnancy. Since the renal threshold for glucose is variable in pregnancy, measurement of urinary glucose concentration is not a satisfactory method of assessment of glycaemia. The method of blood glucose monitoring should be checked in early pregnancy to ensure accuracy and when photoelectric meters are used, they should be calibrated regularly by cross-checking glucose measurement with a hospital laboratory value. The frequency with which it is necessary to carry out home capillary blood glucose testing is flexible, but our patients test a minimum of four times daily. Some patients test six to eight times per day. Such tests are only valuable if a woman is able to perform the procedure reliably and if she has a good understanding of potential problems which can occur and the action necessary if the results are abnormal, even if this is only how to telephone for advice! Women should be advised to check for ketones routinely once a week or on every urine sample if they feel unwell or if blood glucose values are greater than 10 mmol/l. They should be aware of the importance of making contact for medical advice when there is non-fasting ketonuria. An audio glucose meter can allow a person with visual impairment to monitor blood glucose at home. Considerable domestic support is necessary in this situation.

Estimation of glycosylated haemoglobin provides an index of glycaemic control for the few weeks or months prior to sampling, on average reflecting control over the previous 6 to 8 weeks. Prior to and throughout pregnancy it is particularly useful to follow the trend of glycosylated haemoglobin by measuring it at monthly intervals. The local laboratory reference range outwith pregnancy may not be applicable during pregnancy (Venot et al. 1986; Van Dieijen-Visser et al. 1986) and the clinician should not be lulled into a false sense of security by a haemoglobin A_{1C} just above the normal range in the first trimester. Glycosylated albumin estimation may be a more appropriate measurement during pregnancy, in view of the shorter half-life of protein, which may reflect control over the previous 1–2 weeks, but there are few reports of practical experience of this estimation during pregnancy.

Glycosylated protein estimations have some role to play with regard to the prediction of pregnancy outcome. A raised level in the first trimester is associated with an increased incidence of congenital malformation (Miller et al. 1981) and elevated levels in later pregnancy may predict infants large for gestational age, although various other factors contribute to high birthweight (Small et al. 1987). Very rarely abnormal haemoglobins may produce unexpectedly high haemoglobin A_{1C} results and this caused considerable confusion in one of our patients

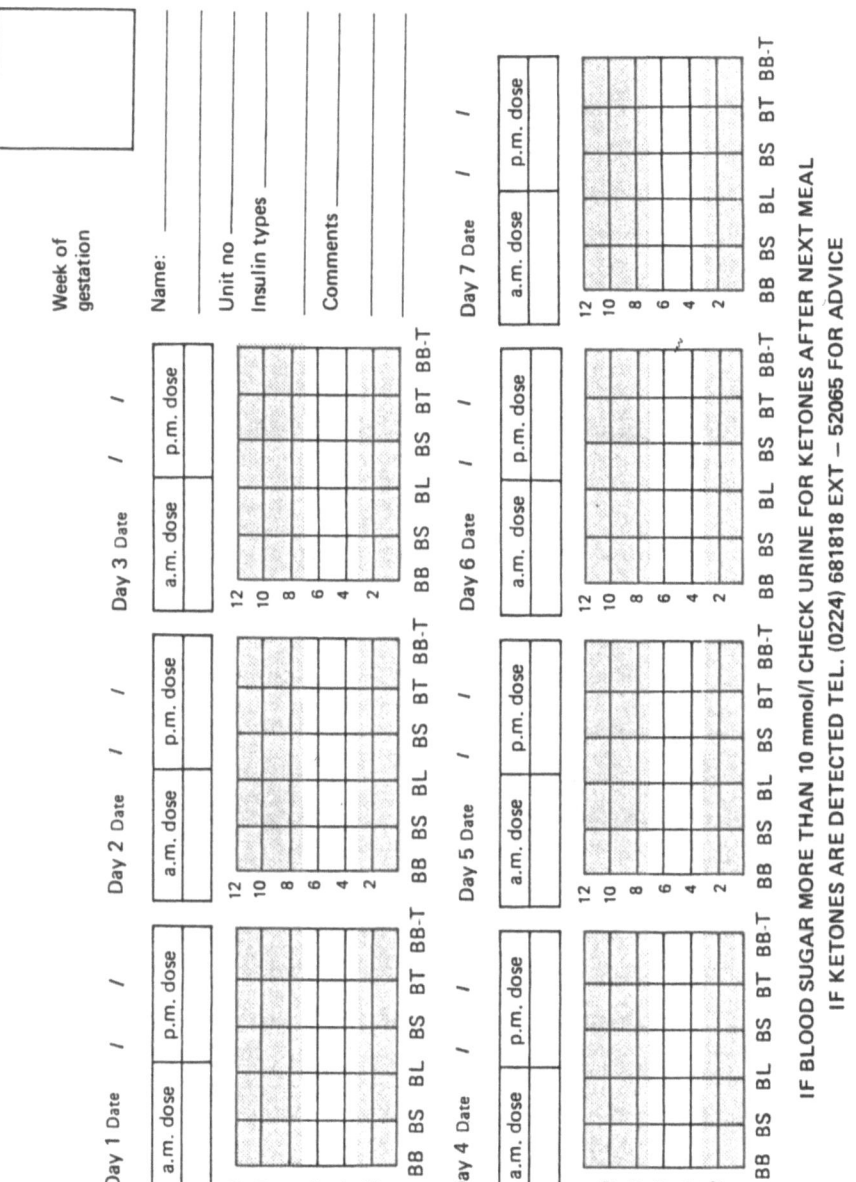

Fig. 14.4. Aberdeen Combined Antenatal/Diabetic Clinic.

managed recently. Glycosylated haemoglobin measured by a colorimetric method had been normal during a previous pregnancy, but haemoglobin A_{1C} measured by an electrophoretic method gave consistently high results, despite normal blood glucose levels.

Other Endocrine Disorders in Diabetic Pregnancy

Thyrotoxicosis and other autoimmune conditions may co-exist with diabetes mellitus and uncontrolled thyrotoxicosis will lead to poor glycaemic control. Recently, we have also managed a case of coincidental primary hyperparathyroidism presenting during pregnancy, and a good result followed second-trimester parathyroidectomy.

Problems Associated with the Complications of Diabetes Mellitus

Cardiovascular Adaptation to Pregnancy and Hypertension

The developing fetus and placenta are not autonomous, but depend on an adequate though not excessive supply of maternal fuels and oxygen. The carefully controlled intrauterine environment depends on flexibility of maternal metabolism and physiology during periods of feeding, fasting and exercise. During pregnancy, cardiac output rises quickly in the first trimester to a level of some 1.5 l/min above the non-pregnant level and this is maintained for the rest of the pregnancy. Arterial blood pressure may be relatively unaffected or there may be a slight reduction in diastolic pressure in mid-pregnancy. The relative constancy of blood pressure, despite the rise in cardiac output, is explained by a fall in peripheral resistance which reflects a tendency to peripheral vasodilation during pregnancy. The autonomic nervous system plays a fundamental role in adaptation of the heart and circulation and it is suggested that cardiovascular adjustment to pregnancy seems to be blunted in diabetic women (Airaksinen et al. 1986).

In addition in women with diabetogenic microvascular disease, the development of significant hypertension during pregnancy is common (Diamond et al. 1985). Clinicians should try to differentiate chronic hypertension from pregnancy-induced hypertension, although both may co-exist. Dr. Diamond and his colleagues found that chronic hypertension was present in older women, most of whom did not have longstanding diabetes. In contrast, pregnancy-induced hypertension was more common in White classes D, F and R (13/30 patients). Chronic hypertension should be diagnosed and treated prior to pregnancy and pregnancy-induced hypertension may be reduced by prepregnancy counselling to optimize metabolic control. Jovanovic has suggested that a blood pressure of 160/90 or lower does not require specific therapy (Jovanovic and Jovanovic 1984). When hypertension becomes more marked, beta adrenoceptor blockers are effective in diabetic pregnancy (Olafson et al. 1986). Thiazide and loop diuretics should be avoided during pregnancy since maternal plasma volume expansion is an important maternal physiological adaptation. The angiotensin-converting enzyme inhibitors, which are effective in the control of hypertension in diabetic subjects, should be avoided during embryogenesis since animal studies have indicated a possible teratogenic effect.

If hypertension develops in pregnancy, glomerular filtration rate (GFR) and effective renal plasma flow (ERPF) decrease to approximately 25% below normal but, since these are 30%–50% above non-pregnant levels, GFR and ERPF may remain above non-pregnant levels. The ability to excrete sodium is usually impaired in the pre-eclamptic patient, although pre-eclampsia can occur in the absence of fluid retention, and when oedema is present plasma volume is usually decreased in comparison to normal pregnancy. Uric acid clearance also decreases and proteinuria is variable. The important factors in the development of proteinuria seem to be the haemodynamic determinants of GFR and the electrostatic properties of the glomerular membrane. Reduced renal plasma flow and loss of the glomerular fixed negative charge on polyanions have been implicated in the pathogenesis of pre-eclampsia. The basement membrane changes associated with diabetes mellitus may explain the increased frequency of pre-eclampsia reported in diabetic pregnancy and, if proteinuria develops, careful in-patient monitoring of maternal blood pressure, proteinuria, renal function and haematology is as necessary as fetal biophysical monitoring is essential.

Diabetic Nephropathy

When diabetic nephropathy is present most authorities would not encourage pregnancy. Although the outlook for that pregnancy may be good if optimal metabolic control is achieved prior to and during pregnancy, long-term maternal health may be disadvantaged, since persistent proteinuria in insulin-dependent diabetes mellitus is associated with a much higher relative risk of renal failure and/or cardiovascular disease than when proteinuria is absent. Although effective means of managing renal failure by chronic ambulatory peritoneal dialysis, haemodialysis and renal transplant therapy may be available, the implications of such therapeutic techniques for a mother and a young family need to be anticipated. Successful pregnancy has been reported following renal transplantation, but advanced diabetic vascular disease puts such pregnancies at significant risk. Ogburn et al. (1986) reviewed nine cases of pregnancy complicated by diabetes and prior renal transplantation and noted maternal and fetal death in a patient with foot and leg ulcers, and pregnancy-induced hypertension in six women.

Series of pregnant women with diabetic nephropathy have been reported by Kitzmiller et al. (1981), Hare and White (1977), Grenfell et al. (1986), Nesler et al. (1985) and Dicker et al. (1986). The pregnancy experience reported extends over many years and includes data collected prior to the advent of modern methods of metabolic or fetal monitoring. Nevertheless, such clinical series give very useful descriptive clinical information on this relatively uncommon problem for many clinicians. From review of these reports it appears that in women with diabetic nephropathy, impaired creatinine clearance does not deteriorate during or after pregnancy any more than would have been predicted outwith pregnancy. Proteinuria increases from the first to the third trimester and one of the factors which appears to predict poor perinatal outcome in proteinuria greater than 3 g/24 h in the first trimester or 10 g/24 h in the third trimester. Proteinuria and creatinine clearance return to prepregnancy levels in the postnatal period. The striking increase in urinary albumin in the presence of diabetic nephropathy in pregnancy presumably relates to the additional physiological adaptations of glomerular permeability during pregnancy. In most series maternal hypertension was associated with proteinuria and correlated negatively with infant birthweight. Hypertension was treated by bedrest, methyldopa, beta-blockers and hydralazine. Supine posture reduced cardiac output and renal plasma flow and resting in the left lateral position to raise renal perfusion, and thereby GFR, was recommended.

With regard to the clinical management of women with nephropathy, if the marked physiological expansion of the intravascular compartment and the presence of underlying impairment (or diminution) of cardiac function leads to congestive cardiac failure, diuretic therapy is essential but otherwise diuretic therapy is to be avoided. In the presence of diabetic nephropathy regular clinical and ultrasonic assessment is essential to monitor fetal growth, which is likely to be retarded. Careful monitoring of blood pressure, weight gain, renal and retinal status is essential and during the third trimester most patients with significant nephropathy are managed as in-patients with regular biophysical *fetal* assessments being performed.

Diabetic Retinopathy

In women with long-standing diabetes it is important to recognize that retinopathy can deteriorate during pregnancy, despite optimal glycaemic control. Following careful studies, Serup (1986) emphasized that retinopathy which progresses during pregnancy often regresses in the puerperium and regular review by an experienced ophthalmologist is necessary. The pathophysiology of the progression of retinopathy during pregnancy and its resolution postpartum is not clear and regular detailed fundoscopy throughout pregnancy is very important. This topic is covered in detail in Chap. 17.

Ischaemic Heart Disease

Ischaemic heart disease is an absolute contraindication to pregnancy (Reece et al. 1986) and occasionally women with longstanding diabetes or middle-aged women with IDDM will present with established ischaemic heart disease. A successful pregnancy has been reported following coronary artery bypass grafting in a diabetic woman (Reece et al. 1986).

Delivery

The timing of delivery in a diabetic woman depends on the progress made during pregnancy but in an uncomplicated situation many women deliver at term.

Diabetes mellitus alone is not an indication for Caesarean section and the mode of delivery would be dictated by obstetric factors if normal blood glucose levels have been achieved. During delivery normal blood glucose levels can be maintained by a continuous intravenous infusion of insulin and dextrose (Jovanovic and Pederson 1983). In our patients 10% dextrose at a rate of 100 ml/h with 1 g of potassium chloride added to each 500 ml is infused by a graduated pump. Biosynthetic human soluble insulin (50 u in 50 ml saline) is infused by adjustable syringe pump and the rate of insulin infusion is altered to maintain plasma glucose between 4 and 7 mmol/l.

Problems in the Future

The last 40 years have seen a continual rise in the numbers of pregnant diabetic women and the epidemiological evidence suggests that this increase will continue. Therapeutic changes for people with diabetes outwith pregnancy, e.g. attempts to modify the immune system with cyclosporin, have implications for the management of diabetic pregnancy, as have the increasing use of pancreatic and renal transplantation (Castro et al. 1986; Pickrell et al. 1988). Although the perinatal mortality in diabetic pregnancy has continued to fall, there is no room for complacency, either on the part of those who are caring for women with diabetes or diabetic women themselves. The partnership of the patient and the various members of her care team demands continued efforts to ensure that optimal results are achieved.

Acknowledgement. Grateful acknowledgement is made to Mrs. Sandra Anderson who typed the manuscript.

References

Airaksinen KEJ, Ikaheimo MJ, Salmela PI, Kirkinen P, Linnaluoto MK, Takkunen JT (1986) Impaired cardiac adjustment to pregnancy in type I diabetes. Diabetes Care 9:376–383

Baker JR, O'Connor JP, Metcalf BA, Lawson MR, Johnston RN (1983) Clinical usefulness of estimation of serum fructosamine concentration as a screening test for diabetes mellitus. Br Med J 287:863–867

Brumfield CG, Huddlestone JF (1984) The management of diabetic ketoacidosis in pregnancy. Clin Obstet Gynaecol 27:50–59

Burrow GN, Hazlett BE, Phillips MJ (1982) A case of diabetes mellitus. N Engl J Med 306:340–343

Castro LA, Baltzer U, Hillebrand G et al. (1986) Pregnancy in juvenile diabetes mellitus under cyclosporin treatment after combined kidney and pancreas transplantation. Transplant Proc 18:1780–1781

Dahlquist G, Rudberg S (1987) The prevalence of microalbuminauria in diabetic children and adolescents and its relation to puberty. Acta Paediatr Scand 76:795–800

Diabetes Epidemiology Research International (1987) Preventing insulin dependent diabetes mellitus: the environmental challenge. Br Med J 295:479–481

Diamond MP, Shadae, M, Hester RA, Vaughan WK, Kautinar B (1985) Complication of insulin dependent diabetic pregnancies by pre-eclampsia and/or chronic hypertension: analysis of outcome. Am J Perinat 2:263–267

Diamond MP, Salzer SL, Vaughan WK et al (1987) Reassessment of White's classification and Pederson's prognostically bad signs of pregnancy in insulin dependent diabetic pregnancies. Am J Obstet Gynecol 156:599–604

Dicker D, Feldberg D, Feleck D, Peleck D, Carpern JA (1986) Pregnancy complicated by diabetic nephropathy. J Perinat Med 14:299–305

Drury MI (1986) Management of the pregnant diabetic patients – are the pundits right? Diabetologia 29:10–12

Duncan JM (1883) On puerperal diabetes. Trans Obstet Soc Lond 1882. 24:256

Grenfell A, Brudenell JM, Doddrige MC, Watkins PJ (1986) Pregnancy in diabetic women who have proteinuria. Q J Med 59(288):379–386

Hare JW, White P (1977) Pregnancy and diabetes complicated by vascular disease. Diabetes 26:953–955

Hare JW, White P (1980) Gestational diabetes and White classification. Diabetes Care 3:294

Jovanovic R, Jovanovic L (1984) Obstetric management when normal glycaemia is maintained in diabetic pregnant women with vascular compromise. Am J Obstet Gynecol 149:617–623

Jovanovic L, Peterson CM (1983) Insulin and glucose requirements during the first stage of labour in insulin dependent diabetic women. Am J Med 75:607–612

Kennedy L, Baynes JW (1984) Non enzymatic glycosylation and the chronic complications of diabetes: an over-view. Diabetologia 26:93–98

Kitzmiller JL, Brown ER, Phillipe M et al. (1981) Diabetic nephropathy and perinatal outcome. Am J Obstet Gynecol 147:741–751

Martin FTR, Heath P, Maurice KR (1987) Pregnancy in women with diabetes mellitus. Fourteen years experience. Med J Aust 146:187–190

Miller E, Hare JW, Cloherty JP et al. (1981) Elevated maternal haemoglobin A1C in early pregnancy and major congenital anomalies in infants of diabetic mothers. N Engl J Med 304:1331–1334

Mølsted-Pedersen L, Kuhl C (1986) Obstetrical management in pregnancy. The Copenhagen experience. Diabetologia 29:13–16

Murphy J, Peters J, Morris P, Hayes TM, Pearson JF (1984) Conservative management of pregnancy in diabetes. Br Med J 288:1203–1206

Mylvaganam R, Stowers JM, Steel JM, et al. (1983) Insulin immunogenicity in pregnancy; maternal and fetal studies. Diabetologia 24:19–25

National Diabetes Data Group (1979) Classification and diagnosis of diabetes and other categories of glucose intolerance. Diabetes 28:1039–1057

Nesler CL, Sinclair SH, Schwartz SS (1985) Diabetic nephropathy in pregnancy. Clin Obstet Gynaecol 28:528–535

Ogburn PL, Kitzmiller JL, Hare JE et al. (1986) Pregnancy following renal transplantation in class T diabetes mellitus. J Am Med Assoc 255:911–915

Olafson P, Montan, S, Sartor G, Sjoberg N (1986) Effects of beta adreno receptor blockade in the treatment of hypertension during pregnancy in diabetic women. Acta Med Scand 220:321–328

Pedersen J, Mølsted-Pedersen L (1965) Prognosis of the outcome of pregnancies in diabetics. Acta Endocrinol (Copenh) 50:70–78

Pickrell MD, Sawers R, Michael J (1988) Pregnancy after renal transplantation: severe intra-uterine growth retardation during treatment with Cyclosporin A. Br Med J 296:825

Pistaiato HI, Haretikinen Sorri KP (1987) Maternal residual beta cell function and the outcome of diabetic pregnancy. Perinat Med 15:83–89

Rayburn W, Piehl E, Jatchen S (1986) Severe hypoglycaemia in pregnancy – its frequency and predisposing factors in diabetic women. Int J Gynaecol Obstet 24:263–268

Rayburn W, Piehl E, Stanfield J, Compton A (1987) Reversing severe hypoglycaemia during pregnancy with glucagon therapy. Am J Perinatol 4:259–261

Reece EA, Egan JFX, Coustan PR et al. (1986) Coronary artery disease in diabetic pregnancy. Am J Obstet Gynecol 154:150–151

Rennie J, Fraser T (1906/7) The islets of Langerhans in relation to diabetes. Biochem J 2:7–19

Rewers M, Laporte RA, Walczek M, Dmochowski IK, Bojaczynska E (1987) An apparent 'epidemic' of youth onset insulin dependent diabetes mellitus in mid western Poland. Diabetes 36:106–113

Robertson G, Wheatley T, Robinson RE (1986) Ketoacidosis in pregnancy: an unusual presentation of diabetes mellitus. Case reports. Br J Obstet Gynaecol 93:1088–1090

Ryan EA, O'Sullivan MJ, Skyler JS (1985) Insulin action during pregnancy: studies with the euglycaemic clamp technique. Diabetes 34:380–389

Serup L (1986) Influence of pregnancy on diabetic retinopathy. Acta Endocrinol [Suppl] (Copenh) 277:122–124

Small M, Cameron A, Lunan CB, McCuish AC (1987) Macrosomia in pregnancy complicated by insulin dependent mellitus. Diabetes Care 10:594–599

Stewart-Brown S, Haslum M, Butler N (1983) Evidence for increasing prevalence of diabetes mellitus in childhood. Br Med J 286:1855–1857

Stubbs SM, Brudenell JM, Pyke DA, Watkins PJ, Stubbs WA, Alberti KGMM (1980) Management of the pregnant diabetic: home or hospital with or without glucose meters. Lancet I:1122–1124

Van Dieijen-Visser MP, Salemans T, Van Wersceh JWJ, Schellekens LA, Brombacher PJ (1986) Glycosylated serum proteins and glycosylated haemoglobin in normal pregnancy. Ann Clin Biochem 23:661–666

Venot J, Beauchamp MO, Ardilouze JL et al. (1986) A longitudinal study of haemoglobin A1C levels during normal pregnancy. Diabete Metab 12:268–271

15. Intensified Insulin Treatment in Diabetic Pregnancy

C. Kühl and B. Møller-Jensen

Introduction

Since dedicated centres for the control and treatment of pregnant diabetic women were established in the late 1940s, the perinatal mortality rate for infants of diabetic mothers (IDMs) has decreased remarkably (Table 15.1) and is now approaching that seen in infants of non-diabetic mothers (Pedersen 1977; Gabbe 1981). The frequency of neonatal morbidity in IDMs has also declined significantly in the same period (Mølsted-Pedersen and Kühl 1986a). The explanation for these favourable results is probably multifactorial but is most likely related to a) the coordinated centralized management by a diabetologist, an obstetrician and a neonatologist, (b) optimization of the maternal metabolic control during pregnancy and (c) early detection and treatment of obstetric, fetal and neonatal complications (Mølsted-Pedersen and Kühl 1986b).

Table 15.1. Perinatal mortality among 2117 infants of diabetic mothers in seven periods in the Copenhagen series

Period	Total no. of infants	Perinatal mortality (%)
1946–1955	285	22.1
1956–1965	561	18.5
1966–1969	255	12.9
1970–1972	231	7.4
1973–1975	259	4.6
1976–1978	294	4.4
1979–1980	232	2.6

The importance of good metabolic control during diabetic pregnancy has been emphasized for many years. Karlsson and Kjellmer (1972) reported a positive correlation between the perinatal mortality rate and the mean maternal blood glucose level during the last 1–2 months of pregnancy; the perinatal mortality rate in IDMs decreased from about 24% in the group with a mean blood glucose above 150 mg/100 ml (8.3 mmol/l) to about 15% in the intermediary group and about 4% in the group with a mean blood glucose below 100 mg/100 ml (5.6 mmol/l). In a review of major clinical studies, Jovanovic and Peterson (1982) found a similar clear correlation between mean maternal blood glucose levels and perinatal mortality.

Improved metabolic control during diabetic pregnancy has also led to a decrease in neonatal morbidity as demonstrated recently by Landon et al. (1987) who examined 75 pregnant diabetic women belonging to White's classes B–D (White 1949). The patients measured at least four daily blood glucose values for a minimum of 16 weeks. The patients were subsequently divided into two groups, one with a mean capillary blood glucose equal to or less than 110 mg/100 ml (6.1 mmol/l), the other with a mean value greater than 110 mg/100 ml. IDMs belonging to the former group, when compared to infants of mothers in the other group, spent significantly fewer days in the neonatal intensive care unit and had a significantly lower frequency of neonatal hypoglycaemia and respiratory distress syndrome. The mean birthweight was similar in the two groups but significantly more infants were large for gestational age in the group born to mothers who had a mean level above 110 mg/100 ml.

Jovanovic et al. (1981) obtained impressive results in a group of 52 diabetic women (White's classes B–F) on intensified insulin therapy combined with seven daily home blood glucose measurements and careful dietary instructions. Clinical follow-up was initiated before the 12th week of gestation and maintained throughout pregnancy. Apart from one case of asymptomatic hypoglycaemia no neonatal morbidity was seen. The results were even better than in a control group of non-diabetic but otherwise comparable pregnant women.

Congenital Malformations

Congenital malformations are seen more often in IDMs than in infants of non-diabetic mothers (Pedersen 1977; Mills 1982). The malformations observed in IDMs tend to be multiple, more severe and more often lethal than those seen in the normal population (Kucera 1971). Unfortunately, a reduction in the frequency of congenital malformations equal to that seen for the perinatal mortality and the neonatal morbidity rates has not been observed in IDMs (Pedersen 1978). In the Copenhagen series, in the two periods 1966–1972 and 1973–1977, the rates of severe congenital anomalies in IDMs of mothers belonging to White's classes B–F were 4.2%–6.7% and 3.1%–7.6%, respectively (Table 15.2). Congenital malformations are now the leading cause of perinatal death in IDMs in most centres.

Human organogenesis is completed within the first 7 weeks of gestation (Mills et al. 1979) and it has been suggested that major congenital malformations are induced during this early period of pregnancy. Although the aetiology of the malformations in IDMs is still not completely known, evidence does exist that tight metabolic control from the time of conception and throughout early pregnancy might lead to a decline in the frequency of congenital anomalies in

Table 15.2. Rate of severe congenital malformations (CM) in infants of diabetic mothers in two periods in the Copenhagen series

White classes	1966–1972		1973–1977	
	Total no. of infants	Infants with severe CM(%)	Total no. of infants	Infants with severe CM(%)
B+C	192	4.2	130	3.1
D+F	180	6.7	145	7.6

IDM. In view of this and in retrospect, it is probably not surprising that the malformation rate has remained high since, until very recently, optimized metabolic control was not initiated prior to but during pregnancy.

A national survey carried out in the UK in 1979–1980 showed an unexpectedly high over-all incidence of 7.1% congenital malformations in IDMs (Lowy et al. 1986). In 40% of the diabetic mothers no blood glucose values were recorded during the first trimester of pregnancy, suggesting that no or inadequate attention was paid to the diabetes in the early pregnancy. In this group of women, the malformation rate of the infants was twice as high as that found in infants born to diabetic mothers who had at least one reported blood glucose value during the first trimester.

Measurement of HbA_{1c} in early pregnancy is a method of retrospective assessment of the tightness of glycaemic control during the important period of embryogenesis. HbA_{1c} was measured before the 14th week of pregnancy in 116 insulin-dependent diabetic women, 15 of whom had given birth to infants with major congenital anomalies (Miller et al. 1981). The mean maternal HbA_{1c} value was significantly lower in the group of women who delivered babies without malformations than in the group of women who delivered babies with malformations (8.4%±1.6% (SD) and 9.5%±1.0%, respectively). Similar results were found by Ylinen et al. (1984) who examined HbA_{1c} before the end of the 15th week of pregnancy in 142 insulin-dependent diabetic women. In pregnancies resulting in malformed children, the mean initial HbA_{1c} was significantly higher than in pregnancies without malformations (9.5%±1.8% vs 8.0%±1.4%). In contrast to Miller et al. (1981), Ylinen et al. (1984) also found a positive correlation between the rate of malformations and the mean initial HbA_{1c} value. Congenital malformations occurred in six out of 17 (35.5%) pregnancies with an HbA_{1c} value equal to or greater than 10%, in eight out of 62 (12.9%) pregnancies with HbA_{1c} values between 8.0% and 9.9% and in only three out of 63 (4.8%) pregnancies with HbA_{1c} below 8.0%.

Numerous in vivo and in vitro animal experiments have been performed in order to elucidate the aetiology of congenital malformations in IDMs. In the pregnant rat model, an increased frequency of skeletal malformations could be produced by a maternal diabetic state induced by streptozotocin before the rats conceived (Eriksson et al. 1982). The malformations could be prevented by insulin treatment of the pregnant rat (Eriksson et al. 1982), and experiments with interrupted insulin treatment of the pregnant diabetic rats confined the teratogenic period to gestational days 2–7, corresponding to gestational weeks 2–4 in human pregnancy (Eriksson et al. 1983).

In vitro investigations have mainly been performed using the whole embryo culture system where a teratogenic effect on mouse embryos of human diabetic serum (Sadler 1980a) and of high glucose levels in otherwise normal human serum (Sadler 1980b) has been shown. Also in the whole mouse embryo culture system, 3-OH-butyrate, which is another potentially teratogenic factor in diabetic pregnancy, has been shown to induce dose-related rates of malformations (Horton and Sadler 1983). A synergistic action of glucose and 3-OH-butyrate has also been demonstrated (Lewis et al. 1983). A detailed review of animal models and possible teratogenic mechanisms of diabetes and diabetes-like conditions has recently been published by Eriksson (1984).

Further strong evidence in support of the hypothesis that non-optimal metabolic control around the time of conception and in the very early pregnancy may predispose to congenital malformations in IDMs came from a large study conducted in East Germany (Fuhrmann et al. 1983). In a total of 420 insulin-dependent diabetic pregnancies, 23 (5.5%) infants with congenital malformations were delivered. Intensive insulin treatment was started before conception in 128 of the women and only one (0.8%) IDM with a congenital malformation was seen in this group. The remaining 292 women, all of whom began intensive metabolic control only after the 8th week of gestation, delivered 22 (7.5%) malformed babies. This difference is highly significant.

The East German results have been corroborated by a recent study of 75 pregnant insulin-dependent diabetic women (Goldman et al. 1986). Forty-four of these women had attended a preconception clinic where intensified insulin therapy had been instituted. HbA_{1c} in the first trimester was significantly lower in this group than in a control group who registered during pregnancy (7.4%±0.3% vs 10.4%±0.5%). In the former group no congenital malformations were found whereas in the "non-attenders", three (9.6%) infants were malformed.

The importance of good diabetic control starting in the preconception period and continuing throughout the gestation has thus clearly been demonstrated. Conventional insulin therapy, i.e. one or two daily insulin injections, seldom leads to a satisfactory degree of metabolic compensation. In most cases an intensive treatment regimen, i.e. multiple daily insulin injections or continuous subcutaneous insulin infusion (CSII), is needed. A prerequisite for the success of intensified insulin treatment is measurement of blood glucose values at home, a method that has been available since the late 1970s.

When planning to optimize the metabolic control in diabetic women who plan to become pregnant or already are pregnant, one should consider how quickly this optimization should be brought about. Laatikainen et al. (1987) followed 40 pregnant diabetics from before the 12th week of gestation. The patients were randomized to either CSII treatment or conventional insulin therapy (CT, 1–4 daily insulin injections). Nine of the 22 patients allocated to the CSII group refused CSII treatment and were hence followed as the CT group. The mean of home- and hospital-measured blood glucose values did not differ between the groups at any time during pregnancy. Mean HbA_{1c} was also similar in both groups. Ophthalmological examinations were performed on all patients at entry, during the first and the third trimesters and 3–6 months after pregnancy. The difference in the number of patients with progressing retinopathy in the two groups was not significant. However, two patients in the CSII group developed acute ischaemic retinal lesions which progressed to proliferative retinopathy despite laser treatment. In these two patients, the rate of decrease in HbA_{1c} was among the fastest and most pronounced of the patients studied. Rapid normalization of blood glucose has also been shown to lead to initial deterioration of retinopathy in non-pregnant insulin-dependent diabetic patients (Dahl-Jørgensen et al. 1985). These results favour a quite gradual rather than a rapid improvement of the metabolic control which therefore most conveniently should be implemented in the prepregnancy period.

At the Copenhagen Centre for Pregnant Diabetics, we have studied the influence of optimized pre- and postconceptional metabolic control by means of CSII on the course and outcome of diabetic pregnancy. Preliminary results of the study have been published elsewhere (Kühl et al. 1984; Møller-Jensen et al. 1985).

Copenhagen Study of Continuous Subcutaneous Insulin Infusion (CSII) Treatment in Diabetic Pregnancy

In the period May 1982–June 1985 all insulin-dependent diabetic women attending Hvidöre Hospital (a specialized clinic for diabetes care near Copenhagen) and planning pregnancy were offered treatment by means of CSII. Nineteen women, White's classes B–F, have subsequently conceived and completed pregnancies during CSII treatment. Seven patients who refused CSII treatment were enrolled in the control group together with 17 diabetic women who entered the study before the 14th week of pregnancy. These women also belonged to White's classes B–F. Further data on the patients appear in Table 15.3.

Table 15.3. Copenhagen study of continuous subcutaneous insulin infusion (CSII) treatment in diabetic pregnancy: patient characteristics

	Age (years)	Weight (kg)	Duration of insulin treatment (years)	White class
CSII (19)	27.3 (27–37)	64.3 (54–78)	10.5 (1–23)	B–F
CT (24)	25.8 (19–37)	61.5 (53–79)	10.3 (3–23)	B–F

Values in parentheses are ranges.

Study Design

Continuous subcutaneous insulin infusion (CSII) treatment (Auto-Syringe AS–6C pumps, Auto-Syringe Inc., Hooksette, New Hampshire; insulin Actrapid HM, Hovo, Denmark) was initiated during a short hospitalization at least 2 months before the conception. The patients were seen after discharge in the outpatient clinic every 2–4 weeks. Seven-point home blood glucose profiles were obtained by means of a reflectance meter at least twice weekly and the insulin dose was adjusted accordingly.

The control group was treated by conventional insulin injections. However, ethical considerations, based on evidence of a deleterious effect of poor metabolic control on the outcome of pregnancy, prompted us to institute at least three daily insulin injections in eight of the control patients in the first trimester and in two additional patients in the second trimester. Four patients refused to perform home blood glucose monitoring. In the remaining 20 patients, twice-weekly blood glucose profiles formed the basis for adjustments in insulin dose.

HbA_{1c}, plasma triglycerides and 3-OH-butyrate were measured monthly in both groups and fasting plasma free insulin concentrations were measured once in each trimester.

Regarding the general principles for control during pregnancy and induction of labour, the patients followed the usual principles of the Copenhagen Centre (Pedersen 1977).

Results

HbA_{1c} decreased significantly from early to late pregnancy in both groups (Table 15.4), but a mean value within normal limits was only seen in the CT group in late prepregnancy. There were no significant differences between the mean HbA_{1c} values in the two groups at any time during pregnancy.

Fasting plasma free insulin concentrations (Table 15.5) were significantly higher in the CSII group than in the CT group throughout pregnancy.

Table 15.4. Copenhagen study of continuous subcutaneous insulin infusion (CSII) treatment in diabetic pregnancy: maternal HbA_{1c} (%) during diabetic pregnancy

	Overall	Early	Late	P (early vs late)
CSII (19)	6.6±0.1	7.1±0.3	6.2±0.2	<0.05
CT (24)	6.7±0.1	7.3±0.4	6.1±0.2	<0.05
P	NS	NS	NS	

Normal range: 4.1%–6.1% (non-pregnant). Results are expressed as mean±SEM. NS, not significant.

Table 15.5. Copenhagen study of continuous subcutaneous insulin infusion (CSII) treatment in diabetic pregnancy: fasting plasma free insulin (nmol/l)

Trimester	1	2	3
CSII (19)	0.17±0.04	0.11±0.02	0.16±0.02
CT (24)	0.07±0.01	0.07±0.01	0.09±0.01
P	<0.05	<0.01	<0.01

Results are expressed as mean±SEM.

Table 15.6. Copenhagen study of continuous subcutaneous insulin infusion (CSII) treatment in diabetic pregnancy: fasting plasma 3-OH-butyrate (mmol/l)

Week of pregnancy	0–12	13–24	25–36	37+
CSII (19)	0.20±0.02	0.14±0.01	0.19±0.03	0.12±0.03
CT (24)	0.39±0.06	0.30±0.07	0.28±0.06	0.18±0.04
P	<0.005	<0.05	NS	NS

Results are expressed as mean±SEM. NS, not significant.

Table 15.7. Copenhagen study of continuous subcutaneous insulin infusion (CSII) treatment in diabetic pregnancy: fasting plasma tryglycerides (mmol/l)

Week of pregnancy	0–12	13–24	25–36	37+
CSII (19)	0.71±0.05	1.12±0.07	2.12±0.15	2.18±0.19
CT (24)	0.91±0.10	1.31±0.13	2.36±0.18	3.00±0.34
P	NS	NS	NS	NS

Results are expressed as mean±SEM. NS, not significant.

Fasting plasma 3-OH-butyrate concentrations (Table 15.6) were significantly lower in the CSII group than in the CT group in the first and the second trimesters. A trend towards lower values was also seen in the third trimester in the CSII group but this difference did not reach statistical significance.

Fasting plasma trigylceride concentrations tended to be lower in the CSII group than in the CT group throughout pregnancy (Table 15.7) but the differences were not significant.

The mean pregnancy length was 257 d in the CSII group and 260 d in the CT group (NS). Nineteen living infants (one pair of twins) in the CSII group had a mean birthweight of 3229±205 g which was similar to the mean birthweight of 3388±160 g in the 24 infants in the CT group. In the CSII group, one late intrauterine death due to cardiac malformations occurred in a White class C woman who became pregnant before good metabolic control was obtained (Møller-Jensen et al. 1985). One case of severe intrauterine growth retardation and a case of mild hypospadia which did not require treatment were also seen in the CSII group. The mothers belonged to White's classes D and F, respectively. No malformations were seen in the CT group. One infant in the CSII group and three infants in the CT group were delivered preterm because of pre-eclamptic toxaemia. No severe neonatal morbidity was observed in either group.

Apart from one case of ketoacidosis due to patient non-compliance in the preconceptional period no major therapy-related complications were encountered during CSII treatment. All but three patients preferred to continue with this treatment after delivery.

Conclusions

CSII treatment has been shown to lead to near-normoglycaemia in non-pregnant (Dahl-Jørgensen et al. 1985) and pregnant (Hertz et al. 1984) insulin-dependent diabetic patients. In spite of the patients being highly motivated, this goal was not reached in all CSII treated women in our study, as reflected in the mean HbA_{1c} values during pregnancy. The failure to obtain normoglycaemia might be due to our unselected patient material. As judged by HbA_{1c}, a surprisingly similar degree of good metabolic control was seen in the CSII and CT groups. However, it should be remembered that 10 patients in the CT group were on thrice-daily insulin injections, the indication for which was unsatisfactory metabolic control during treatment with twice-daily injections. When evaluating the other metabolic parameters, the higher fasting plasma free insulin concentrations found during pregnancy in the CSII group as compared to the CT group might reflect a better insulinization during the early morning hours and the corresponding lower fasting plasma 3-OH-butyrate concentrations observed in the CSII group during the first two trimesters might seem favourable in view of in vitro animal studies showing a teratogenic effect of 3-OH-butyrate (Horton and Sadler 1983). Therefore it may well be that CSII treatment does offer a true advantage over intensified conventional insulin therapy in the treatment of diabetic women who either plan to become pregnant or already are pregnant.

Discussion

Our results regarding comparison of CSII treatment and intensified conventional treatment of pregnant diabetic women are in accordance with the results published by other investigators. Coustan et al. (1986) examined 22 pregnant insulin-dependent women who were randomized to either CSII treatment or intensive conventional insulin therapy using two to four daily injections. All patients measured blood glucose at home six to seven times daily and the target blood glucose level was 50–120 mg/100 ml (2.8–6.7 mmol/l). In contrast to our results, all patients had glycosylated haemoglobin levels within the normal range after 8 weeks of treatment and only three patients had blood glucose levels outside the target range. However, no differences were found between the groups regarding mean home-monitored blood glucose values. Inpatient evaluations with hourly blood glucose measurements were done for each patient and the mean amplitude of glycaemic excursions was calculated. No difference was found between the groups at any time of measurement. The outcome of pregnancy was favourable in all patients. The study concluded that with similar attention paid, the method of insulin administration is not critical for the achievement of tight metabolic control.

In another study (Carta et al. 1986), CSII treatment (eight patients) was compared to intensified conventional treatment (four daily injections of soluble insulin; seven patients) in pregnant insulin-dependent diabetics entering the study before the 11th week of pregnancy. No significant differences were found between the groups regarding mean blood glucose or HbA_{1c} during pregnancy. Non-fatal cardiac malformations were found in two infants, one in each group. In the CSII case, maternal normoglycaemia had been obtained before conception and continued throughout pregnancy. The authors concluded that although CSII treatment seemed safe and effective it could not be considered superior to intensified conventional treatment of pregnant diabetic women.

CSII treatment is thus feasible and may lead to an excellent degree of metabolic control during diabetic pregnancy. However, if the same care is offered to the patients, a similar degree of optimal diabetes control can be obtained with multiple injection regimens. It is normally rather difficult to persuade the patients to take four or more injections a day if they have to use conventional syringes, but with the recently introduced insulin pens, multiple injections have become much more convenient (Berger et al. 1985). CSII treatment is expensive and resource consuming and many patients find it inconvenient to wear a quite bulky device 24 h/d (Saurbrey et al. 1988). In view of this, multiple injection therapy using the pen system might be preferred by many pregnant diabetic women.

While optimized metabolic control before and during diabetic pregnancy certainly has improved the prognosis of these pregnancies, another issue of concern is now the possible deleterious effects of hypoglycaemia. An increased frequency of hypoglycaemic reactions might be expected when normoglycaemia is aimed at in diabetic patients. An inverse relation between the median blood glucose concentration and the frequency of biochemical hypoglycaemia (capillary blood glucose concentration below 3 mmol/l) has thus been demonstrated (Thorsteinsson et al. 1986). Until recently no harmful effects of hypoglycaemia on the outcome of diabetic pregnancy had been reported (Pedersen 1977) but recent information probably necessitates re-evaluation of this issue.

Ellington (1987) studied 9.5-day-old rat embryos which were either cultured for 48 h in a control medium or in media with low or very low glucose concentrations. At the end of the culture period the medium glucose concentrations were considerably lower than the starting concentrations. After the 48-h culture period, embryos from glucose-depleted media had significantly smaller crown–rump lengths, a lower total protein content and fewer somites than embryos cultured in the control (i.e. "normoglycaemia") media. Furthermore, most of the embryos cultured at the low glucose concentrations had severe dysmorphic lesions especially involving the head and branchial arches. The deleterious effects of exposure to low glucose concentrations on embryonic development appeared not to be reversible since embryos cultured for 24 h in the low glucose media followed by 24 h in the control medium developed just as poorly as those exposed to a glucose-deficient medium for the entire 48 h.

Deleterious effects of "hypoglycaemia" have also been demonstrated in the mouse embryo. Sadler and Hunter (1987) showed an inverse relationship between the glucose concentration of the culture medium and the malformation rate in mouse embryos. The culture media were prepared from normoglycaemic and hypoglycaemic rat sera. When growth in media prepared from hypoglycaemic serum supplemented with glucose to make concentrations equal to normoglycaemic serum, the embryos had a normal development. This indicates that possible counter-regulatory factors in the serum did not produce the malformations and suggests that it was the glucose deficiency which caused the teratogenic insults.

General Conclusion

Optimization of metabolic control is essential during diabetic pregnancy. The optimization should be started in the preconception period for three reasons: (a) there is increasing evidence that (near-) normalization of blood glucose in the very first weeks of pregnancy leads to a reduction in the frequency of malformations in IDMs; (b) patient education and cooperation are prerequisites for maintenance of optimal metabolic control. Often a deterioration of the diabetes regulation is seen in the initial "learning" phase. When intensified insulin regimens are started in the preconception period, conception can be delayed until the patient has become an "expert"; and (c) in the preconception period a sufficient amount of time can be spent on the improvement of the metabolic control in order to minimize the risk of a rapid progression of diabetic retinopathy (if present).

There is no universal agreement as to how strictly a diabetic woman who is pregnant or wants to become pregnant should be controlled. Normoglycaemia is certainly not a realistic goal in all patients. It may simply not be achievable in some patients, and in other patients it is not to be recommended due to lack of awareness of hypoglycaemia. As documented in the literature, the prognosis for the diabetic pregnancy is good even if blood glucose is not completely normalized. In our opinion, the target blood glucose level should be somewhat individualized meaning that one should aim at the best possible metabolic control for each patient. When setting this target it must be taken into consideration what the risk of repeated hypoglycaemic attacks is likely to be, and also whether the blood glucose level strived for might adversely influence the patient's social life.

References

Berger AS, Saurbrey N, Kühl C, Villumsen J (1985) Clinical experience with a device that will simplify insulin injections. Diabetes Care 8:73–76

Carta Q, Meriggi E, Trossarelli GF et al. (1986) Continuous subcutaneous insulin infusion versus intensive conventional insulin therapy in type 1 and type 2 diabetic pregnancy. Diabete Metab 12:121–129

Coustan DR, Albert Reece E, Sherwin RS (1986) A randomized clinical trial of the insulin pump vs intensive conventional therapy in diabetic pregnancies. J Am Med Assoc 255:631–636

Dahl-Jørgensen K, Brinchmann-Hansen O, Hanssen KF, Sandvik L, Aagenaes Ø, Aker Diabetes Group (1985) Rapid tightening of blood glucose control leads to transient deterioration of retinopathy in insulin-dependent diabetes mellitus: the Oslo study. Br Med J 290:811–815

Ellington SKL (1987) Development of rat embryos cultured in glucose-deficient media. Diabetes 36:1372–1378

Eriksson UJ (1984) Congenital malformations in diabetic animal models – a review. Diabetes Res 1:57–66

Eriksson UJ, Dahlström E, Larsson KS, Hellerström C (1982) Increased incidence of congenital malformations in the offspring of diabetic rats and their prevention by maternal insulin therapy. Diabetes 30:1–6

Eriksson UJ, Dahlström E, Hellerström C (1983) Diabetes in pregnancy; skeletal malformations in the offspring of diabetic rats after intermittent withdrawal of insulin in early gestation. Diabetes 32:1141–1145

Fuhrmann K, Reiher H, Semmler K, Fischer F, Fischer M, Glöckner E (1983) Prevention of congenital malformations in infants of insulin-dependent diabetic mothers. Diabetes Care 6:219–223

Gabbe SG (1981) Diabetes mellitus in pregnancy: have all the problems been solved? Am J Med 70:613–618

Goldman JA, Dicker D, Feldberg D, Yeshaya A, Samuel N, Karp M (1986) Pregnancy outcome in patients with insulin-dependent diabetes mellitus with preconceptional diabetic control: a comparative study. Am J Obstet Gynecol 155:293–297

Hertz RH, King KC, Kalhan SC (1984) Management of third-trimester diabetic pregnancies with the use of continuous subcutaneous insulin infusion therapy: a pilot study. Am J Obstet Gynecol 149:256–260

Horton WE, Sadler TW (1983) Effects of maternal diabetes in early embryogenesis. Alternations in morphogenesis produced by the ketone body, B-hydroxybutyrate. Diabetes 32:610–616

Jensen BM, Kühl C, Mølsted-Pedersen L, Saurbrey N, Fog-Pedersen J (1986) Preconceptional treatment with insulin infusion pumps in insulin-dependent diabetic women with particular reference to prevention of congenital malformations. Acta Endocrinol [Suppl 277] (Copenh) 112:81–85

Jovanovic L, Peterson CM (1982) Optimal insulin delivery for the pregnant diabetic patient. Diabetes Care [Suppl 1] 5:24–37

Jovanovic L, Druzin M, Peterson CM (1981) Effect of euglycemia on the outcome of pregnancy in insulin-dependent diabetic women as compared with normal control subjects. Am J Med 71:921–927

Karlsson K, Kjellmer I (1972) The outcome of diabetic pregnancies in relation to the mothers blood sugar level. Am J Obstet Gynecol 112:213–220

Kucera J (1971) Rate and type of congenital anomalies among offspring of diabetic women. J Reprod Med 7:61–70

Kühl C, Møller-Jensen B, Saurbrey N, Mølsted-Pedersen L, Pedersen JF (1984) Intensified insulin treatment in diabetic pregnancy. Diabetes Educator 10:60–63

Laatikainen L, Teramo K, Hieta-Heikurainen H, Koivisto V, Pelkonen R (1987) A controlled study of the influence of continuous subcutaneous insulin infusion treatment on diabetic retinopathy during pregnancy. Acta Med Scand 221:367–376

Landon MB, Gabbe SG, Piana R, Mennuti MT, Main EK (1987) Neonatal morbidity in pregnancy complicated by diabetes mellitus: predictive value of maternal glycemic profiles. Am J Obstet Gynecol 156:1089–1095

Lewis NJ, Akazawa S, Freinkel N (1983) Teratogenesis from B-hyroxybutyrate during organogenesis in rat embryo organ culture and enhancement by subteratogenic glucose. Diabetes [Suppl 1] 32:11A

Lowy C, Beard RW, Goldschmidt J (1986) Congenital malformations in babies of diabetic mothers. Diabetic Medicine 3:458–462

Miller E, Hare JW, Cloherty JP et al. (1981) Elevated maternal hemoglobin A$_{1c}$ in early pregnancy and major congenital anomalies in infants of diabetic mothers. N Engl J Med 304:1331–1334

Mills JL (1982) Malformations in infants of diabetic mothers. Teratology 25:385–394

Mills JL, Baker L, Goldman AS (1979) Malformations in infants of diabetic mothers occur before seventh gestational week. Diabetes 28:292–293

Møller-Jensen B, Kühl C, Mølsted-Pedersen L (1985) Fatal congenital malformations in infant of insulin pump treated diabetic mother. Acta Endocrinol [Suppl] 273:73 (Abstract)

Mølsted-Pedersen L, Kühl C (1986a) Pregnancy and diabetes. In: Alberti KGMM, Krall LP (eds) The diabetes annual, 2. Elsevier, Amsterdam New York Oxford, pp 185–196

Mølsted-Pedersen L, Kühl C (1986b) Obstetrical management in diabetic pregnancy: the Copenhagen experience. Diabetologia 29:13–16

Pedersen J (1977) The pregnant diabetic and her newborn. Munksgaard, Copenhagen

Pedersen J (1978) Congenital malformations in newborns of diabetic mothers. In: Sutherland HW, Stowers JM (eds) Carbohydrate metabolism in pregnancy and the newborn. Springer-Verlag, Berlin Heidelberg New York, pp 264–276

Sadler TW (1980a) Effects of maternal diabetes on early embryogenesis: I. The teratogenic potential of diabetic serum. Teratology 21:339–347

Sadler TW (1980b) Effects of maternal diabetes on early embryogenesis: II. Hyperglycemia-induced exencephaly. Teratology 21:349–356

Sadler TW, Hunter ES (1987) Hypoglycemia: how little is too much for the embryo? Am J Obstet Gynecol 157:190–193

Saurbrey N, Arnold-Larsen S, Møller-Jensen B, Kühl C (1988) Comparison of continuous subcutaneous insulin infusion with multiple insulin injections using the NovoPen. Diabetic Medicine 5:150–153

Thorsteinsson B, Pramming S, Lauritzen T, Binder C (1986) Frequency of daytime biochemical hypoglycaemia in insulin-treated diabetic patients: relation to daily median blood glucose concentrations. Diabetic Medicine 3:147–151

White P (1949) Pregnancy complicating diabetes. Am J Med 7:609–616

Ylinen K, Aula P, Stenman U-H, Kesäniemi-Kuokkanen T, Teramo K (1984) Risk of minor and major fetal malformations in diabetics with high haemoglobin A$_{1c}$ values in early pregnancy. Br Med J 289:345–346

16. Nephropathy in Pregnancy

J. G. Klebe, C. E. Mogensen and T. Christensen

Microalbuminuria in Diabetic Pregnancy: An Early Marker of Complications?

Introduction

Management of diabetic pregnancy is one of the areas of diabetology where the benefits of modern diabetes treatment are most clearly seen (Freinkel et al. 1985). Since the Second World War perinatal mortality in the Western World has decreased from around 30%–40% to a few per cent, at least in large specialized centres with centralization of control of the diabetic pregnancy (Pedersen 1977; Freinkel et al. 1985).

There are, however, still unsolved problems compared with normal pregnancy (L. M. Pedersen et al. 1964; L. M. Pedersen 1974; J. Pedersen 1977; Fuhrmann et al. 1984; Klebe et al. 1986; Reece and Hobbins 1986).

Pregnancy may induce additional damage to the microvascular system of the pregnant diabetic woman, especially in the kidney and the retina (Kitzmiller et al. 1981).

Thus, the interaction between pregnancy and the vascular system of diabetic women remains complicated, sometimes with devastating effects, more commonly deleterious for the fetus than for the child-bearing woman. Renal and vascular damage, including blood pressure elevation, is often involved and therefore sensitive methods for measuring elevated urinary protein excretion, especially albumin, so-called microalbuminuria (Viberti et al. 1982a; Mogensen and Christensen 1984; Mogensen 1987), might be useful in the early prediction of complications in diabetic and also non-diabetic pregnancy. This is the case in the non-pregnant diabetics (Viberti et al. 1982b; Parving et al. 1982; Mathiesen et al. 1984; Mogensen and Christensen 1984; Vigstrup and Mogensen 1985; Feldt-Rasmussen 1986; Feldt-Rasmussen et al. 1986) where microalbuminuria is a sensitive marker of generalized subclinical vascular disturbance and damage (Feldt-Rasmussen 1986), and it predicts overt nephropathy (Parving et al. 1982; Viberti et al. 1982b; Mathiesen et al. 1984; Mogensen and Christensen 1984) as well as proliferative retinopathy (Vigstrup and Mogensen 1985).

Patients and Methods

We studied consecutively 97 insulin-dependent diabetic patients referred to the Diabetic Pregnancy Unit at Aarhus Kommunehospital. One patient was pregnant twice. When pregnancy was recognized patients were referred for initial hospitalization for a few days for blood glucose stabilization, general examination and White classification. In many cases patients were seen earlier for prepregnancy advice. The patients were controlled at least every second week until the 32nd week. Thereafter monitoring was performed weekly. When attending the clinic for general obstetric control, analyses of s-oestriol and human placental lactogen (HPL), ultrasound examinations of crown–rump length and biparietal diameter were performed. In addition, blood glucose, blood pressure and urinary albumin excretion (UAE) (on 24-h urine samples collected at home) were determined (Miles et al. 1970). The UAE were available from the initial hospitalization until delivery and the puerperium and 3 months later. All patients performed self-monitoring of blood glucose six times daily at least twice weekly. HbA_{1c} was assayed nearly every month by cation-exchange chromatography (Poulsen and Jespersen 1986) and at approximately the same intervals creatinine clearance was measured, also on 24-h urine samples collected at home. After the 32nd week values of two albumin excretion rates were used in the calculation, and non-stress cardiotocography was performed weekly.

Urinary Albumin Excretion (UAE) in Normal Pregnancy

No increase in UAE is seen in normal pregnancy, either early or late. In our laboratory 330 normal pregnant women showed values of 3.0 $\mu g/min \pm 1.8$ in week 20 (geometric mean±tolerance factor) (Fig. 16.1) corresponding to or lower than non-pregnant normals (Miles et al. 1970; Mogensen 1986); also no increase was

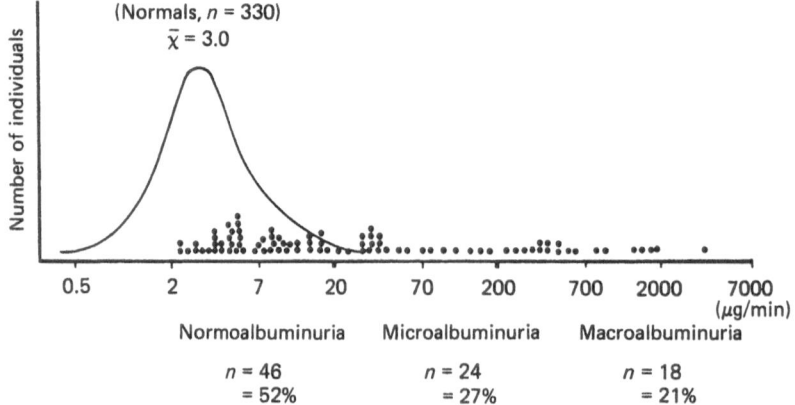

Fig. 16.1. Urinary albumin excretion rate in normal and diabetic pregnancies (week 16–21). The *solid line* shows the distribution curve for normal pregnancies (*n*=330), the *dots* indicate diabetics (*n*=88).

seen in the different trimesters or late in pregnancy (weeks 38–41) in normal women with a normal urine flow with 5.5 μg/ml$\pm$1.6 in morning urine samples (n=35) expressed as μg/min.

Urinary Albumin Excretion (UAE) in Diabetic Pregnancy

Classification of the Pregnant Diabetic Woman. Table 16.1 shows the patients divided according to the White classification and urinary albumin excretion. White's class B included 22 patients with insulin-dependent diabetes; 13 with short duration of diabetes and nine with insulin-dependent gestational diabetes. Nineteen patients in White's class B had normoalbuminuria. In White's class C eight of 10 patients had mostly normoalbuminuria; the 46 White's class D patients are a more mixed group with 28 patients with normoalbuminuria and 16 patients with initial microalbuminuria. All six patients in White's class F had macroalbuminuria. Ten patients in White's class F/R with both proliferative retinopathy and overt nephropathy almost all had macroalbuminuria. In contrast to White's class F, F/R, the four patients in White's class R with solitary proliferative retinopathy had the same pattern as White's class C–D.

Table 16.1. Patients classified according to the White classification and according to renal involvement in diabetes

White class	Albuminuria at admission			
	Normo	Micro	Macro	Total
B	19	2		21
C	8	2		10
D	28	16	2	46
F			6	6
F/R		1	9	10
R	3	1		4
Total	58	22	17	97

Besides the White's classification we used, with small modifications, a newly proposed classification system for renal involvement in insulin-dependent diabetics, collectively elaborated by Belgian, Danish and British groups active in the study of renal involvement in diabetes (Mogensen et al. 1985). According to this system the 97 patients were classified (Table 16.2). Subdivided according to the new classification, group I included patients with diabetes diagnosed during pregnancy. Group II comprised patients with normal UAE around week 16 (<20 μg/min). This group had to be subdivided into groups IIa, IIb and IIc, since a number of patients later in pregnancy showed values higher than 20 μg/min (IIb), and one patient even values over 200 μg/min (IIc). Group III included patients with microalbuminuria early in pregnancy (UAE 20.1–200 μg/min): group IIIa patients had stable UAE, (200 μg/min); group IIIb comprised patients who later in pregnancy showed macroalbuminuria. Group IV patients had clinical proteinuria, which corresponds to approximately >200 μg/min in UAE.

Figure 16.2 shows the UAE in the different White's classes in the three trimesters, the puerperium and 3 months later. It appears from Fig. 16.2 that

Table 16.2. 97 pregnant diabetics subdivided according to a new classification. The patient with two pregnancies was grouped as IIb and IIc

		Total number
I	Diabetes diagnosed in pregnancy	9
IIa	Normoalbuminuria	32
IIb	Normo→microalbuminuria	13
IIc	Normo→macroalbuminuria	1
IIIa	Microalbuminuria	22
IIIb	Micro→macroalbuminuria	2
IV	Macroalbuminuria	18
Total		97

patients in White's classes B and C react equally, with a slight reduction of the UAE in the second trimester, moderate raised values in the third trimester, marked elevation in the puerperium and normalization 3 months later. White's class D had the same pattern but with UAE values on a higher level. Surprisingly, White's class R (the pregnant women with proliferative retinopathy as the sole complication) react in the same manner with values between White's classes C and D. Class F, F/R could be subdivided according to nephrotic syndrome. White's class F, F/R without nephrotic syndrome patients show results similar to patients in the other White classes but in macroalbuminuric levels. Patients with nephrotic syndrome, however, react in a different way. They had the highest UAE, which was increasing throughout pregnancy, but with a slight reduction after delivery. A further reduction was found 3 months later but in these patients the highest UAE persisted.

Figure 16.3 shows the longitudinal course of UAE in pregnant women according to the new classification. Mean values are shown, with the exception of data from eight gestations in seven patients with complicated pregnancies. Two

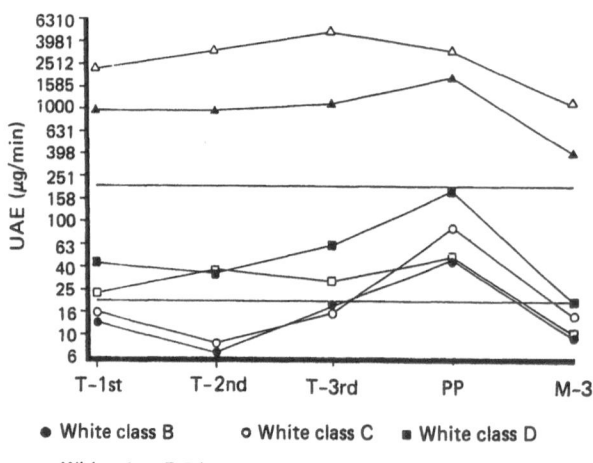

Fig. 16.2. Urinary albumin excretion in diabetic pregnancy according to White's classification.

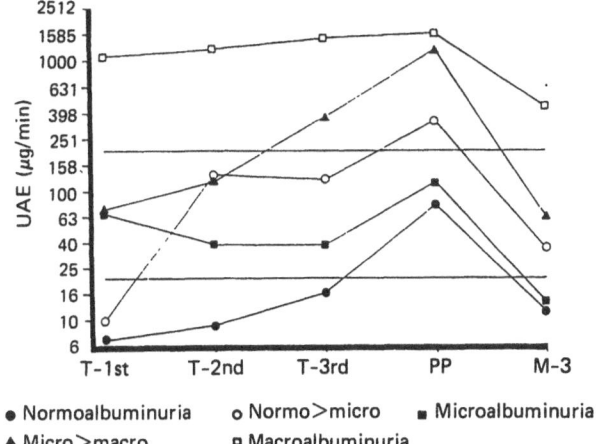

Fig. 16.3. Urinary albumin excretion rate in diabetic pregnancy according to the new classification system.

patients in group IIb, one in group IIc and the one in group IV developed pre-eclampsia. In addition, one patient in group IV with heavy proteinuria early in pregnancy developed a marked decline in creatinine clearance and an increase in blood pressure. In six pregnancies (one in group IIa, two in group IIb, one in group IIc, one in group IIIa and one in group IV) early or late intrauterine death was recorded (Fig. 16.4). Intrauterine death was preceded in four of the pregnancies by a gradual and considerable increase in UAE over the course of several weeks. In two pregnancies in one patient fetal death and late abortion occurred.

In one patient in group IIa with intrauterine death no change in UAE was seen. No complications were seen during the course of pregnancy except psychological and social, and this demise at week 38 remains unexplained.

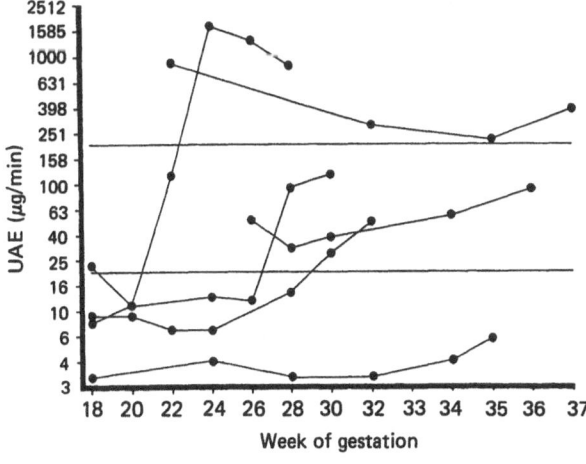

Fig. 16.4. Urinary albumin excretion rate in diabetic pregnancy with late abortion or fetal death.

The patient in group IV without increasing UAE was a neglector, developed pre-eclampsia and was admitted with intrauterine death.

As shown in Table 16.2, 14 of 46 patients (45%) changed from normoalbuminuria to microalbuminuria during pregnancy which is a phenomenon generally not seen in normal pregnancy (Fig. 16.1). Patients with microalbuminuria usually remained stable, unless pre-eclampsia or intrauterine death occurred. In group IV UAE and clinical proteinuria were also stable as seen in Fig. 16.3.

β_{+2}-Microglobulin Excretion

No significant increase was seen in β_{+2}-microglobulin excretion in pregnancies presenting with intrauterine death (257→252 ng/min, 66→183 ng/min, 81→59 ng/min).

Blood Pressure and Serum Creatinine in the Course of Pregnancy

The mean arterial pressure (MAP), defined as diastolic plus one-third of pulse pressure, had a tendency to increase in all groups, but this increase only becomes significant in group IIb which was characterized by an increase in UAE during pregnancy. Throughout all the groups, I, IIa, IIb, IIc, IIIa, IIIb and, IV, initial MAP increased.

A significantly increased serum creatinine was, not unexpectedly, seen in group IV. The level is above the reference value for non-diabetic women in pregnancy. White's class F, F/R had elevated serum creatinine values which had not returned completely to normal levels 3 months after birth. Patients with nephrotic syndrome had the most pronounced increase of their serum creatinine values but with a normalization 3 months after birth. One patient showed a marked decline in creatinine clearance and a concomitant increase in blood pressure and an increase in protein excretion, when expressed as a percentage of glomerular filtration rate (GFR).

Urinary Tract Infection

Significant bacteriuria was seen in few patients. There was no association with changes in UAE.

Discussion of Urinary Albumin Excretion

This consecutive study shows that marked abnormalities in urinary albumin excretion were seen in diabetic pregnancy, both early and late in its course. In many patients an abnormal increase in UAE was seen during pregnancy namely in 45% of patients with normal values around week 20. Generally such increases were not seen in normal pregnancy (Pedersen et al. 1982; Irgens-Moeller et al. 1986; Lopez-Espinoza et al. 1986), which is in accord with our normal material. In several cases, changes in UAE in the subclinical range were associated with a complicated course of pregnancy. The four pregnancies in three patients with late abortion or intrauterine death showed a gradual and marked increase in UAE in the preceding weeks. No increase was seen in β_2-microglobulin excretion and the increase is therefore likely to be of glomerular origin. No concomitant decrease in creatinine clearance was seen.

The increase in UAE may represent a form of subclinical pre-eclampsia with development of microalbuminuria and later macroalbuminuria, which is more than 200 μg/min. Decreased placental blood flow is seen in diabetic pregnancy (Nylund et al. 1982) as in pre-eclampsia, a condition which is also associated with increased frequency of late intrauterine death (Redman 1984; Gregorini et al. 1986). Pre-eclampsia is seen more often in diabetic than in non-diabetic pregnancy (Pedersen 1977). In fact, four patients in groups IIb, IIc and group IV did develop the clinical picture of pre-eclampsia.

Hyperfiltration is one of the physiological responses to pregnancy which is also found in diabetes (Sims 1961). The hyperfiltration process may induce microalbuminuria, e.g. mediated by increased transglomerular pressure. Both abnormaltiies are seen in association with poor metabolic control of diabetes, e.g. even at clinical diagnosis (Mogensen 1971; Parving et al. 1976; Vittinghus and Mogensen 1982). We found no significant association between UAE and creatinine clearance, and patients in this study were generally well controlled, as documented from the mean blood glucose and the HbA_{1c} values (mean $6.6\% \pm 1.04$).

A proper statistical evaluation of complications in diabetic pregnancy is generally difficult. This applies to our study also because of the rather small number of patients with complications among the 97 pregnancies. However, the gradual increase in UAE starting in the subclinical range certainly seems to be a sensitive marker of a more poor prognosis. In this study intervention was not attempted because we had no experience with measurement of UAE at the start of the project. Early treatment may be a possibility. The most obvious modality of intervention would be the discontinuation of physical work by the patient and in addition possibly the recommendation of bed rest, since that may at least partially restore sufficient blood flow to the kidney, uterus and placenta. Antihypertensive treatment could also be considered (Redman 1984; Gregorini et al. 1986).

A toxic or haemodynamic effect induced by pregnancy is likely to be the major cause of the increase in UAE from the normal to subclinical elevation and later to frank proteinuria. In some cases this phenomenon seems to result in late intrauterine death. However, many of the patients with initially low UAE may show some structural glomerular changes which also may be involved in the temporarily enhanced albumin excretion during pregnancy. In many centres, including our own, diabetic pregnancy is usually terminated around week 38. On the other hand, in several centres the treatment policy has changed and pregnancy is not terminated. The issue is not resolved and there is no consensus but it might be possible that if subdivision of patients with respect to UAE is done, the pregnancy may need to be terminated only in patients with increasing UAE. Studies are needed to evaluate such a policy in diabetic women. In all patients good metabolic control, absence of a large fetus and the presence of a normal pelvis are clearly important factors if pregnancy is to be allowed to continue.

We recommend that further large-scale studies on the prognostic value of UAE in diabetic pregnancy should be carried out. New prognostic markers with possible therapeutic implications are clearly needed so that the frequency of deleterious complications in diabetic pregnancy can be reduced to a level not higher than in normal pregnancy. Urinary albumin excretion may in conjunction with established obstetric parameters qualify as one marker in this respect. A rapid, non-expensive and sensitive immunoassay is now available (Harmoingn et al. 1985).

In this study a number of patients (18%) showed evidence of diabetic nephropathy on referral. Only one of these patients, and none from the other groups, showed a marked deterioration in renal function, as measured by creatinine clearance, during pregnancy. This reduced renal function persisted after pregnancy.

In the absence of heavy proteinuria, hypertension and reduced renal function pregnancy does not seem to accelerate renal disease in diabetes (Kitzmiller et al. 1981; Nesler et al. 1985), which is in accordance with our finding and in addition studies on the effect of pregnancy on other glomerular diseases (Backer et al. 1985; Hayslett 1985; Katz and Lindheimer 1985).

The White's classification, namely grouping diabetic patients according to complication and duration of disease, is widely used in most centres. This classification is very useful but additional information may be obtained when classifying patients according to UAE. Thus patients starting with normal excretion rates who later develop increased UAE may be more prone to complications. This will not be detected using the White's classification. It should also be borne in mind that many patients, e.g. in White's class D, show a normal albumin excretion rate throughout pregnancy and thus they will not be prone to the development of complications. The present classification of diabetic patients in pregnancy is in accordance with a new classification system regarding renal changes in non-pregnant patients (Mogensen et al. 1985), and this system may also be useful in pregnant women with diabetes.

Renal Size in Diabetic Pregnancy

Introduction

In normal non-pregnant women the renal size is influenced by several factors. Nephrosclerosis will end in diminished renal size together with renal end-stage failure. In contrast, elevated levels of growth hormone (Corvilain and Abramow 1962), diabetes with malregulation (Viberti et al. 1982a; Feldt-Rasmussen et al. 1986; Mogensen 1986) and hyperfiltration will increase renal size (Mogensen and Andersen 1975; Christensen 1984; Feldt-Rasmussen 1986).

In normal pregnancy the placenta synthesizes different hormones, some with growth-hormone-like function. These hormones could be responsible for the renal hyperfiltration. In pregnancy the cardiac output is increased and so also is the central venous pressure which influences renal perfusion. Furthermore, in normal pregnancy there is a marked change of insulin receptors throughout pregnancy which influences the blood glucose regulation (Hjøellund et al. 1986). These factors are similar to those which in the non-pregnant produce renal enlargement. It is unknown if these biochemical and haemodynamic alterations operate in this way in normal pregnancy.

Impaired renal function is seen in some pregnant women with diabetes (Nesler et al. 1985). Because it is unknown if decreased renal function is connected with changes in renal size, we studied the influence of human placental lactogenic hormone, glucose regulation and hyperfiltration on renal volume throughout pregnancy. Furthermore we investigated the validity of the White classification in relation to the renal volume and especially in pregnant women with overt nephropathy. As there still is doubt about whether or not pregnancy may induce, worsen or accelerate diabetic nephropathy, we extended the study to include measurement of renal volume 3 months after delivery.

Methods

Renal volume was determined by means of ultrasonography. Static ultrasound equipment (Brüel & Kjœr) with a built-in volume programme was applied. With the patients in the prone position the longitudinal axis of the kidney was registered and the renal space/area was marked with intervals of 1 cm (Rasmussen et al. 1978). The total renal volume of the two sides was corrected to 1.73 m^2 prepregnancy body surface. We measured the renal volume in the women who attended for a prepregnancy consultation, and again in the first, second and third trimesters, in the puerperium and after a further 3 months. As the investigation is ongoing we are presently in the process of measuring the renal volume again 1 year after delivery.

Renal Volume in Normal Pregnancy

Twenty-four healthy pregnant women aged 20–30 years with uncomplicated pregnancies form the control group. In the non-pregnant women the renal volume was 225 ml. In the first trimester the renal volume was estimated to be 236.8±35.9 ml (mean±SD) and in the second trimester the corresponding values had increased to 252.6±21.8 ml. In the third trimester the values were 292.3±44.8 and after delivery there was a reduction to 223.9±15.4 ml.

Renal Volume in Diabetic Pregnancy:

In non-pregnant diabetic women the renal size is enlarged to 275 ml (Christensen 1984). Figure 16.5 shows the renal volume according to the White classification.

White's class B patients, which includes women with short duration of their diabetes without vascular complications and patients with insulin-dependent gestational diabetes, had mean renal volumes of 230 ml before pregnancy which increased during pregnancy to 360 ml, with reductions to 300 ml after birth, and nearly to normal values at 250 ml 3 months later.

Patients in White's class C react in the same way but on higher levels with maximal values of 390 ml, a reduction to 350 ml after birth and return to average diabetic values of 275 ml 3 months after delivery.

The renal size in White's class R in pregnancy was nearly similar to White's class C-D.

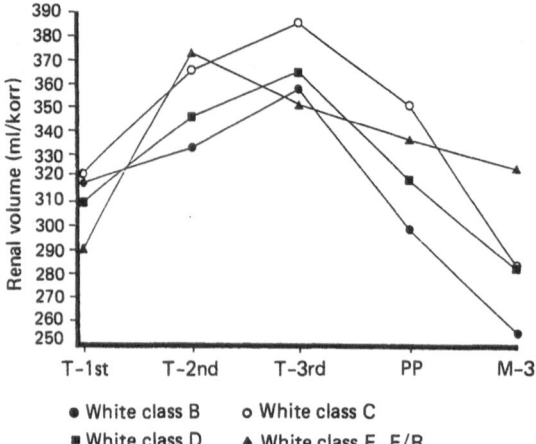

Fig. 16.5.   Renal volume changes in diabetic pregnancy according to White's classification.

In White's class D the prepregnancy renal volume was 270 ml. Throughout pregnancy the values increased to a maximum of 370 ml followed by a reduction after delivery and return to average diabetic levels 3 months later.

White's class F, F/R included patients with small and large renal volumes. After subdivision of White's class F, F/R on the basis of nephrotic syndrome, patients without nephrotic syndrome showed only a minor elevation of the renal volume during pregnancy (see Fig. 16.6). After birth and 3 months later the renal

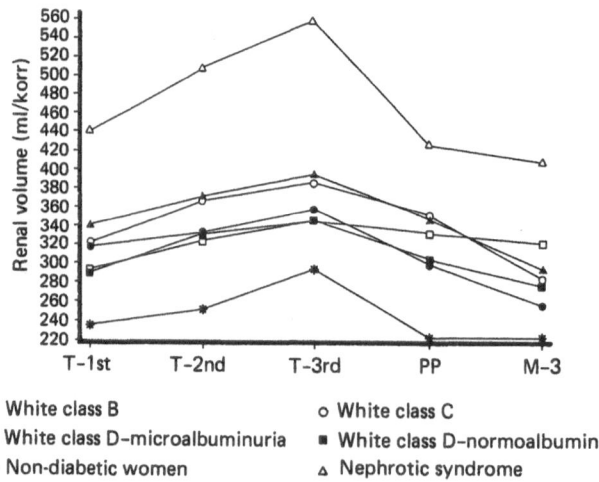

Fig. 16.6.   Renal volume changes in diabetic pregnancy in the different White's classes after subdivision according to urinary albumin excretion and nephrotic syndrome.

volumes were still enlarged compared with prepregnancy levels. In contrast, White's class F with nephrotic syndrome showed not only the largest renal volumes and most enlargement throughout pregnancy and a marked decrease of renal volume after delivery, but also 3 months later this group had still the largest renal volume, by more than 400 ml.

Discussion of Renal Volume

In normal pregnancy the renal size increases by approximately 20%. However, shortly after delivery a return to normal values occurs. The reason for such changes is unknown. Probably both biochemical and haemodynamic factors play a role in the mechanism of this renal enlargement. Hyperfiltration due to an increased filtration pressure gradient or biochemical changes caused by the different placental hormones may lead to an alteration in molecular structure and size of components of the glomerulus. Since there is no difference in the renal size of multiparae and primiparae, and the changes in the renal volume together with other renal parameters return to normal after delivery, it is assumed that pregnancy in normal women has no deleterious effect on renal function.

Proteinuria is the main marker for renal disease in diabetes. About 40% do develop nephropathy according to a long-term follow-up study from the Steno Memorial Hospital (Parving et al. 1982). A patient with a GFR of 100 ml/min can expect, with a mean decline of 3.5 ml/min per month, that end-stage renal failure will be reached after 30 years. If progression is rapid, end-stage renal failure may be reached in 10 years. This is always accompanied by a reduction in renal size. Therefore, the pregnant population will include diabetics with normal renal function, a large group with incipient nephropathy and some women with overt nephropathy. Incipient nephropathy will result in increased glomerular filtration with renal enlargement.

Our investigation of renal volume in pregnancy shows pregnant women with normal, with enlarged and some with reduced renal volumes. White's class B women with initial normal renal volume react with the same pattern as normal non-diabetic pregnant women but on a higher level. As soon as the duration of the diabetes is more than 10 years the kidney reacts with more pronounced enlargement but still returns to the diabetic level. Patients in White's class R, which is usually included in White's class F/R, react in the same way as those in White's class C-D, indicating that proliferative retinopathy as a single complication has no deleterious influence on renal function. Patients in White's class D, a more complex group including both patients with duration of their diabetes >20 years and those with benign retinopathy and only short duration of their diabetes, seemed to have slightly reduced renal volume initially and less response during pregnancy possibly due to incipient nephropathy. Our investigation shows that White's class F, F/R patients have to be divided on the basis of those with and without nephrotic syndrome. Pregnant women with overt nephropathy without nephrotic syndrome had reduced responses of the renal volume throughout pregnancy with nearly no reduction of renal size after birth and only a minor reduction 3 months later, implying that pregnancy may worsen existing overt nephropathy. Pregnant women with nephrotic syndrome who had the lowest HbA$_{1c}$ values throughout pregnancy exhibited the largest renal volume in the first trimester with the most pronounced enlargement of renal volume to over double the magnitude of diabetic prepregnancy values implying that glomerular hyperfiltration must be partly responsible for these changes. Since there is only a slight reduction of the kidney size 3 months later hyperfiltration is probably dangerous for the kidney and possibly causes permanent damage to the kidney. Further follow-up studies of renal volume will elucidate this problem.

Relation Between Kidney Size and Microalbuminuria in Diabetic Pregnancy

In diabetic pregnancy there is a connection between UAE and the renal volume (Fig. 16.6). However, a subdivision according to the White classification is necessary to give more detailed information. Pregnant women with normoalbuminuria and with short duration of their diabetes had the smallest renal size which reacted in a way similar to that of pregnant women without diabetes. Women in White's class C, only 20% of whom had microalbuminuria, had more pronounced increases of their renal volumes throughout pregnancy. Subdivision of White's class D patients into those with and without microalbuminuria is necessary too. Women in White's class D with normoalbuminuria had renal volumes of 290 ml in the first trimester and a normal increase occurred in pregnancy with return to normal diabetic levels (275 ml) 3 months later. They reacted in the same manner as patients with short duration of their diabetes. However, those in White's class D microalbuminuria exhibited large renal volumes (340 ml) in the first trimester, with increased values of 390 ml in the third trimester followed by a reduction after delivery without a return to normal renal volume 3 months later. Most of the patients with macroalbuminuria belong to White's class F, F/R. Subdivision on the basis of the presence or absence of nephrotic syndrome is necessary. Patients with macroalbuminuria without nephrotic syndrome had relatively small renal volumes, small increases of renal volumes throughout pregnancy, minor decreases of the renal volume after delivery and almost no further decrease of renal volume 3 months later. Patients with nephrotic syndrome however, had the most pronounced UAE values with the exception of one patient with nearly end-stage renal failure. They also had the largest renal volumes in the first trimester, the most pronounced increases of renal volume throughout pregnancy followed by a marked reduction after delivery but with no return to renal volume normal values 3 months later, which infers that nephrotic syndrome in pregnancy causes deterioration in renal function.

Final Conclusions

Complications still occur in diabetic pregnancy, namely higher malformation rates, higher perinatal mortality and morbidity in spite of centralization of care and control before and during pregnancy in diabetic units. On the basis of quantification of UAE, pregnant diabetic women can be allocated into three groups, namely those with normoalbuminuria, those with microalbuminuria and those with macroalbuminuria which are associated with the development of complications during pregnancy including blood pressure elevation, pre-eclampsia and occasional fetal death. Persistent macroalbuminuria is always a bad sign and heavy increasing proteinuria can lead to end-stage renal failure.

In normal pregnancy the increasing renal volume and the microalbuminuria occurring in relation to delivery normalizes in the puerperium. There is no difference between the renal volume of primiparae and multiparae. Therefore, we assume that normal pregnancy has no permanent deleterious influence on renal function.

In the diabetic pregnancy the renal volume enlarges throughout pregnancy with the maximal increase in kidney size in the third trimester. Shortly after delivery the renal size is diminished, and 3 months later in uncomplicated diabetic women renal size is nearly normalized. However, in patients with microalbuminuria and macroalbuminuria the renal size does not return to normal 3 months after delivery which could imply that pregnancy in patients with incipient or overt nephropathy can cause permanent deterioration in the renal function.

White's class R with proliferative retinopathy as the only complication has a good prognosis in respect of renal function.

Good concordance was found between White's classification and UAE. This investigation shows that the White classification still is useful but a subdivision according to the albumin excretion and nephrotic syndrome will give more detailed information of prognostic value.

On the basis of our results of UAE we propose a new additional classification system for forecasting obstetrical complications in pregnancy. The measurement of microalbuminuria could be of value therefore in the management of diabetic pregnancy as an early marker of later complications.

References

Backer GJ, Fairley KF, Whitworth JA (1985) Pregnancy exacerbates glomerular disease. Am J Kidney Dis 6:266–272

Christensen JS (1984) On the pathogenesis of the increased glomerular filtration rate in short-term insulin-dependent diabetes. Laegeforeningens forlag Thesis

Corvilain J, Abramow M (1962) Some effects of human growth hormone on renal hemodynamics and on tubular phosphate transport in man. J Clin Invest 41:1230–1235

Feldt-Rasmussen B (1986) Increased transcapillary escape rate of albumin in type 1 (insulin-dependent) diabetic patients with microalbuminuria. Diabetologia 29:282–286

Feldt-Rasmussen B, Mathiesen E, Deckert T (1986) Effect of two years of strict metabolic control on the progression of incipient nephropathy in insulin-dependent diabetes. Lancet II:1300–1344

Freinkel N, Dooley SL, Metzger BE (1985) Care of the pregnant woman with insulin-dependent diabetes mellitus. N Engl J Med 313:96–101

Fuhrmann K, Reiher H, Semmler K, Glockner E (1984) The effect of intensified conventional insulin therapy before and during pregnancy on the malformation rate in offspring of diabetic mothers. Exp Clin Endocrinol 83:173–177

Gregorini G, Perico N, Remuzzi G (1986) Pathogenesis of preeclampsia. Martinus Nijhoff, Boston, pp 13–33

Harmoingn A, Ala-Houhala I, Vuorien P (1985) Rapid and sensitive immunoassay for albumin determination in urine. Clin Chim Acta 149:269–274

Hayslett JP (1985) Pregnancy does not exacerbate primary glomerular disease. Am J Kidney Dis 6:273–277

Hjøellund E, Pedersen O, Espersen T, Klebe JG (1986) Impaired insulin receptor binding and postbinding defects of adipocytes from normal and diabetic pregnant women. Diabetes 35:598–603

Irgens-Moeller L. Hemmingsen L, Holm J (1986) Diagnostic value of micro-albuminuria in pre-eclampsia. Clin Chim Acta 157:295–298

Katz AI, Lindheimer MD (1985) Does pregnancy aggravate primary glomerular disease? Am J Kidney Dis 6:261–265

Kitzmiller JL, Brown ER, Phillippe N et al. (1981) Diabetic nephropathy and perinatal outcome. Am J Obstet Gynecol 141:741–751

Klebe JG, Espersen T, Allan J (1986) Diabetes mellitus and pregnancy. A seven-year material of pregnant diabetics, where control during pregnancy was based on a centralized ambulant regime. Acta Obstet Gynecol Scand 65:235–240

Lopez-Espinoza I, Dhar H, Humphreys S, Redman CWG (1986) Urinary albumin excretion in pregnancy. Br J Obstet Gynaecol 93:176–181

Mathiesen ER, Oxenboell B, Johansen K, Svendsen PAA, Deckert T (1984) Incipient nephropathy in type 1 (insulin-dependent) diabetes. Diabetologia 26:406–410

Miles DW, Mogensen CE, Gundersen HJG (1970) Radioimmunoassay for urinary albumin using a single antibody. Scand J Clin Lab Invest 26:5–11

Mogensen CE (1971) Urinary albumin excretion in early and long-term juvenile diabetes. Scand J Clin Lab Invest 28:183–193

Mogensen CE (1986) Microalbuminuria and kidney function. Notes on methods, interpretation, and classification. In: Clarke WL, Larner J, Pohl SL (eds) Methods in diabetes research, vol. 2: Clinical Methods. John Wiley, New York, 612

Mogensen CE (1987) Microalbuminuria as a predictor of clinical diabetic nephropathy. Nephrology forum. Kidney Int 31:673–689

Mogensen CE, Andersen MJF (1975) Increased kidney size and glomerular filtration rate in untreated juvenile diabetes: normalization by insulin treatment. Diabetologia 11:221–224

Mogensen CE, Christensen CK (1984) Predicting diabetic nephropathy in insulin-dependent patients. N Engl J Med 311:89–93

Mogensen CE, Chachati A, Christensen CK et al. (1985) Microalbuminuria: an early marker of renal involvement in diabetes. Uremia Invest 9:85–95

Nesler CL, Sinclair SH, Schwartz SS, Gabbe SG (1985) Diabetic nephropathy in pregnancy. Clin Obstet Gynecol 28:528–535

Nylund L, Lunell NO, Lewander R, Persson B, Sarby B (1982) Uteroplacental blood flow in diabetic pregnancy: measurements with indium 113m and a computer-linked gamma camera. Am J Obstet Gynecol 144:298–302

Parving H-H, Noer I, Deckert T et al. (1976) The effect of metabolic regulation on microvascular permeability to small and large molecules in short-term juvenile diabetics. Diabetologia 12:161–166

Parving H-H, Oxenbcill B, Svendsen PAA, Christiansen JS, Andersen AR (1982) Early detection of patients at risk of developing diabetic nephropathy. A longitudinal study of urinary albumin excretion. Acta Endocrinol (Copenh) 100:550–555

Pedersen EB, Rasmussen AB, Johannesen P et al. (1982) Urinary excretion of albumin, beta-2-microglobulin and light chains in preeclampsia, essential hypertension in pregnancy and normotensive pregnant and non-pregnant control subjects. Scand J Clin Lab Invest 41:777–784

Pedersen J (1977) The pregnant diabetic and her newborn, 2nd edn. Munksgaard, Copenhagen

Pedersen LM (1974) The transverse diameter of the pelvic inlet in diabetic women in relation to age at onset of diabetes. Acta Endocrinol (Copenh) 75 (Suppl 182):65–72

Pedersen LM, Tygstrup J, Pedersen J (1964) Congenital malformation in newborn infants of diabetic women. Lancet I:1124–1126

Poulsen JH, Jespersen J (1986) A comparison of the determination of glucosylated haemoglobin by isoelectric focusing and cation-exchange chromatography on minicolumns. Scand J Clin Lab Invest 46:259–263

Rasmussen SN, Haase L, Kjeldsen H, Hancke S (1978) Determination of renal volume by ultrasonic scanning. J Clin Ultrasound 6:160–164

Redman CWG (1984) The definition of pre-eclampsia. Scand J Clin Lab Invest 44 (Suppl 169):7–14

Reece EA, Hobbins JC (1986) Diabetic embryopathy: pathogenesis, prenatal diagnosis and prevention. Obstet Gynecol Surv 41:325–335

Sims EAH (1961) Serial studies of renal function in pregnancy complicated by diabetes mellitus. Diabetes 10:190–197

Viberti GC, Mackintosh D, Bilous RW, Pickup JC, Keen H (1982a) Proteinuria in diabetes mellitus: role of spontaneous and experimental variation of glycaemia. Kidney Int 21:714–720

Viberti GC, Hill RD, Jarrett RJ, Argyropoulos A, Mahmud U, Keen H (1982b) Microalbuminuria as a predictor of clinical nephropathy in insulin-dependent diabetes mellitus. Lancet I:1430–1432

Vigstrup J, Mogensen CE (1985) Proliferative diabetic retinopathy: at risk patients identified by early detection of microalbuminuria. Acta Ophthalmol Scand 63:530–534

Vittinghus E, Mogensen CE (1982) Graded exercise and protein excretion in diabetic man and the effect of insulin treatment. Kidney Int 21:725–729

17. Pregnancy and Diabetic Retinopathy

J. V. Forrester, H. M. A. Towler and D. W. M. Pearson

Introduction

In 1950 Beetham reported on the occurrence of retinopathy in a group of 200 pregnant diabetics. He found that diabetic retinopathy deteriorated during pregnancy, and his results were supported by data from further studies (Oakley 1953; Stephens et al. 1963). In 12 patients with proliferative retinopathy, Beetham observed that all experienced visual deterioration and four progressed to blindness. Later studies by White (1965) confirmed that both haemorrhagic and proliferative retinopathy worsened during pregnancy and that there was a tendency towards regression of the retinopathy (i.e. improvement) after delivery, an observation made anecdotally in two cases of longstanding diabetes by Lawrence in 1948. Beetham (1950) advocated that patients with proliferative retinopathy should avoid pregnancy, and terminations should be offered to pregnant diabetics on the basis that more than 50% of patients with any degree of retinopathy had a reduced chance of a successful pregnancy and all patients with proliferative retinopathy at the onset of pregnancy experienced perinatal mortality plus visual loss.

Since these early reports, there have been marked improvements in the management of diabetic pregnancies with less nephropathy and hypertension and increased infant survival. In addition, the dogma relating to progression of the retinopathy has been challenged, mainly as a result of recent information on the natural history of diabetic retinopathy. It has become clear that diabetic retinopathy is a function of the duration of diabetes, with much less importance being attributable to other factors. In addition, untreated proliferative diabetic retinopathy is likely to progress over several weeks in the absence of other conditions such as pregnancy. Presently there is a better understanding of the pathogenesis of diabetic retinopathy which has led to a clearer recognition of the various clinical types of retinopathy and of the "at risk" individual.

Clinical Manifestations of Diabetic Retinopathy

Diabetic retinopathy is initially a disease of the retinal microvasculature, ultimately leading to retinal damage. There are two broad classes of retinopathy, background diabetic retinopathy (BDR) and proliferative diabetic retinopathy (PDR) (Table 17.1). After several years of diabetes, minimal BDR manifests as the occasional microaneurysm, eventually progressing to dot and blot haemorrhages and hard exudates which may involve the macula and cause reduced vision (Fig. 17.1a). This condition usually exists for years. For as yet unknown reasons, BDR may abruptly progress to preproliferative retinopathy manifested by numerous cotton wool spots or soft exudates (retinal microinfarcts), flame-shaped retinal haemorrhages and venous abnormalities (beading, intraretinal microvascular abnormalities, IRMA) (Fig. 17.1b). Fluorescein angiography reveals widespread areas of retinal underperfusion (ischaemia) (Fig. 17.1c). Finally, frank new vessels appear on the disc (NVD) (Fig. 17.1d) or elsewhere in the retina (NVE) (Fig. 17.1e) which produce preretinal or subhyaloid haemorrhages, and subsequently intravitreal haemorrhages, with sudden visual loss. Reparative processes in the vitreous produce contraction of the vitreous gel causing repeated intravitreal bleeding and eventual traction retinal detachment. Traction retinal detachment can also be caused by preretinal or epiretinal fibroglial reaction (gliosis) and represents the "burnt-out" stage of PDR (Fig. 17.1f).

Table 17.1.   Diabetic retinopathy: clinical types

1. Background	(a) Minimal – occasional microaneurysm
	(b) Moderate – haemorrhages, hard exudates
	(c) Marked – includes maculopathy
2. Preproliferative	(a) Venous changes – beading etc.
	(b) Ischaemic changes – soft exudates
	(c) Intraretinal microvascular abnormalities (IRMA)
3. Proliferative	(a) Flat new vessels – disc (NVD)
	– elsewhere (NVE)
	(b) Forward new vessels – vitreous haemorrhage
	(c) Gliosis of retina
	(d) Traction retinal detachment

Pathogenesis of Diabetic Retinopathy

Endothelial cell damage is probably the initial event in the pathogenesis of diabetic retinopathy (for review see Forrester 1987). Pathologically the earliest sign is loss of mural cells (pericytes) from the retinal vessels (Cogan et al. 1961; Ashton 1983). Although the function of pericytes in retinal vessels is at present unclear, they probably have a contractile role similar to arterial smooth-muscle cells in larger vessels, and may contribute towards the regulation of capillary blood flow. More recently they have been shown to exert a regulatory role over endothelial cell proliferation in vitro (Orlidge and D'Amore 1987) and may therefore assist in maintaining the normally low endothelial cell turnover. Loss of

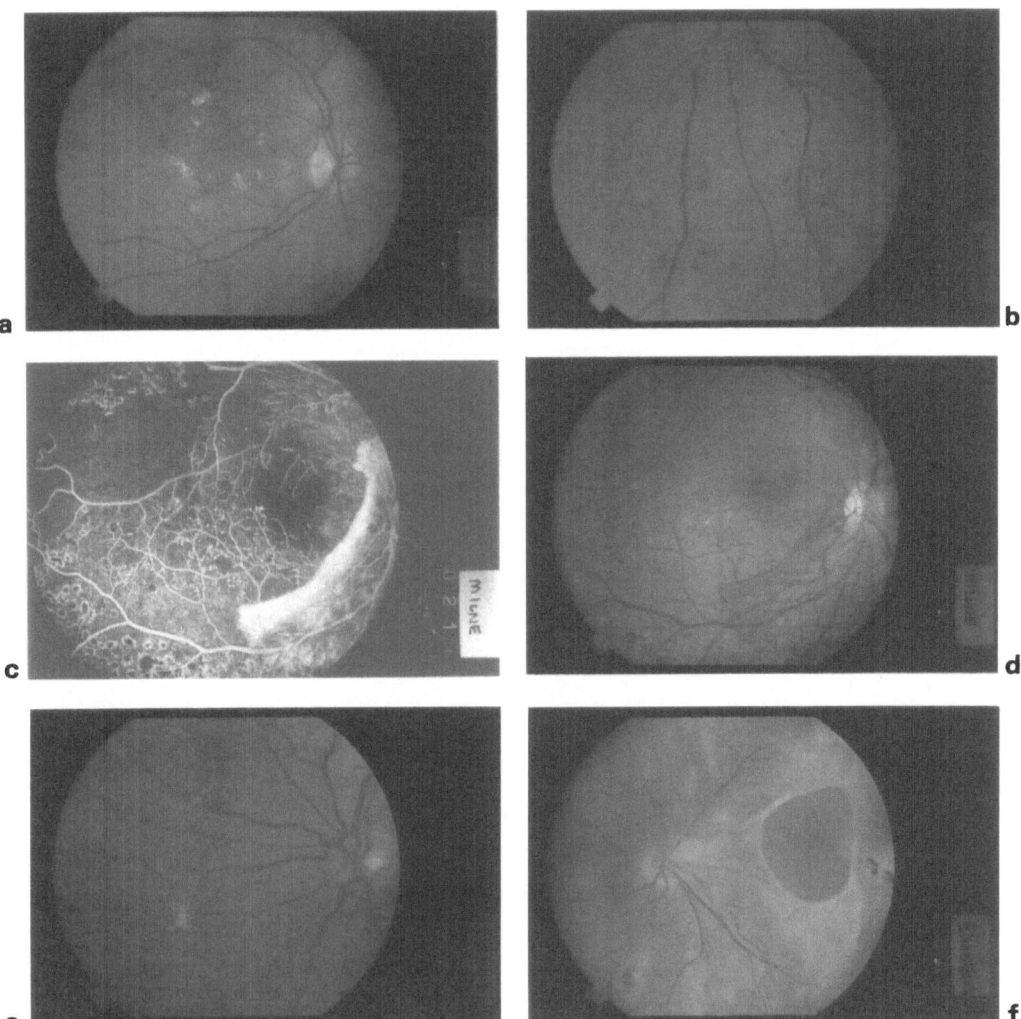

Fig. 17.1a–f. a, Background diabetic retinopathy; **b**, preproliferative – ischaemic; **c**, preproliferative – venous beading; **d**, proliferative – NVD; **e**, proliferative – NVE; **f**, fluorescein angiography: ischaemia. Colour reproduction sponsored by Lipha Pharmaceuticals Ltd.

pericytes is thought to have a permissive effect for the development of local microvascular dilatation leading to microaneurysms. In addition, the endothelium, which has been damaged as a result of prolonged hyperglycaemia and hyperlipidaemia, by mechanisms possibly involving aldose reductase (Kennedy et al. 1983), becomes permeable to proteins and other plasma constituents (exudates and haemorrhages).

Retinal neovascularization occurs later, almost as a secondary event. The damaged endothelium loses its non-thrombogenic properties on its luminal surface and intravascular microthrombi ensue. Retinal ischaemia is a prerequisite for diabetic neovascularization and new vessels develop within retinal tissue that is relatively well perfused. Neovascularization can therefore be viewed as a modified "repair mechanism" and is similar to other forms of angiogenesis which require alteration in growth control of vascular endothelium.

Angiogenesis involves a series of discrete changes in existing vasculature (D'Amore 1987). Alterations in the vascular basement membrane associated with changes in the shape of endothelial cells permit the cells to invade and adhere to the extracellular matrix. In a suitable environment the cells migrate away from the vessel and form cords of advancing cells within the tissues (Folkman 1982). Meanwhile cells downstream of the leading cells undergo proliferation and contribute to the advancing cord of cells. We have shown that retinal capillary endothelial (RCE) cells and pericytes migrate preferentially on a fibronectin-rich matrix, while proliferation of RCE cells may occur in both fibronectin and collagen as long as there is a source of growth factors, e.g. from serum or from damaged tissue (McIntosh et al. 1988). Eventually, the cord of cells undergoes tube formation while its leading tip orients towards and fuses with a similar neighbouring cord of cells to form a capillary loop.

The initial degradation of the vascular basement membrane is believed to result from plasmin-mediated conversion of procollagenase to the active enzyme collagenase (Taylor and Weiss 1985) which is then free to act on the collagenous matrix of the basement membrane. Plasmin is generated locally from plasminogen which itself is catalysed by plasminogen activator (PA) released from the endothelial cell. Normally plasminogen activator activity is regulated by plasminogen activator inhibitor (PAI-1) but these relationships may be disturbed in diabetes (Brownlee and Cerami 1981).

Angiogenesis generally is under the control of local and systemic factors. The requirement for growth factors in retinal angiogenesis was first proposed by Michaelson (1948) who suggested that there was a diffusable factor in ischaemic retina which stimulated angiogenesis. Recently, two forms of angiogenic factors have been identified in retina: (a) heparin-binding growth factors (Baird et al. 1985), similar to acidic and basic fibroblast growth factor (Mr 14–18 K) and (b) a low-molecular-weight angiogenic factor (Elstow et al. 1985) which has not yet been characterized.

The remarkable structural similarity between local retina-derived heparin-binding growth factor (HBGF) and hypothalamus-derived growth factor has provided an important link between systemic, particularly hormonal, factors and locally produced factors in the initiation of angiogenesis (D'Amore and Klagsburn 1984). Indeed it has been suggested that release of HBGF from the hypothalamus into the circulation may initiate or perpetuate PDR. Other associations between the hypothalamic–pituitary axis and diabetic retinopathy are long established. For instance, growth-hormone-deficient diabetic dwarfs appear to be protected from retinopathy in spite of prolonged duration of hyperglycaemia (Merimee et al. 1970). Growth hormone contains a diabetogenic fragment (Lostroh and Krahl 1974) which is released from the single-chain molecule after limited proteolysis with pepsin (Lohstroh and Krahl, 1976). The effects of the peptide are long-lasting, even after a single dose of 30–40 mmol in mice. These effects are relevant to periods of increased growth activity (e.g. puberty, pregnancy) and may account for an increased association with PDR during these times. Exercise-induced elevated growth hormone levels have been found in patients with longstanding diabetes both with (Lundbaeck et al. 1970; Passa et al. 1974) and without retinopathy (Sundkvist et al. 1984) and have been correlated with elevated Factor VIII-related antigen (VIII R:Ag) and plasmino-gen activator levels (Sundkvist et al. 1984), evidence which points towards a microangiopathic effect.

The physiological effect of growth hormone are mediated through a second group of hormones, insulin-like growth factors (IGF) or somatomedins. Growth hormone causes release of IGF-I (somatomedin C), a 70-amino-acid molecule (Jansen et al. 1983), from stores in the liver whence it initiates growth of peripheral tissues. IGF-I is also secreted by a variety of other tissues and cells and may therefore have an autocrine or paracrine function, i.e. by acting locally at sites of secretion (Mathews et al. 1986). Conflicting data on the levels of plasma IGF-I in diabetes have been reported (Cohen et al. 1977; Nash 1979; Winter et al. 1979). Amiel et al. (1984) reported that in young diabetics IGF-I levels were reduced in spite of elevated levels of growth hormone, and the reduced IGF-I correlated with poor metabolic control. They suggested that hypersecretion of growth hormone was caused by a negative feedback mechanism relating to reduced synthesis of IGF-I by the liver. Similar studies in rats have indicated that low levels of IGF-I are due to a postreceptor mechanism involving resistance to growth hormone stimulation (Maes et al. 1986). In contrast, Merimee et al. (1983) found that patients with PDR, particularly of the accelerated variety, had elevated levels of IGF-I. Amiel et al. (1984) suggested that this may have been a secondary effect consequent upon tightened metabolic control in patients with worsening retinopathy. However, further studies have shown that IGF-I levels are elevated in the vitreous of eyes from patients with PDR compared with non-diabetic vitreous (Grant et al. 1986). Locally elevated IGF-I could stimulate angiogenesis, particularly since IGF-1 has been shown to be chemotactic for retinal capillary endothelial cells in vitro (Grant et al. 1987).

Other hormones, including pregnancy hormones, disturb carbohydrate meta-bolism and may therefore have a direct or indirect synergistic effect on diabetic retinopathy. During pregnancy the anterior lobe of the pituitary hypertrophies and there are increased levels of ACTH and aldosterone (Cugini et al. 1987). In addition, during the later stages of pregnancy, placental production of progester-one and oestrogen greatly increases. Although oestrogen has no significant effect on carbohydrate metabolism (it may even have a slight hypoglycaemic effect) (Kalkhoff 1975), progesterone impairs glucose tolerance and increases the insulin requirement for good diabetic control in pregnancy (Kalkhoff et al. 1970). This effect may in part be due to "insulin resistance" or may be a direct inhibitory effect on insulin release from the pancreas (Neilsen 1984). Whether these effects on glucose metabolism affect retinopathy is not clear, but pregnant diabetics with retinopathy have higher levels of serum progesterone during the first and second trimesters compared with pregnant diabetics without retinopathy (Larinkari et al.

1982). Such patients also have elevated levels of placental lactogen (HPL) compared with control pregnant diabetics without retinopathy. This may have a more direct influence on PDR since HPL substitutes for growth hormone during the later stages of pregnancy and generates elevated levels of IGF-I (Bala et al. 1981; Teale and Marks 1986). Diabetic placental tissue expresses greater levels of both IGF-I mRNA (Mills 1985) and IGF-II (Shen et al. 1986). Human placental lactogen may generate IGF-I release in an autocrine manner similar to the effects of growth hormone (Strain et al. 1987).

Numerous other serum and platelet release factors are elevated in diabetics and also in pregnancy, and are directly associated with retinopathy. These include fibrinogen and Factor VIII antigen (Almer et al. 1975), beta-thromboglobulin and platelet factor 4 (Borsey et al. 1980; Sacchi et al. 1985) while endothelial cells may secrete decreased levels of the anti-thrombogenic agent, prostacyclin (Paton et al. 1982). Plasma fibronectin levels are decreased in diabetics while tissue fibrinectin appears to be increased (Labat-Robert et al. 1984). This may be important for PDR since fibronectin is a requirement for capillary endothelial cell migration (McIntosh et al. 1988). Diabetics with severe retinopathy have increased blood viscosity which may be in part due to elevated fibrinogen (Dintenfass 1977) plus platelet abnormalities. Hyperlipidaemia (Kohner and Oakley 1975) and hypertension, even of short duration (West 1978), may contribute to the progression of retinopathy and clearly the latter is important to pregnant diabetics with or without renal disease and pre-eclampsia.

Pregnancy is also associated with marked changes in blood volume and flow through the tissues. In addition, hyperglycaemia causes changes in haemodynamics (Parving et al. 1983; Yoshida et al. 1983) and these have been implicated in the microangiopathy not only in the eye but also in the kidney (Zatz et al. 1985). The increased blood flow in vessels which are unable to compensate due to impaired autoregulation (Rhie et al. 1982; Kastrup et al. 1986) may be sufficient to initiate a sequence of events leading to retinal ischaemia and subsequent PDR.

There are thus many possible mechanisms whereby diabetics in pregnancy are more likely to develop deteriorating background retinopathy and to precipitate PDR.

Epidemiology of Diabetic Retinopathy

The clinical evidence for deterioration in diabetic retinopathy during pregnancy has, however, come under scrutiny in recent years. This is because reliable epidemiological data on the natural history of diabetic retinopathy have accrued in the last 5 years (Rand et al. 1985; Kuniman et al. 1986; Krolewski et al. 1986). It is now clear that the single most important risk factor for the development of retinopathy in type I diabetes is duration of diabetes. The incidence of background retinopathy accumulates in a linear manner after an initial retinopathy-free phase of about 4–5 years (Palmberg et al. 1981; Klein et al. 1984; Kuniman et al. 1986) and reaches a prevalence of about 90% after 15 years of diabetes. Chronic exposure to endothelial-cell-damaging factor(s) provided this is above some as yet unknown threshold, is clearly sufficient to initiate background retinopathy (Krolewski et al. 1986). The relationship of duration of diabetes to PDR is less clear. Onset of PDR occurs later than background retinopathy (around 10 years later on average) and there is a progressive increase in the number of cases with a prevalence of about 60% after 40 years (Klein et al. 1984). However, although there is a linear rise in yearly incidence rate of PDR after approximately 7–8 years, after 15 years the annual rate of new cases remains the same (Krolewski et al. 1986). Therefore, while all patients are susceptible to PDR, some additional factor is required which upregulates the intensity of exposure to the retinopathy-inducing factor, thereby initiating PDR. This additional factor could be one of several events which are not known to alter the risk of PDR e.g. puberty, pregnancy, hypertension, renal disease, poor glycaemic control, etc. Therefore a specific retinopathy-worsening effect of pregnancy per se need not apply in order to cause deterioration.

Similar studies on the development of retinopathy in childhood and adolescence have shown the same correlation with duration of diabetes although the initial lag phase is slightly longer (5 years) (Burger et al. 1986). In addition, the risk of early retinopathy decreases with the earlier age of onset of diabetes. These data suggest that growth affords some protection against the development of retinopathy and are therefore relevant to retinopathy in pregnancy since most pregnant diabetics who are at risk of PDR have developed diabetes in childhood or adolescence (see below).

Epidemiology of Diabetic Retinopathy in Pregnancy

Data from the initial studies by Beetham (1950) and White (1965) were gathered at a time when epidemiological information on the natural history of diabetic retinopathy was not available. Several recent studies have examined this problem and conflicting reports have emerged regarding the question of whether diabetic retinopathy worsens during pregnancy. It is important to define the nature of the retinopathy before attempting to provide answers. There are several aspects of the problem to be addressed; e.g. does pregnancy (a) induce retinopathy, (b) worsen background retinopathy, (c) worsen proliferative retinopathy or (d) convert background to proliferative retinopathy? The available data now suggest that pregnancy per se does not induce retinopathy in otherwise normal eyes.

Three recent prospective studies of retinopathy, one of which included a control non-pregnant group of patients, indicate that deterioration of background retinopathy occurs during pregnancy (Moloney and Drury 1982; Van Ohrt 1984; Serup 1986) while other studies did not detect this change (Cassar et

Table 17.2. Diabetic retinopathy worsens during pregnancy: a review of published data

		Background	PDR
Cassar	1978	No	No
Horvat	1980	No	No
Moloney	1982	Yes	Yes
Price	1984	No	Yes
Van Ohrt	1984	Yes	No
Serup	1986	Yes	No

al. 1978; Horvat et al. 1980) (Table 17.2). In contrast, few studies have found that progression of PDR occurs at a greater rate during pregnancy than would be expected in non-pregnant diabetics with PDR. Data on the conversion of background retinopathy to PDR are difficult to establish. In a retrospective analysis of 197 pregnant diabetics in Aberdeen during 1979–1987 we have detected seven patients who progressed from background retinopathy (White class D) to PDR (White class R) (Table 17.3). All of these patients plus four other patients who had PDR prior to pregnancy, had had diabetes for at least 10 years (Table 17.4) with onset during adolescence or childhood. The percentage of cases with PDR from this population of patients with 10 years or longer duration of diabetes was 10.6%. The predicted prevalence of PDR in a population of this size is 11.4% after 10 years of diabetes (Krolewski et al. 1986) which is not significantly different. These data suggest that pregnancy per se may not increase the risk of PDR. However, this does not preclude the possibility that pregnancy acts as one of several triggering events which can convert background retinopathy to PDR (see above).

Table 17.3. Diabetic retinopathy in pregnancy: Aberdeen experience (1979–1987)

No. of patients	White[a] class	Retinopathy at onset	Progression to PDR
35	A	None	None
67	B	None	None
58	C	None	1 (IRMA)
32	D	Background	7
5	F/R	PDR	—

[a] White (1965); classified at first visit to combined pregnancy/diabetic clinic.

Table 17.4. Proliferative diabetic retinopathy in pregnancy (Aberdeen, 1979–1987)

Patient no.	Duration of diabetes (years)	Age at diagnosis
1	22	2
2	24	7
3	15	10
4	15	10
5	14	12
6	22	4
7	17	11
8	16	15
9	29	6
10	26	8
11	25	6

The apparent progression of background retinopathy during pregnancy (see Table 17.2) requires an explanation, as does the finding from prospective studies that these changes regress after pregnancy (Moloney and Drury 1982; Van Ohrt 1984; Serup 1986). Recent data have shown that rapid tightening of glycaemic control in diabetes causes initial deterioration in retinopathy, evidenced by ischaemic changes in the retina (Lauritzen et al. 1983; Kroc Collaborative Study 1984; Dahl-Jorgensen et al. 1985; Engerman and Kern 1987; Helve et al. 1987) although the long-term results suggest that tight control is beneficial. Phelps et al. (1986) correlated glycaemic control with retinopathy during pregnancy and suggested that the deterioration in background retinopathy was due to tighter control and not to the pregnancy. It is normal practice in most prepregnancy diabetic clinics to "improve" overall diabetic control, and this correlation therefore seems logical. Analysis of previous studies (e.g. Moloney and Drury 1982) indicates that ischaemic changes significantly correlated with more normal blood sugar levels and indeed, the first report by Lawrence (1948) of deterioration of retinopathy during pregnancy occurred in a woman who underwent a period of "diabetic stabilization".

It is not known how better diabetic control initially worsens retinopathy. However, poorly controlled diabetics are known to have elevated plasma growth hormone (GH) levels but reduced IGF-I values. When the diabetes is normalized, GH levels also return to normal while there is a compensatory overproduction of IGF-I (Amiel et al. 1984). This may temporarily increase the likelihood of retinopathy (see above, role of IGF-I in retinopathy).

The conclusions from these studies are that deterioration of background retinopathy during pregnancy is probably due to rapid tightening of diabetic control, while the development of PDR in pregnancy is only likely to occur in patients with existing background retinopathy who have had diabetes for at least 10 years duration. Proliferative diabetic retinopathy developing during pregnancy will take its natural course if untreated as in non-pregnant diabetics, i.e. it progresses over a matter of weeks to severe visual loss with blindness in at least 50% of cases. Proliferative diabetic retinopathy therefore requires active intervention.

Approach to Management of Diabetic Retinopathy in Pregnancy

Beetham (1950) proposed that termination of pregnancy was indicated in diabetics whose retinopathy was progressing, because all patients experienced visual loss and the incidence of perinatal deaths was very high. However, although there was no adequate therapy for PDR, White (1965) challenged this advice and suggested that termination was not indicated. Recent epidemiological data plus improvements in therapy for PDR and survival of diabetic neonates have radically altered the approach to the management of diabetic retinopathy in pregnancy.

Patients with diabetes for longer than 10 years and with background retinopathy should be regularly monitored by ophthalmoscopy throughout the pregnancy. Care should be taken to avoid a too rapid improvement in the control of their diabetes in the prepregnancy clinic. If ischaemic changes develop in the retina, fluorescein angiography may be of value in determining the extent of retinal involvement which might predict the risk of PDR. Preproliferative changes should be carefully sought, e.g. venous beading and dilatation, intraretinal microvascular abnormalities (IRMA), macular oedema, etc.

Frank new vessels on the disc (NVD) or elsewhere (NVE) should be treated urgently and aggressively with laser energy panretinal ablation (PRA) while they are still flat, i.e. on the retinal surface. Panretinal ablation may require 2000–4000 500-micron laser burns to induce regression of NVD or NVE, and if this is not sufficient, treated areas of retina should be retreated. Such therapy is no less effective in PDR during pregnancy than in PDR in other patients (Hercules et al. 1980; Price et al. 1984). Unfortunately, some of these patients may experience persistent loss of central vision, which is due to ischaemic maculopathy with or without oedema and which generally does not respond to laser therapy, although it may improve after delivery (Sinclair et al. 1984).

Forward new vessels indicate that vitreous detachment has occurred, i.e. that the vitreous gel has separated from the retinal surface and has drawn the immature adherent retinal vessels forward into the vitreous cavity. Vitreous detachment is often incomplete and continued traction on the vessels is likely to produce vitreous haemorrhage. Partial vitreous detachment has been shown to be a significant factor for progression of PDR compared with no vitreous detachment or with complete vitreous detachment (Takahashi et al. 1981). There is also the dilemma of whether or not to treat forward NV with PRA since induced regression of the vessels will cause counter-traction with areas of vessel–vitreous adhesion. Thus the treatment itself at this stage may cause vitreous haemorrhage.

The inexorable progression of PDR with partial vitreous detachment leads to traction on the retina which may encroach on the macula. An unstable retinopathy of this nature with extensive preretinal gliosis probably requires vitrectomy. Such conditions should be treated prior to pregnancy. If they develop during pregnancy they usually occur late in the last trimester and can be treated surgically after delivery since some degree of spontaneous regression (or stabilization) due to complete vitreous detachment will occur in this period.

Conclusion

The traditional concept of pregnancy inducing deterioration of diabetic retinopathy should be reviewed in the light of recent epidemiological data. Progression of ischaemic retinopathy may be due to tightening of diabetic control in pregnancy and usually reverts to normal after delivery. The incidence of PDR is probably not greater than can be expected within this age group of diabetics of long duration. Progression of PDR during pregnancy also follows a predictable pattern and is dependent more on vitreous changes than on other factors. Proliferative diabetic retinopathy with flat NVD or NVE should therefore be treated as aggressively in pregnant as in non-pregnant individuals.

Hormonal factors are probably important in determining that pregnancy can act as a secondary trigger for PDR. Similar changes occur during puberty and may be aggravated by the action of progesterone or carbohydrate metabolism. Progesterone-containing oral contraceptives may have a similar effect on retinopathy in diabetics and their use in such patients should be carefully monitored.

Acknowledgements. This work was supported by a grant from the British Diabetic Association to Professor J. V. Forrester. Lipha Pharmaceuticals contributed generously to the preparation of the colour illustrations.

References

Almer L-O, Pandolfi M, Milsson IM (1975) Diabetic retinopathy and the fibrinolytic system. Diabetes 24:529–541

Amiel SAJ, Sherwin RS, Hintz RL, Gertner JM, Press CM, Tamborline WV (1984) Effect of diabetes and its control on insulin-like growth factors in the young subject with Type I diabetes. Diabetes 33:1175–1179

Ashton N (1983) Pathogenesis of diabetic retinopathy. In: Little HL, Jack RL, Patz A, Forsham PH (eds) Diabetic retinopathy. Thieme-Stratton, New York, pp 85–97

Baird A, Esch F, Gospodarowicz D, Guillemin R (1985) Retina- and eye-derived endothelial growth factors: partial molecular characterisation and identity with acidic and basic fibroblast growth factors. Biochemistry 24:7855–7860

Bala RM, Lopatka J, Leung A et al. (1981) Serum immunoreactive somatomedin levels in normal adults, pregnant women at term, children at various ages and children with constitutionally delayed growth. J Clin Endocrinol Metab 52:508–512

Beetham WP (1950) Diabetic retinopathy in10pregnancy. Trans Am Ophthalmol Soc 48:205–211

Borsey DQ, Dawes J, Fraser DM, Prowse CV, Elton RA, Clarke BF (1980) Plasma betathromboglo-bulin in diabetes mellitus. Diabetologia 18:353–357

Brownlee M, Cerami A (1981) The biochemistry of the complications of diabetes mellitus. Annu Rev Biochem 50:385–432

Burger W, Hovener G, Dusterhus R, Hartmann R, Weber B (1986) Prevalence and development of retinopathy in children and adolescents with Type I (insulin dependent) diabetes mellitus. A longitudinal study. Diabetologia 29:17–22

Cassar J, Kohner EM, Hamilton AM, Gordon H, Joplin GF (1978) Diabetic retinopathy and pregnancy. Diabetologia 15:105–111

Cogan DG, Toussaint D, Kuwabara T (1961) Retinal vascular patterns. IV. Diabetic retinopathy. Arch Ophthalmol 66:366–378

Cohen MP, Jasti K, Rye DL (1977) Somatomedin in insulin dependent diabetes mellitus. J Clin Endocrinol Metab 60:648–657

Cugini P, Letizia C, Murano G (1987) Increased serum aldosterone in diabetic pregnancy. Diabetologia 30:166–168

Dahl-Jorgensen K, Brinchmann-Hansen O, Hanssen KF, Sandvik L, Aagenaes O (1985) Rapid tightening of blood glucose control leads to transient deterioration of retinopathy in insulin dependent diabetes mellitus: the Oslo Study. Br Med J 290:811–815

D'Amore P (1987) Mechanisms of angiogenesis. Annu Rev Physiol 49:453–464

D'Amore PA, Klagsburn M (1984) Endothelial cell mitogens derived from retina and hypothalamus: biochemical and biological similarities. J Cell Biol 99:1545–1549

Dintenfass L (1977) Blood viscosity factors in severe non diabetic and diabetic retinopathy. Biorheology 14:151–157

Elstow SF, Schor AM, Weiss JB (1985) Bovine retinal angiogenesis factor is a small molecule (molecular mass <600). Invest Ophthalmol Vis Sci 26:74–79

Engerman RL, Kern TS (1987) Progression of incipient diabetic retinopathy during good glycemic control. Diabetes 36:808–812

Folkman J (1982) Angiogenesis: initiation and control. Ann NY Acad Sci 401:212–227

Forrester JV (1987) Mechanisms in the formation of new vessels in the retina. Diab Med 4:423–431

Grant M, Russel B, Fitzgerald C, Merimee TJ (1986) Insulin-like growth factors in the vitreous. Studies in control and diabetic subjects with neovascularisation. Diabetes 35:416–420

Grant M, Jordan R, Merimee TJ (1987) Insulin-like growth factor 1 modulates endothelial cell chemotaxis. J Clin Endocrinol Metab 65:370–371

Helve E, Laatikainen L, Merennines L, Koivisto VA (1987) Continuous insulin infusion therapy in patients with Type 1 diabetes. Acta Endocrinol 115:313–319

Hercules B, Wozencroft M, Gayel IJ, Jeacock J (1980) Peripheral retinal ablation in the treatment of proliferative diabetic retinopathy during pregnancy. Br J Ophthalmol 64:87–93

Horvat M, MacLean H, Goldberg L, Crock GW (1980) Diabetic retinopathy in pregnancy: a 12 year prospective survey. Br J Ophthalmol 64:398–403

Jansen M, van Schaik FMA, Ricker AT et al. (1983) Sequence of cDNA encoding human insulin-like growth factor I precursor. Nature 306:609–611

Kalkhoff RK (1975) Effects of oral contraceptive agents on carbohydrate metabolism. J Steroid Biochem 6:949–956

Kalkhoff RK, Jacobson M, Lemper D (1970) Progesterone, pregnancy and the augmented plasma insulin response. J Clin Endocrinol Metab 31:24–28

Kastrup J, Rorsgaard S, Parving HH, Lassen MA (1986) Impaired regulation of cerebral blood flow in long-term Type 1 (insulin-dependent) diabetic patients with nephropathy and retinopathy. Clin Physiol 6:549–559

Kennedy A, Frank RN, Varma SD (1983) Aldose reductase activity in retinal and cerebral microvessels and cultured microvascular cells. Invest Ophthalmol Vis Sci 24:1250–1258

Klein R, Klein BEK, Moss SE, Davis MD, De Mets DL (1984) The Wisconsin Epidemiological Study of Diabetic Retinopathy when age at diagnosis is less than 30 years. Arch Ophthalmol 102:520–526

Kohner EM, Oakley NW (1975) Diabetic retinopathy. Metabolism 24:1085–1102

Kroc Collaborative Study (1984) Blood glucose control and the evolution of diabetic retinopathy and albuminuria. N Engl J Med 311:365–372

Krolewski AS, Warram JH, Rand LI, Christlieb AR, Busick EJ, Kahn CR (1986) Risk of proliferative diabetic retinopathy in juvenile-onset Type I diabetes: a 40 year follow-up study. Diabetes Care 9:443–452

Kuniman MW, Welborn TA, McCann VJ, Stanton KG, Constable IJ (1986) Multiple factors in the prediction of risk of proliferative diabetic retinopathy. N Engl J Med 313:1433–1438

Labat-Robert J, Leutenegger M, Llopis G, Ricard Y, Derouette J-C (1984) Plasma and tissue fibronectin in diabetes. Clin Physiol Biochem 2:39–48

Larinkari J, Laatikainen L, Ranta T, Moronen P, Pesonen K, Laatikainen T (1982) Metabolic control and serum hormone levels in relation to retinopathy in diabetic pregnancy. Diabetologia 22:327–332

Lauritzen T, Frost-Larsen K, Larsen H-W, Decker T (1983) Steno Study Group. Effect of one year of near-normal blood glucose levels on retinopathy in insulin-dependent diabetics. Lancet I:200–204

Lawrence RD (1948) Acute retinopathy without hyperpiesis in diabetic pregnancy. Br J Ophthalmol 32:461–465

Lostroh AJ Krahl ME (1974) A hyperglycemic peptide from pituitary growth hormone: preparation with pepsin and assay in ob/ob mice. Proc Natl Acad Sci USA 71:1244–1246

Lostroh AJ, Krahl ME (1976) Diabetogenic peptide from human growth hormone: partial purification from peptic digest and long-term action in ob/ob mice. Proc Natl Acad Sci USA 73:4706–4710

Lundbaeck K, Christiansen MJ, Jensen VA et al. (1970) Diabetes, diabetic angiopathy and growth hormone. Lancet II:131–133

Maes M, Underwood LE, Ketelslegers J-M (1986) Low serum somatomedin-C in insulin-dependent diabetes: evidence for a post-receptor mechanism. Endocrinology 118:377–382

Mathews LS, Morstedt G, Palmitter RD (1986) Regulation of insulin-like growth factor I gene expression by growth hormone. Proc Natl Acad Sci USA 83:9343–9347

McIntosh L, Muckersie L, Forrester JV (1988) Retinal capillary endothelial cells prefer different substrates for growth and migration. Tissue Cell 20 (in press)

Merimee TJ, Fineberg SE, McKusick VA et al. (1970) Diabetes mellitus and ateliotic dwarfism; a comparative study. J Clin Invest 49:1096–1102

Merimee TJ, Zapf J, Froesch ER (1983) Insulin-like growth factors: studies in diabetics with and without retinopathy. N Engl J Med 309:527–530

Michaelson IC (1948) The mode of development of retinal vessels. Trans Ophthalmol Soc UK 68:137–180

Mills NC, Gyves MT, Ilan J (1985) Mol Cell Endocrinol 39:61–69

Moloney JBM, Drury MI (1982) The effect of pregnancy on the natural course of diabetic retinopathy. Am J Ophthalmol 93:745–756

Nash H (1979) Growth failure, somatomedin and growth hormone levels in juvenile diabetes mellitus: a pilot study. Aust NZ J Med 45:236–239

Neilsen JH (1984) Direct effect of gonadal and contraceptive steroids on insulin release from mouse pancreatic islets in organ culture. Acta Endocrinol 105:245–250

Oakley W (1953) Prognosis in diabetic pregnancy. Br Med J 1:1413–1415

Orlidge A, D'Amore PA (1987) Inhibition of capillary endothelial cell growth by pericytes and smooth muscle cells. J Cell Biol 105:1455–1462

Palmberg P, Smith M, Waltman S et al. (1981) The natural history of retinopathy in insulin dependent juvenile onset diabetes. Ophthalmology 88:613–618

Parving HH, Viberti GC, Keen H, Christiansen JS, Lassen NA (1983) Haemodynamic factors in the genesis of diabetic macroangiopathy. Metabolism 32:943–949

Passa P, Ganville C, Canivet J (1974) Influence of muscular exercise on plasma level of growth hormone in diabetics with and without retinopathy. Lancet II:72–74

Paton RC, Guillot R, Passa P, Canivet J (1982) Prostacyclin production by human endothelial cells cultured in diabetic serum. Diabete Metab 8:323–328

Phelps RL, Sakol P, Metzger BE, Jampol LM, Freinkel N (1986) Changes in diabetic retinopathy during pregnancy. Correlations with regulation of hyperglycemia. Arch Ophthalmol 104:1806–1810

Price JH, Hadden DR, Archer DB, Harley J (1984) Diabetic retinopathy in pregnancy. Br J Obstet Gynecol 91:11–17

Rand LI, Krolewski AS, Aiello LM, Warram JH, Baker RS, Maki T (1985) Multiple factors in the prediction of risk of proliferative diabetic retinopathy. N Engl J Med 313:1433–1438

Rhie FH, Christlieb AR, Sandor T et al. (1982) Retinal vascular reactivity to norepinephrine and angiotensin II in normals and diabetics. Diabetes 31:1056–1060

Sacchi S, Curci L, Piccinini L et al. (1985) Platelet granule release in diabetes mellitus. Scand J Clin Lab Invest 45:165–168

Serup L (1986) Influence of pregnancy on diabetic retinopathy. Acta Endocrinol (Suppl) 277:122–124

Shen S-J, Wang C-Y, Nebson KK, Jansen M, Ilan J (1986) Expression of insulin-like growth factor II in human placentas from normal and diabetic pregnancies. Proc Natl Acad Sci USA 83:9179–9182

Sinclair SH, Nesler C, Foxman B, Nichols CW, Grabbe S (1984) Macular oedema and pregnancy in insulin-dependent diabetes. Am J Ophthalmol 97:154–167

Stephens JW, Page OC, Hare RL (1963) Diabetes and pregnancy. A report of experience in 119 pregnancies over a period of ten years. Diabetes 12:213–219

Strain A, Hill DJ, Swenne I, Milner RDG (1987) Regulation of DNA synthesis in human fetal hepatocytes by placental lactogen, growth hormone and insulin-like growth factor I/somatomedin C. J Cell Physiol 132:33–40

Sundkvist G, Almer L-O, Lilja B, Pandolfi M (1984) Growth hormone and endothelial function during exercise in diabetics with and without retinopathy. Acta Med Scand 215:55–61

Takahashi M, Trempe CL, Maguire K, McMeel JW (1981) Vitreoretinal relationship in diabetic retinopathy. A biomicroscopic evaluation. Arch Ophthalmol 99:241–245

Taylor CM, Weiss JB (1985) Partial purification of a 5.7 K glycoprotein from bovine vitreous which inhibits both angiogenesis and collagenase activity. Biochem Biophys Res Commun 133:911–916

Teale JD, Marks V (1986) The measurement of insulin-like growth factor 1: clinical applications and significance. Ann Clin Biochem 23:413–424

Van Ohrt (1984) The influence of pregnancy on diabetic retinopathy with special regard to the reversible changes shown in 100 pregnancies. Acta Ophthalmol 62:603–616

West KM (1978) Epidemiology of diabetes and its vascular lesions. Elsevier, New York p. 425

White P (1965) Pregnancy and diabetes: medical aspects. Med Clin North Am 49:1015–1024

Winter RJ, Phillips LS, Klein MN, Traisman HS, Green OC (1979) Somatomedin activity and diabetic control in children with insulin-dependent diabetes. Diabetes 28:952–954

Yoshida A, Feke GT, Morales-Stoppello J, Collas GD, Gioger DG, McMeal JW (1983) Retinal blood flow alterations during progression of diabetic retinopathy. Arch Ophthalmol 101:225–227

Zatz R, Meyer TW, Rennke HG, Brenner BM (1985) Predominance of hemodynamic rather than metabolic factors in the pathogenesis of diabetic glomerulopathy. Proc Natl Acad Sci 82:5963–5967

18. Screening and Management of Gestational Diabetes Mellitus

M. Maresh and R. W. Beard

Screening for Gestational Diabetes

The principal criteria for a screening test are that it should be simple and inexpensive to perform with a high sensitivity and specificity for the condition. In the case of gestational diabetes the screening test is a glucose tolerance test (GTT).

Glycosuria

Almost all women are screened for abnormal glucose tolerance during pregnancy by one means or another. The most basic test is looking for glycosuria, but this will only detect major degrees of abnormality since the renal threshold is about 10 mmol/l. Sutherland et al. (1970) found that 11% of an unselected obstetric population of 1418 women had random glycosuria, but less than 1% of those with glycosuria had an abnormal GTT.

Potential Diabetic Features

The next refinement is to use the presence of "potential diabetic features" as the screening method. The following features are generally agreed upon: first-degree relative with diabetes; obesity (over 20% ideal body weight or maternal weight greater than 90 kg during pregnancy); previous overweight baby (greater than 4.0–4.5 kg); unexplained stillbirth or neonatal death; and a history of latent diabetes (e.g. during pregnancy, illness or oral contraceptive usage). This may lead to an excessive number of glucose tolerance tests being required, 37% of the whole obstetric population according to O'Sullivan et al. (1973) and 35% according to Gillmer et al. (1980). In contrast Hadden (1980) only found 8.5% requiring a GTT in his antenatal population, reflecting a different community mix. Whilst it is impractical to subject one-third of pregnant women to glucose tolerance tests, testing up to 10% should be feasible. However, about one-third of women with abnormal GTTs do not have potential diabetic features (O'Sullivan et al. 1973; Gillmer et al. 1980) and so other methods of screening have been investigated.

Response to Glucose Load

A widely accepted method, although one not widely used in the United Kingdom, is the one proposed by O'Sullivan et al. (1973). It is the method recommended by the Second International Workshop Conference on Gestational Diabetes (1985). A 50-g oral glucose load is given irrespective of time and a 1-h venous plasma glucose of 7.8 mmol/l or more indicates the need for a full GT. This will result in about 8% of women requiring a GTT (Beard et al. 1980). The ideal time for performing this test is at 28 weeks gestation when a venepuncture is usually performed anyway. However, O'Sullivan et al. (1973) in 752 GTTs found that 21% of those with an abnormal GTT had had a normal screen (a test sensitivity of 79%). Lowering the cut-off to 7.4 mmol/l will reduce this, but increase the proportion of women requiring GTTs to 25% (Carpenter and Coustan 1982). In an attempt to decrease the amount of screening it has been suggested that only those over 25 years old should be screened, but this will reduce the overall sensitivity to 74%.

An alternative screening method has been to assess the response to a mixed meal – "the breakfast tolerance test" (Coustan et al. 1987), but the preliminary results do not suggest any significant advantage.

Random Blood Glucose

Rather than give a glucose load Lind (1985) advocated relating the venous blood glucose concentration to the time of the last meal. He established a range of normal values according to the length of time from eating and simplified it by taking the 99th percentile for those who had eaten less than 2 h before (6.4 mmol/l) and those who had eaten more than 2 h before (5.8 mmol/l). He applied this to his population and only 2.3% screened positive. Only 1.3% (34) actually went on to have GTTs but using WHO criteria four had diabetes and 14 impaired glucose tolerance (IGT). Unfortunately no data are available on sensitivity and specificity and a prevalence of IGT of only 0.33% suggests cases were missed. Indeed a study by Jowett et al. (1987) has compared this screening test with a glucose tolerance test and has concluded that sensitivity and specificity make it an unacceptable screening method for either IGT or diabetes. Similar results have been reported by Nasrat et al. (1988).

Potential Diabetic Features and Fasting Blood Glucose

A method of improving the use of "potential diabetic features" by including a fasting glucose concentration has been used for many years by the Copenhagen group (Mortensen et al. 1985). Using a fasting blood glucose cut-off of 4.1 mmol/l produces a sensitivity of over 90% although specificity is reduced. Jowett et al. (1987) applied this method to their data and found similar results (sensitivity 92%, specificity 49%). Before recommending this method it would need to be evaluated further in other populations.

Glycated Haemoglobin and Proteins

A different approach to screening has been to measure glycated haemoglobin which is an indicator of plasma glucose concentrations over the previous 2 months. However, it has not been possible to find a cut-off point that would differentiate between normal and abnormal glucose tolerance (Shah et al. 1982; Artal et al. 1984; Bacigalupo et al. 1984; Cousins et al. 1984; McFarland et al. 1984; Ross 1984; Frisoli et al. 1987). This may be because the fasting glucose concentration may not be elevated or because the short duration of the condition does not give time for increased glycation to be apparent. Glycosylation of serum proteins should be a better indicator since it reflects a shorter period, but the initial promising reports (Roberts et al. 1983) have not been substantiated (McFarland et al. 1984; Ryan et al. 1987).

Conclusion

The 50-g glucose load given to the mother unprepared between 24 and 28 weeks of pregnancy (O'Sullivan et al. 1973) would appear to be the most appropriate method currently available and has been recommended by the Second Internatio-nal Workshop Conference on Gestational Diabetes Mellitus (1985). However, the results of combining fasting glucose and potential diabetic features (Morten-sen et al. 1985) are encouraging and when more data are available confirming the practicality, sensitivity and specificity of this method it may well be a suitable alternative. This is not far removed from combining the fasting test with a 75-g load and making the woman wait 2 h. In countries with a very high prevalence of abnormal GTTs such as in the Middle East this may be the wisest approach.

The Management of Gestational Diabetes

To Treat or Not?

This question has only ever been assessed in a controlled manner by O'Sullivan et al. in Boston. They compared gestational diabetics treated with insulin and dietary advice with those who were just given routine antenatal care. Whilst birthweight was lowered in the treated group, perinatal mortality was not significantly lowered (O'Sullivan et al. 1966). A further study was undertaken but never completed (due to lack of funds) and analysis of the data (O'Sullivan 1975) again showed a decrease in perinatal mortality with treatment, but this result was not statistically significant. With the decrease in perinatal mortality such a study is now impractical, although it would be feasible to look at morbidity indices which were not addressed by O'Sullivan.

Dietary Advice

Whilst widely advocated in Europe, dietary advice has been criticized in the USA because the increased lipolysis associated with dietary restriction will increase ketonaemia. Two studies suggested an association between maternal ketonuria (ketonaemia was not assessed) and a decreased IQ in the infant (Churchill et al. 1969; Stehbens et al. 1977), although subsequent re-analysis of one of these papers could not confirm this association (Naeye and Chez 1981).

Ketonaemia normally increases in the third trimester (Williamson 1975; Maresh et al. 1985) and dietary restriction in gestational diabetes has only a little additional effect, making it of dubious clinical relevance (Maresh et al. 1985). In normal pregnancy the use of high fibre diets reduces the degree of ketonaemia compared with a normal Western diet (Fraser et al. 1988), although studies in gestational diabetes are limited (Fraser 1983).

Whilst dietary restriction clearly will decrease an excessive postprandial hyperglycaemic response it might not be considered a suitable method of decreasing fasting hyperglycaemia. However, it has been shown that the insulin glucose ratio will decline with dietary advice in women with gestational diabetes in the third trimester compared with controls (Maresh et al. 1985), thus helping to attain normoglycaemia.

The current recommendations of the British Diabetic Association are that 50% of energy should be obtained from carbohydrate and that as much fibre as possible should be included in the diet. Although these are general recommendations they should be applied in pregnancy also. The total calories in the diet should be between 1800 and 2000 daily which should be restricted further if the woman is obese.

If the fasting plasma glucose concentrations are under 6 mmol/l then strict adherance to the dietary advice should result in a normal pregnancy outcome. Compliance needs to be assessed by observance of changes in maternal weight, postprandial glucose measurements and regular interviews with a dietician. Glycated haemoglobin concentrations should be measured monthly as an additional check to ensure that the condition is not worsening with gestation. If there is concern about the control, admission to hospital for a glucose profile is advisable. The three-point profile recommended by Rivzi et al. (1980) with blood samples taken before breakfast, before lunch and 2 h after supper is usually sufficient.

Opinions in the USA appear to be changing as shown by a concluding statement at the 1985 International Workshop on Gestational Diabetes: "some caloric restriction in obese women with gestational diabetes may improve glucose homeostasis without an unacceptable degree of ketonaemia".

Insulin Therapy

Since gestational diabetes is associated with decreased insulin action peripherally, supplementary insulin therapy appears logical. However it needs to be

complemented by moderate dietary restriction to prevent excessive fat deposition. Therapy, compared with no treatment, has resulted in a decrease in
overweight babies even allowing for maternal obesity (O'Sullivan et al. 1966).
This was shown further by Coustan and Lewis (1978) although their groups of
treated and untreated patients were not totally comparable. Roversi et al. (1980),
with their regime of using the maximum insulin dose that the mother can tolerate
without becoming hypoglycaemic, reported only a 2% incidence of babies whose
weight was greater than the 90th percentile. Current practice is to limit insulin
therapy to those women whose fasting plasma glucose concentration is persis-
tently raised. This is because recent trials comparing insulin therapy plus dietary
advice with dietary advice alone in the less severe gestational diabetics have not
shown any significant anthropometric or metabolic improvements in the neonate
(Maresh et al. 1985; Persson et al. 1985).

Since the relationship between increasing glucose concentration and poor
pregnancy outcome is well established in the insulin-dependent diabetic (Karlson
and Kjellmer 1972) a cut-off for fasting plasma glucose between 6.0 and 7.0
mmol/l is generally regarded as being a good indication for commencing insulin
therapy. Using 6.0 mmol/l as the threshold will include about 25% of women
diagnosed as being abnormal (Maresh et al. 1986). If the prevalence is about
1.5% in the general antenatal population this will result in only 0.4% of the
population being classified as insulin-requiring gestational diabetics. This is of a
similar order to the number of insulin-dependent diabetics and thus should not
overload the clinical services. Insulin therapy should be adjusted in the same way
as in the insulin-dependent diabetic, i.e. by regular home monitoring of plasma
glucose concentrations (supplemented by inpatient assessment if necessary),
attention to weight gain, monthly glycated haemoglobin estimations and fetal
assessment for the effects of maternal hyperglycaemia.

The actual insulin regimes recommended have varied. O'Sullivan et al. (1966)
used one injection of isophane insulin while Coustan and Lewis (1978) added
soluble insulin to this. Roversi et al. (1980) used multiple injections of soluble
insulin whilst others (Maresh et al. 1985; Persson et al. 1985) have used one or
two doses of intermediate action insulins. Clearly much depends on the
experience and practice of individual units; there are a number of ways of
achieving 24-h normoglycaemia and that with which the unit is most familiar
should be used. Actual dosages will vary from person to person, but are likely to
start with a dose of 10–20 units/d and will be increased according to the response.
Whilst insulin therapy has not been associated with clinical or biochemical
evidence of hypoglycaemia in these studies, management should be conducted by
those who look after the insulin-dependent diabetic. All insulin-treated women
should be warned about the symptoms of hypoglycaemia and how to react to
them.

Oral Hypoglycaemic Drugs

Since these will cross the placenta to the fetus and theoretically cause fetal
hypoglycaemia they have not been widely used in pregnancy. However, the
Aberdeen group (Stowers and Sutherland 1975) have extensive experience using
them and have not found any adverse fetal or perinatal problems, whilst their use

has resulted in an improvement in glucose tolerance. Coetzee and Jackson (1979) from South Africa have reported similarly good results.

The Obstetric Management of Gestational Diabetes

The identification of a woman with gestational diabetes is a therapeutic intervention in itself as the woman will usually be transferred to full hospital antenatal care under the supervision of an obstetrician experienced in managing diabetic pregnancy. He or she must look out for fetal indicators of poor maternal diabetic control just as in women with insulin-dependent diabetes. Regular clinical estimation of fetal size and liquor volume should be supplemented by ultrasound assessment of these indices.

If there is no evidence of excessive fetal growth and if normoglycaemia is being achieved through dietary measures alone, then it is safe to allow the pregnancy to go to term and to await spontaneous labour. If insulin has been required because of fasting hyperglycaemia then the fetus already may have been affected and may be macrosomic. In addition these mothers are often obese which increases birthweight. These babies are thus at risk of a traumatic delivery and a decision about time and mode of delivery has to be taken as carefully as in women with insulin-dependent diabetics. Indeed the only two traumatic deliveries in all those with diabetes over the last 10 years at St Mary's Hospital, London occurred in two obese women with gestational diabetes, both of whom, after having previous normal deliveries, had babies with severe shoulder girdle dystocia. Although one cannot measure shoulder diameters using ultrasound, the lower thoracic or abdominal circumference does relate well to fetal weight.

Measurements of fetal shoulder diameter using computerized axial tomography (CAT) scanning (Kitzmiller et al. 1987) and magnetic resonance imaging (MRI) (Chap. 10) are now being reported and these methods may be incorporated into routine practice. If these measurements are combined with an accurate assessment of the pelvic outlet clinically and radiologically then a rational decision as to whether to perform an elective caesarean can be taken. Even in women with more severe gestational diabetes intervention rarely needs to take place before 38 weeks gestation, thus reducing neonatal morbidity. The increased rate of unexplained mature stillbirths found in women with insulin-dependent diabetes is not found in women with gestational diabetes. The women with more severe gestational diabetes are probably best managed by the same obstetric policy as for women with insulin-dependent diabetes. Since gestational diabetic women are likely to be multiparous, induction of labour is likely to be successful.

Labour can be managed in a conventional manner with the exceptions that dextrose should not be given as an intravenous fluid and that plasma glucose concentrations should be measured 2 hourly. A reflectance meter is ideal for this, provided that the staff are familiar with its use. If the glucose levels rise to over 7.0 mmol/l and delivery is not imminent then insulin should be given. There are various regimes which can be used, but the use of an intravenous insulin infusion pump (delivering at a rate of about 1 unit/h) with a dextrose infusion is ideal (e.g. Beard and Maresh 1988) provided attention is paid to the possibility of the pump being accidentally turned off. The presence of moderate to large amounts of ketones in the urine is also best managed with a dextrose and insulin infusion. A secondary arrest pattern on the partogram should be managed by early recourse to abdominal delivery.

Postnatal Management

After delivery, insulin should be withheld since the rapid decline in placental hormones leads to the loss of the pregnancy-associated insulin resistance. Glucose control should be checked by daytime measurements before discharge from hospital. Breast feeding should be encouraged. A GTT should be performed after about 6 weeks. Should this be normal then the patient should be advised that in future pregnancies, abnormal glucose tolerance is likely to reappear. If it does not this is likely to be related to a change in maternal weight or to the non-reproducibility of the GTT. All women who have had gestational diabetes, particularly those who are overweight, should be encouraged to keep to their diet for the rest of their lives regardless of whether their GTT is normal or not, since it is likely that they can diminish the substantial risk of developing either overt diabetes or an abnormal GTT. Clearly those women with an abnormal GTT after pregnancy are going to require continuing diabetic care.

References

American Diabetes Association Second International Workshop Conference on Gestational Diabetes (1985) Summary and recommendations. Diabetes 34 [Suppl 2]:123–126

Artal R, Mosley GM, Dorey FJ (1984) Glycohemoglobin as a screening test for gestational diabetes. Am J Obstet Gynecol 148:412–414

Bacigalupo G, Langner K, Saling E (1984) Glycosylated haemoglobin (HbA1), glucose tolerance and neonatal outcome in gestational diabetic and non diabetic mothers. J Perinat Med 12:137–145

Beard RW, Gillmer MDG, Oakley NW, Gunn PJ (1980) Screening for gestational diabetes. Diabetes Care 3:468–471

Beard RW, Maresh M (1988) Diabetes. In: de Swiet M (ed) Medical disorders in obstetric practice, 2nd edn. Blackwell Scientific Publications, Oxford (in press)

Carpenter MW, Coustan DR (1982) Criteria for screening tests for gestational diabetes. Am J Obstet Gynecol 144:768–773

Churchill JA, Berendes HW, Nemore J (1969) Neuropsychological deficits in children born of diabetic mothers. Am J Obstet Gynecol 105:257–267

Coetzee EJ, Jackson WPU (1979) Metformin in management of pregnant insulin-dependent diabetes. Diabetologia 16:241–245

Cousins L, Dattel BJ, Hollingsworth DR, Zettner A (1984) Glycosylated hemoglobin as a screening test for carbohydrate intolerance in pregnancy. Am J Obstet Gynecol 150:455–460

Coustan DR, Lewis SB (1978) Insulin therapy for gestational diabetes. Obstet Gynecol 51:306–310

Coustan DR, Widness JA, Carpenter MW, Rotondo L, Pratt DC (1987) The breakfast tolerance test: screening for gestational diabetes with a standardised mixed nutrient meal. Am J Obstet Gynecol 157:1113–1117

Fraser RB (1983) High fibre diets in pregnancy. In: Campbell DM, Gillmer MDG (eds) Nutrition in pregnancy. Royal College of Obstetricians and Gynaecologists, London, pp 269–277

Fraser RB, Ford FA, Lawrence GF (1988) Insulin sensitivity in third trimester pregnancy. A randomized study of dietary effects. Br J Obstet Gynaecol 95:223–229

Frisoli G, Naranjo L, Shehab N (1987) Glycohemoglobins in normal and diabetic pregnancy. Am J Perinat 3:183–187

Gillmer MDG, Oakley NW, Beard RW, Nithyanawthan R, Cawston M (1980) Screening for diabetes during pregnancy. Br J Obstet Gynaecol 87:377–382

Hadden DR (1980) Screening for abnormalities of carbohydrate metabolism in pregnancy 1966–1977: the Belfast experience. Diabetes Care 3:440–446

Jowett NI, Samanta AK, Burden AC (1987) Screening for diabetes in pregnancy: is a random blood glucose enough? Diabetic Medicine 4:160–163

Karlson K, Kjellmer I (1972) The outcome of diabetic pregnancies in relation to the mother's blood sugar level. Am J Obstet Gynecol 112:213–217

Kitzmiller JL, Mall JC, Gin GD, Hendricks SK, Newman RB, Scheer L (1987) Measurement of fetal shoulder width with computed tomography in diabetic women. Obstet Gynecol 70:941–945

Lind T (1985) Antenatal screening using random blood glucose values. Diabetes 34 [Suppl 2]:17–20

McFarland KF, Murtiashaw M, Baynes JW (1984) Clinical value of glycosylated serum protein and glycosylated haemoglobin levels in the diagnosis of gestational diabetes mellitus. Obstet Gynecol 64:516–518

Maresh MJA, Gillmer MDG, Beard RW, Alderson CS, Bloxham B, Elkeles RS (1985) The effect of diet and insulin on metabolic profiles of women with gestational diabetes mellitus. Diabetes 34 [Suppl 2]:88–93

Maresh MJA, Gillmer MDG, Elkeles RS, Beard RW (1986) Is gestational diabetes a clinical problem? Presentation at the 23rd British Congress of Obstetrics and Gynaecology

Mortensen HB, Mølsted-Pedersen L, Kuhl C, Backer P (1985) A screening procedure for diabetes in pregnancy. Diabete Metabol 11:249–253

Naeye RL, Chez RA (1981) Effects on maternal acetonuria and low pregnancy weight gain on children's psychomotor development. Am J Obstet Gynecol 139:189–193

Nasrat AA, Johnstone FD, Hasan SAM (1988) Is random plasma glucose an efficient screening test for impaired glucose tolerance in pregnancy? Br J Obstet Gynaecol (in press)

O'Sullivan JB, Gellis SS, Dandrow RV, Tenney BO (1966) The potential diabetic and her treatment in pregnancy. Obstet Gynecol 27:683–689

O'Sullivan JB, Mahan CM, Charles D, Dandrow RV (1973) Screening criteria for high-risk gestational diabetic patients. Am J Obstet Gynecol 116:895–900

O'Sullivan JB (1975) Prospective study of gestational diabetes and its treatment. In: Sutherland HW, Stowers JM (eds) Carbohydrate metabolism in pregnancy and the newborn. Churchill Livingstone, Edinburgh, pp 195–204

Persson B, Stangenberg M, Hansson U, Nordlander E (1985) Gestational diabetes mellitus: comparative evaluation of two treatment regimens, diet versus insulin and diet. Diabetes 34 [Suppl 2]:101–105

Rivzi J, Gillmer MDG, Oakley NW, Beard RW (1980) Evaluation of plasma glucose control in pregnancy complicated by gestational diabetes. Br J Obstet Gynaecol 87:383–387

Roberts AB, Baker JR, Court DJ, James AG, Henley P, Ronayne ID (1983) Fructosamine in diabetic pregnancy. Lancet II:998–999

Ross I (1984) Glycosylated haemoglobin in the detection of gestational diabetes in an unselected population. In: Sutherland HW, Stowers JM (eds) Carbohydrate metabolism in pregnancy and the newborn. Churchill Livingstone, Edinburgh, p. 206–208

Roversi GD, Gargiulo M, Nicolini U et al. (1980) Maximum tolerated insulin therapy in gestational diabetes. Diabetes Care 3:489–494

Ryan EA, Stark R, Crockford PM, Suthijumroon A (1987) Assessment of value of glycosylated albumin and protein in detection of gestational diabetes. Diabetes Care 10:213–216

Shah BD, Cohen AW, May C, Gabbe SG (1982) Comparison of glycohemoglobin determination and the one hour oral glucose screen in the identification of gestational diabetes. Am J Obstet Gynecol 144:774–777

Stehbens JA, Baker GL, Kitchell M (1977) Outcome at ages 1, 3 and 5 years of children born to diabetic women. Am J Obstet Gynecol 127:408–413

Stowers JM, Sutherland HW (1975) The use of sulphonylureas biguanides and insulin in pregnancy. In: Sutherland HW, Stowers JM (eds) Carbohydrate metabolism in pregnancy and the newborn. Churchill Livingstone, Edinburgh, pp 205–220

Sutherland HW, Stowers JM, McKenzie C (1970) Simplifying the clinical problem of glycosuria in pregnancy. Lancet I:1069–1071

Williamson DH (1975) Regulation of the utilisation of glucose and ketone bodies by brain in the perinatal period. In: Camerini-Davalos RA, Cole HS (eds) Early diabetes in early life. New York, Academic Press, p 200

19. A Prospective Multicentre Study to Determine the Influence of Pregnancy upon the 75-g Oral Glucose Tolerance Test (OGTT)

The Diabetic Pregnancy Study Group of the European Association for the Study of Diabetes

Co-ordinator: Professor T. Lind
MRC Human Reproduction Group,
Princess Mary Maternity Hospital,
Great North Road, Newcastle-upon-Tyne, NE2 3BD

Computing: Dr. P. R. Philips
Health Care Research Unit,
University of Newcastle-upon-Tyne,
21 Claremont Place, Newcastle-upon-Tyne NE2 4AA

Centres Taking Part

Aberdeen, Scotland
(H. W. Sutherland)

Copenhagen, Denmark
(L. Mølsted-Pedersen, C. Kuhl)

Newcastle, England
(T. Lind)

Zagreb, Yugoslavia
(A. Drazancic)

London, England
(M. Maresh)

Southampton, England
(M. Hatem)

Vienna, Austria
(A. Pollak)

Belfast, N. Ireland
(D. R. Hadden)

Bonn, West Germany
(O. Bellmann)

Misda, Malta
(E. S. Grech, C. Savona-Ventura)

Berlin, East Germany
(K. Fuhrmann)

Introduction

During 1980 the World Health Organization (WHO) suggested criteria for diagnosing diabetes mellitus and impaired glucose tolerance (IGT) based upon blood glucose concentrations following a 75-g oral glucose load; in 1985 a second WHO study group substantially endorsed these recommendations after some minor modifications. For reasons not explained, the first report (1980) suggested that the criteria used to diagnose diabetes and IGT in the general population could be applied to pregnant women (p. 11); the second report (1985) endorsed this view using the argument that the application of set diagnostic criteria to large groups of pregnant and non-pregnant individuals would make it possible to determine more specifically the effect of lesser degrees of glucose intolerance upon maternal and child health. However this report did not acknowledge the fact that pregnancy causes postprandial blood glucose values to remain elevated for longer periods of time; hence more mothers are likely to exceed any timed postprandial value and thus be labelled "glucose intolerant" while only displaying the extremes of physiological adaptation.

The aim of this study was to determine the range of responses of women throughout pregnancy to a 75-g oral glucose load. To ensure that the data were reasonably representative of a Westernized antenatal population 11 centres throughout Europe were asked to take part. The majority of the doctors contacted were members of the Diabetic Pregnancy Study Group (DPSG) which is part of the European Association for the Study of Diabetes (EASD). They were asked to perform the 75-g OGTTs under the clinical and laboratory conditions prevailing in everyday practice using the test procedures suggested by the WHO (1980, 1985). As the interpretation of the results was to be based upon WHO criteria the minimum number of blood tests required per test was two: fasting and at 2 h. Many centres provided additional data from blood glucose levels at 30, 60 and 90 min.

One of the problems in any study covering a wide geographical area is that local factors may affect the glucose response independently of pregnancy itself. For example one centre (Malta) had a high incidence of diabetes in the general population which was reflected in the number of women with a history of a first-degree relative having this condition. Another centre (Copenhagen) reported that the majority of mothers smoked cigarettes while Zagreb had a large proportion of mothers who had had more than one previous early pregnancy loss. However if any organization is going to recommend criteria for diagnosing diabetes on a worldwide basis then the possible effects of these regional variations must be understood. Our study population will therefore be described in detail by centre before the data are reviewed for the group as a whole.

The Population Studied

The only specified reason for the exclusion of anyone from the trial was known diabetes mellitus though one centre (Southampton) prospectively excluded anyone with a first-degree relative with diabetes. The possible effect of this will be discussed below.

Gestation at Testing

Ideally we would have liked to study women during each trimester of pregnancy as traditionally defined: up to 97d, 98–188 d and 189 d or more. However few mothers actually attended their first antenatal clinic such that they could be recruited to the project and the test completed within 97 d. Computer analysis showed that 167 tests were within 117 d of the patient's last menstrual period (LMP) and this has been used to define our early pregnancy group. Thereafter 513 tests were performed between 118 and 195 d and 507 tests from 196 d to term

(Table 19.1). These numbers are slightly in excess of the numbers of mothers studied as will be discussed below.

Types of Blood Sample Obtained

Because of the emphasis that the tests should be undertaken under the clinical conditions prevailing in each centre's everyday practice there were differences in the type of blood sample obtained. One centre reported capillary plasma concentrations while the remainder measured either capillary whole blood or venous plasma concentrations; in two centres both values were reported. One centre determined glucose concentrations in both venous plasma and venous whole blood (Table 19.1). Because some mothers could be put into more than one test group, i.e. capillary whole blood and venous plasma the numbers of test results available exceed the number of patients.

Number of Tests Undertaken

In Berlin some of the patients who were tested during the first and second trimesters agreed to have further tests during the remaining trimester; in this way 149 women yielded 327 test results. In the total study population there were 1009 women offering data from 1187 separate tests; when the tests offering two types of blood sample were included, 1296 data sets became available for analysis (Table 19.1).

Maternal Characteristics

The mean and range values for the age, height, weight and body mass index (BMI) of the mothers are shown by centre in Table 19.1. Because age and weight could change in the course of pregnancy the values at the time of testing were used. One centre (Southampton) did not record maternal weight at testing but at the time of booking. For purposes of general comparison the Southampton weight data are given in Table 19.1 but not used for calculation of BMI.

Social Details

Smoking Habit

The majority of mothers taking part were non-smokers in the group as a whole; in Copenhagen 60% smoked but the number of women studied was small (Table 19.2). Smoking was not permitted immediately prior to, or in the course of a test at any centre.

Family History of Diabetes

With the exception of Southampton no attempt was made to exclude people from the study because of a family history of diabetes. The numbers of patients studied

Table 19.1. The mean and range values for various maternal characteristics in the population studied shown by centre and for the group as a whole. Because age and weight increase progressively throughout pregnancy the values for age, weight and body mass have been given for the third trimester in the group as a whole

Centre	Number of tests by gestation (d)			Type of blood sample	Age at test (years)		Height (cm)		Test weight (kg)		Body mass kg/m²	
	<117	118–195	196+		Mean	Range	Mean	Range	Mean	Range	Mean	Range
Aberdeen	—	110	2	CP	27	18–38	161	147–178	68	52–113	26	21–42
Belfast	—	83	17	VP	27	18–39	159	145–175	65	47–101	26	19–40
East Berlin	89	133	105	CWB	25	17–37	165	146–178	65	47–98	24	19–33
Bonn	—	5	55	CWB;VP	31	17–43	165	149–179	80	60–127	29	22–47
Copenhagen	—		25	CWB;VP	29	23–36	166	150–175	67	48–80	24	19–30
London	11	31	—	VP	27	19–41	163	151–177	67	52–90	25	20–33
Newcastle	18	21	24	VP;VWB	29	22–36	163	147–183	68	43–104	25	18–36
Southampton	25	21	174	VP	26	15–38	162	138–184	(64	43–90)[a]	NS	NS
Valetta	2	50	61	VP	28	18–42	158	140–177	68	48–103	28	18–41
Vienna	12	29	39	CWB	25	17–35	165	146–180	62	46–84	23	17–32
Zagreb	10	30	5	CWB	28	20–48	166	156–178	68	48–109	25	17–40
Whole group	167	513	507		27	15–43	162	138–184	70	46–127	26	18–47

C, capillary; V, venous; P, plasma; WB, whole blood
[a]Maternal weights in Southampton were recorded at first visit and not at testing.

Table 19.2. Percentage of non-smokers and those with a family history of diabetes together with the previous pregnancy outcomes in the individual centres as well as for the group as a whole

Centre	% Non-smoking	% with FH of diabetes			Distribution (%) of previous pregnancies					
					<28 weeks			>28 weeks		
		0	1°	2°	0	1	2	0	1	2
Aberdeen	83	79	5	16	76	20	4	62	28	10
Belfast	60	87	8	5	84	14	2	30	35	35
East Berlin	92	90	1	9	76	22	2	49	40	11
Bonn	NR	NR	NR	NR	63	20	17	32	37	31
Copenhagen	40	100	0	0	64	36	0	72	24	4
London	68	95	3	2	57	31	12	57	33	10
Newcastle	94	91	3	6	78	18	4	48	44	8
Southampton	70	100	0	0	71	20	9	64	22	14
Valetta	68	61	29	10	89	10	1	45	35	20
Vienna	77	100	0	0	73	18	9	56	34	10
Zagreb	96	100	0	0	43	24	33	27	60	13
Group mean	75	89	5	6	76	17	6	51	34	15

FH, family history; NR, not recorded

in individual centres are too small for the incidence of diabetes to be calculated with confidence but for the group as a whole 5% had a parent or sibling with diabetes. The exception was Malta where 29% of mothers had an affected first-degree relative; this is a feature of that particular population but the majority are not insulin dependent (Table 19.2).

Previous Pregnancy Loss Prior to 28 Weeks Gestation

The majority of those studied had never lost a pregnancy prior to 28 weeks and of those who had the greater proportion had only experienced one such loss. The exception was Zagreb where one-third of the women had had two or more abortions; it seems probable that many of these were therapeutic terminations and not indicative of reproductive inefficiency (Table 19.2).

Previous Pregnancies Going Beyond 28 Weeks

A large proportion of the women studied were primigravidae; of the parous women the majority had only had one previous baby but in two centres about one-third of the participants had had two or more babies (Belfast and Bonn; Table 19.2).

Outcome of Present Pregnancy

Gestation at Delivery

Sonar facilities were available in all of the centres taking part and virtually all of the mothers were scanned during the first half of pregnancy to help confirm the duration of pregnancy; the gestation at delivery is therefore the best estimate possible. The babies born very preterm were the consequence of spontaneous labour while those going beyond 42 weeks were eventually induced for genuine postmaturity. The mean and range values for gestation at delivery for each centre are shown in Table 19.3 together with the data for the group as a whole.

Birthweights

Because the majority of women from each centre delivered at term, the upper range of birthweights is similar for each centre (Table 19.3). On the other hand some extremely small babies were delivered as a consequence of spontaneous early labour. In the UK the dividing line between an abortion and a live birth or stillbirth is 28 weeks gestation. This caused the occurrence of a 980-g abortion but a 550-g stillbirth because the latter delivered at 29 weeks.

Method of Delivery

For the purposes of classification vaginal delivery includes vertex and breech presentations, forceps delivery includes the use of the ventouse while Caesarean section embraces elective and emergency operations. Spontaneous abortions are also given in Table 19.3 but because the great majority of women were not asked to take part until after 10 weeks gestation and after a sonar scan confirmed a viable fetus the numbers with this complication are very small.

With relatively small numbers of women in each centre one or two extra being delivered by, for example, Caesarean section, can have a marked effect upon the percentage distribution. However the figures for the group as a whole are reasonably representative being based upon more than 1000 cases.

Infant Outcome

There were seven stillbirths and one neonatal death in the whole study group; the details are given in Table 19.4.

Test Procedure

The Test

The guidelines suggested by the WHO (1980, 1985) were followed; a 75-g oral glucose load was given with the blood sampling intervals being timed from the start of the drink.

Table 19.3. The mean and range values for length of gestation and birthweight, together with the method of delivery and infant outcome for the mothers in each centre and for the group as a whole

Centre	Gestation at delivery (d)		Birthweight (g)		Method of delivery (%)			Outcome of present pregnancy (numbers)				
	Mean	Range	Mean	Range	Vaginal	Forceps	C/S	LB	SB	NND	Ab	NS
Aberdeen	280	193–306	3355	980–4640	75	17	8	109	1	1 (1)	1	—
Belfast	281	246–302	3447	2270–4540	77	14	9	100(4)	0	0		—
East Berlin	279	143–313	3359	1390–4670	90	4	6	139	1	0	2	7
Bonn	273	203–294	3301	550–4740	67	8	25	58	1	0		1
Copenhagen	281	246–311	3347	2260–4170	84	0	16	25	0	0		—
London	279	230–307	3377	2100–4080	70	18	12	40	0	0		1
Newcastle	279	245–311	3451	2660–4500	71	21	8	98	1	0		1
Southampton	272	210–294	3348	1620–4650	74	15	11	216	0	0		6
Valetta	278	243–295	3373	1530–4200	86	7	7	112	1	0		—
Vienna	274	196–292	3341	1750–4460	94	0	6	77	1	0		1
Zagreb	272	230–293	3326	1700–4030	91	0	9	44	1	0		—
Total	278	143–313	3367	550–4740	81	9	10	921	7	1	3	17

Number in parentheses indicates infants with anomalies.
Ab, abortion; LB, live birth; C/S, caesarean section; SB, stillbirth; NND, neonatal death; NS, not stated.

Table 19.4. Clinical details of the seven stillbirths and one neonatal death occurring in the total group

Infant outcome	Gestation (d)	Weight (g)	Comment
Stillbirth			
1	240	2850	Unexplained IUD at autopsy
2	254	2350	Severe accidental haemorrhage
3	203	550	Missed abortion delivering after 28 weeks
4	263	2740	Unexplained IUD at autopsy
5	275	1530	Growth-retarded IUD. Nil found at autopsy
6	196	—	Missed abortion delivering after 28 weeks
7	265	2690	Unexplained IUD at autopsy
Neonatal death			
1	285	3740	Multiple heart defects

IUD, intrauterine death

Assay Methods

All centres employed autoanalyser techniques using glucose oxidase or hexoki-nase enzyme methods for the determination of blood glucose.

Assay Comparability

Six samples of freeze-dried serum were prepared in Newcastle and sent to each centre for assay. The tubes were simply labelled 1–6 with no indication of the likely glucose concentration; tubes 4, 5 and 6 were actually aliquots from the same sample. Six centres assayed the samples soon after receiving them (Table 19.5); in two centres there was a prolonged delay before the samples were analysed and the values were so low that glucose degradation seemed probable. In three instances the participating doctors had moved to other centres. As there cannot be a "correct" answer, the individual values have been compared to the mean concentration for each sample. It appears that the centres would assay to within 0.5 mmol/l of the mean over the range 2–9 mmol/l.

Table 19.5. Glucose determinations on six serum samples assayed "blind" by six of the centres in the study

Centre	Glucose (mmol/l)					
	Sample 1	Sample 2	Sample 3	Sample 4[a]	Sample 5[a]	Sample 6[a]
Belfast	6.8 (−0.5)	5.1 (−0.2)	8.7 (0.1)	2.2 (0.5)	2.2 (0.5)	2.1 (0.6)
East Berlin	5.7 (0.6)	4.6 (0.3)	8.9 (−0.1)	2.0 (0.7)	2.1 (0.6)	2.1 (0.6)
Copenhagen	5.9 (0.4)	4.7 (0.2)	8.8 (0)	2.6 (0.1)	2.4 (0.3)	2.3 (0.4)
Newcastle	6.2 (0.1)	4.7 (0.2)	8.7 (0.1)	3.2 (−0.5)	3.3 (−0.6)	3.2 (−0.5)
Valetta	6.9 (−0.6)	5.5 (−0.6)	9.3 (−0.5)	2.8 (−0.1)	2.9 (−0.2)	2.9 (−0.2)
Vienna	6.2 (0.1)	—	8.6 (0.2)	3.6 (−0.9)	3.2 (−0.5)	3.6 (−0.9)
Mean	6.3	4.9	8.8	2.7	2.7	2.7
± ISD	0.47	0.37	0.25	0.6	0.5	0.63

Figures in brackets show difference from mean value. Overall mean difference = 0.008 ± 0.47
[a] Aliquots of the same sample.

Relation of Venous and Capillary Blood Glucose Levels

The WHO reports (1980, 1985) published criteria for the interpretation of the OGTT and imply that a definite relation exists between the glucose concentrations in say, venous plasma and capillary whole blood. While in physiological terms such a relation will exist the question is whether it is sufficiently constant to allow the comparison of data from different centres when some report venous plasma values and others capillary whole blood concentrations. In our series some centres measured venous plasma glucose, others capillary whole blood and one used capillary plasma; it thus seemed important to determine whether a relation did exist such that interpolation from the value of one blood sample to another type was practicable.

Capillary Whole Blood and Venous Plasma

Five centres sent data from 147 paired samples and the concentrations were found to be very similar. Another way to compare possible differences is to subtract the venous plasma value from its paired capillary whole blood value; the mean difference was virtually zero indicating no consistent difference between these sample types under everyday clinical and laboratory conditions. These data are shown in Table 19.6.

Capillary and Venous Whole Blood

Two centres offered data from 66 paired samples; the mean value of the differences between these pairs was significantly different from zero indicating that in general capillary whole blood values were above venous whole blood values. However there were wide variations in the individual values as can be seen from the data in Table 19.6.

Capillary and Venous Plasma

Two centres measured glucose concentrations in such pairs on 79 occasions. Physiologically it would be expected that capillary plasma concentrations would be higher than the venous plasma levels, the difference reflecting tissue uptake. The data did reveal such a difference both in the mean values and the mean of the differences between sample types but again there were wide individual variations (Table 19.6).

Plasma and Whole Blood Values Within Samples

As plasma levels can always be expected to be higher than the whole blood concentration in the same sample assay, precision can be tested on such pairs. There were 73 capillary samples upon which whole blood (CWB) and plasma (CP) concentrations were measured and 36 pairs of venous blood similarly assayed. The correlation coefficient (r) between CWB and CP was 0.94, the

Table 19.6. Data on the relation between plasma and whole blood glucose concentrations in paired samples of capillary and venous blood. Thus Belfast determined glucose levels on VP, VWB, CP and CWB allowing the relations between all samples to be examined while Newcastle determined VP and CWB levels on simultaneously paired blood samples

Centre	n	Glucose concentration (mmol/l)						
		VP	CWB	CWB–VP diff	VWB	CWB–VWB diff	CP	CP–VP diff
Belfast	36	4.6 ± 0.71	4.7 ± 0.70	0.07 ± 0.44	4.2 ± 0.58	0.53 ± 0.44	5.1 ± 0.87	0.45 ± 0.49
East Berlin	30	—	4.6 ± 0.80	—	4.5 ± 0.63	0.06 ± 0.50	—	—
Copenhagen	43	5.1 ± 1.19	4.8 ± 1.1	−0.15 ± 0.70	—	—	5.3 ± 1.2	0.24 ± 0.52
Newcastle	15	4.9 ± 0.53	4.3 ± 0.51	−0.56 ± 0.46	—	—	—	—
Valetta	13	4.0 ± 0.35	4.2 ± 0.68	0.15 ± 0.57	—	—	—	—
Zagreb	40	3.8 ± 0.64	4.3 ± 0.63	0.55 ± 0.26	—	—	—	—
Mean ± SD		4.5 ± 0.97 (n = 147)	4.6 ± 0.82 (n = 177)	0.08 ± 0.6 (n = 147)	4.3 ± 0.62 (n = 66)	0.31 ± 0.52 (n = 66)	5.21 ± 1.03 (n = 79)	0.33 ± 0.51 (n = 79)

VP, venous plasma; CWB, capillary whole blood; VWB, venous whole blood; CP, capillary plasma; diff, difference in concentration between the samples indicated

plasma values almost always being higher than those for the whole blood. For venous blood the correlation (r) was 0.91 and in every case the plasma value was higher than that for whole blood. As it is physiologically improbable that whole blood glucose concentrations will be higher than those for plasma from the same sample it implies that under everyday situations laboratories may occasionally be up to 1.0 mmol/l out in their estimates.

Change in Haematocrit

Another variable likely to affect whole blood glucose calculations is haematocrit. To investigate this the centres were asked to determine venous haematocrit (using automatic blood counter measurements of red cell count and mean cell volume) and capillary haematocrit by microcentrifugation. Data from 175 venous blood samples and 150 paired capillary samples were obtained and the mean values with their standard deviations from the three trimesters of pregnancy are shown in Table 19.7. Data from a non-pregnant control group are also shown.

Table 19.7. Haematocrit values in 175 venous blood samples and 150 paired capillary samples obtained throughout pregnancy together with values from a non-pregnant control group (numbers of observations in brackets)

Gestation (d)	Venous haematocrit (%)	(n)	Capillary haematocrit (%)	(n)	Haematocrit difference (%)	(n)
0[a]	34 ± 5	(28)	38 ± 5	(27)	3.6 ± 2.7	(27)
<117	34 ± 7	(30)	38 ± 3	(24)	2.9 ± 3.4	(24)
118–195	34 ± 4	(61)	37 ± 4	(58)	2.6 ± 3.1	(58)
196+	34 ± 4	(57)	36 ± 4	(41)	1.9 ± 3.0*	(41)

* Significantly lower than non-pregnant ($P<0.05$).
[a] 0 = Non-pregnant control group.

The venous haematocrit did not change during any stage of pregnancy relative to the non-pregnant value but the capillary haematocrit decreased progressively as pregnancy advanced. The difference between capillary and venous haematocrits within the paired samples ($n=150$) was examined: in the non-pregnant women the mean difference was 3.5% (±2.7% SD) which was significantly greater than the difference by the third trimester (1.9%±3%; $P<0.05$).

Conclusions Concerning Methodology

While theoretically a relation can be expected between the glucose concentrations in different types of blood samples there are too many variables influencing this relation for any "conversion factor" from the glucose concentration in one type of sample to another to be realistic. Ideally tests using say, venous plasma samples would be interpreted against criteria determined from similar samples, and so on. We have shown that under everyday clinical conditions the glucose concentrations in capillary whole blood and venous plasma are virtually the same. A practical solution would be to use one or other of these sample types wherever possible and apply the same "cut-off" values to both.

Oral Glucose Tolerance Test (OGTT) Results

Seven centres provided venous plasma glucose values, five reported capillary whole blood levels and one gave capillary plasma values (Table 19.1). One centre also provided venous whole blood concentrations but these were too few to report upon and will not be considered further. All centres offered fasting and 2-h glucose data with the majority also reporting 30-, 60- and 90-min values. A minority also provided 180-min concentrations.

Venous Plasma Glucose Values

Mean Concentrations

There were 56 tests performed during the first 117 d of pregnancy, 211 tests in the interval between 118 and 195 d and 356 tests during the last stage of pregnancy. The mean values and one standard deviation at each test time during early, mid and late pregnancy are given in Table 19.8. The progressive increase in glucose concentrations as pregnancy advances in both venous plasma and capillary whole blood is clearly shown, the levels at 60, 90, 120 and 180 min being significantly higher during the last trimester than during the first. Particular attention is drawn to the 2-h value of 6.3±1.4 mmol/l during late pregnancy. This is discussed in more detail below.

Centile Values

The 5th, 10th, 20th, 50th, 80th, 90th and 95th centile values were calculated for each trimester of pregnancy; for purposes of illustration the 5th, 50th and 95th centile values for the third trimester are shown in Fig. 19.1. If 2-h concentrations between 8 and 11 mmol/l are indicative of impaired glucose tolerance (IGT) then about 15% of pregnant women will fall into this category during the third trimester if venous plasma values are used. The 95th centile value for the fasting venous plasma concentration during the second trimester was influenced by a "cluster" of patients from one centre who had unusual test responses (Table 19.9). Thirteen women recorded a fasting level of 6.9 mmol/l or more during the second trimester of whom 12 came from Belfast and one from Malta; of these five were normal (2-h value less than 8.0 mmol/l), seven were classed as having 1GT (2-h value 8–11 mmol/l) and one was diabetic. They thus formed the top 5% of the 211 values available; by comparison the 95th centile value for the 196 women having second-trimester fasting values measured on capillary whole blood was only 4.7 mmol/l and for the 110 capillary plasma samples was 5.1 mmol/l. Indeed

Table 19.8. Mean (± SD) blood glucose values during a 75-g oral glucose tolerance test (OGTT) according to sample type and stage of pregnancy

Pregnancy (d)	Fasting	Sampling time (min)				
		30	60	90	120	180
Venous plasma glucose (mmol/l)						
<117	4.2 ± 0.4	6.6 ± 1.0	5.6 ± 1.5	5.4 ± 1.6	4.8 ± 1.3	3.7 ± 0.95
(*n*)	(55)	(31)	(55)	(31)	(55)	(26)
118–195	4.8 ± 1.0	7.6 ± 1.7	6.9 ± 1.8	6.3 ± 1.7	6.0 ± 1.5	3.8 ± 1.2
(*n*)	(211)	(190)	(163)	(143)	(209)	(55)
196+	4.2 ± 0.6	7.0 ± 1.5	7.5 ± 1.8*	7.3 ± 1.8*	6.3 ± 1.4*	5.3 ± 1.5*
(*n*)	(354)	(182)	(291)	(121)	(353)	(104)
Capillary whole blood glucose (mmol/l)						
<117	3.9 ± 0.6	6.8 ± 1.0	6.4 ± 1.2	5.7 ± 1.0	5.3 ± 1.1	3.5 ± 1.0
(*n*)	(111)	(110)	(111)	(101)	(111)	(89)
118–195	3.8 ± 0.5	6.8 ± 1.1	6.6 ± 1.3	6.0 ± 1.2	5.5 ± 1.1	3.8 ± 1.1
(*n*)	(196)	(191)	(196)	(161)	(196)	(137)
196+	3.8 ± 0.5	6.9 ± 1.1	7.5 ± 1.4*	6.5 ± 1.4*	6.0 ± 1.2*	4.7 ± 1.4*
(*n*)	(228)	(174)	(229)	(168)	(229)	(185)
Capillary plasma glucose (mmol/l)						
118–195	4.5 ± 0.3	8.2 ± 1.2	7.7 ± 1.5	7.0 ± 1.3	6.4 ± 1.0	—
(*n*)	(110)	(110)	(110)	(110)	(110)	

* Difference from values at <117 d significant (*P*<0.001).

only one other woman had a fasting value in excess of 6.9 mmol/l in the whole series and it seems reasonable to suggest that the 95th centile value for venous plasma fasting glucose in a general antenatal population is more likely to be about 5 mmol/l.

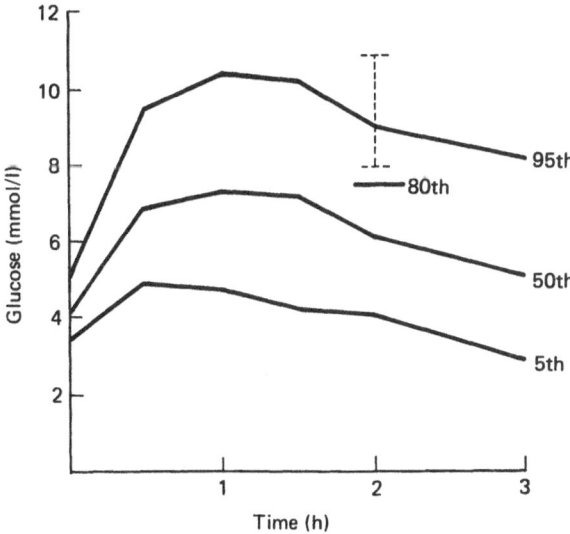

Fig. 19.1. 5th, 50th and 95th centile values for venous plasma glucose concentrations during the third trimester of pregnancy. The *dotted line* indicates the range 8–11 mmol/l suggested as diagnostic of impaired glucose tolerance (IGT) by the WHO.

Table 19.9. The 5th, 50th and 95th centile values at timed intervals following a 75-g oral glucose load for venous plasma and capillary whole blood samples throughout pregnancy (number of observations in brackets)

Centile	Sample time (min)				
	Fasting	30	60	90	120
Venous plasma concentration (mmol/l)					
<117 d	(55)	(31)	(55)	(31)	(55)
5th	3.6	5.2	3.3	2.8	2.6
50th	4.2	6.2	5.4	5.2	4.7
95th	4.9	9.1	7.8	8.7	6.8
118–195 d	(211)	(190)	(163)	(143)	(209)
5th	3.7	5.0	4.3	4.0	3.8
50th	4.6	7.4	6.9	6.3	5.7
95th	6.9	10.6	10.1	9.0	9.0
196+ d	(354)	(182)	(291)	(121)	(353)
5th	3.5	4.9	4.7	4.2	4.2
50th	4.1	6.8	7.3	7.2	6.1
95th	5.2	9.4	10.5	10.4	9.0
Capillary whole blood (mmol/l)					
<117 d	(111)	(110)	(111)	(101)	(111)
5th	2.9	5.2	4.3	4.4	3.4
50th	3.8	6.9	6.3	5.6	5.3
95th	4.8	8.9	8.7	7.6	7.3
118–195 d	(196)	(191)	(196)	(161)	(196)
5th	3.0	5.2	4.7	4.2	3.8
50th	3.8	6.7	6.5	5.8	5.5
95th	4.7	8.6	8.7	7.9	7.2
196+ d	(228)	(174)	(229)	(168)	(229)
5th	3.1	5.2	5.2	4.4	4.1
50th	3.8	6.9	7.3	6.5	5.9
95th	4.5	8.9	10.2	8.8	8.2

Capillary Whole Blood Glucose Values

Mean Concentrations

There were 111 tests performed within the first 117 d of pregnancy, 196 between 118 and 195 d and 229 tests during later pregnancy. The data are given in Table 19.8 and again demonstrate the progressive increase in glucose levels as pregnancy advances, the third-trimester values at 60, 90, 120 and 180 min being significantly above the early pregnancy values. However, these concentrations are not markedly different from the venous plasma levels and on occasion are somewhat lower supporting the suggestion that there is no marked difference between venous plasma and capillary whole blood concentrations.

Centile Values

The same centile values were calculated for capillary whole blood; the values are lower at 2 h but nevertheless over 5% of the women would be classified as having IGT on their 2-h values (Table 19.9).

Capillary Plasma Glucose Values

Only Aberdeen reported capillary plasma levels but over 100 women were tested during the second trimester; as would be expected the mean values at each sample time were higher than for either venous plasma or capillary whole blood. The standard deviations for all types of blood samples (Table 19.8) indicate there would be considerable overlap of values from the different sample types.

Factors Possibly Influencing the 75-g Oral Glucose Tolerance Test (OGTT) Response

To determine whether a family history of diabetes, the smoking habit of the mother or her parity affected the response to an oral glucose load the possible influences of these factors were analysed during each trimester of pregnancy.

Family History of Diabetes

Only those women with a parent or sibling with diabetes were compared to those without any diabetes in the family. The data were analysed by trimester and sample type (i.e. CWB or VP); no clinically significant differences were found. The data for the third trimester are given in Table 19.10. Removing Southampton from the data set did not cause any significant change.

Smoking Habit

Whether or not the patient was a cigarette smoker during pregnancy did not appear to influence the test responses at any stage; the third-trimester data given in Table 19.10 illustrate this.

Parity

To keep the numbers in each group as large as possible women in their first pregnancy were compared to women of all parities but no blood glucose differences emerged (Table 19.10).

Characteristics of Women with a 2-h Value of 8 mmol/l or More

If a specified cut-off value is to be used to define a person as "glucose intolerant" then the possible influences of other variables such as a family history of diabetes, maternal age, body mass, parity and infant birthweight need to be assessed. The

Table 19.10. Mean (± SD) glucose values at fasting, 60 and 120 min during late pregnancy according to blood sample type, whether the mother had a family history of diabetes, whether a smoker and her parity

Group	Number	Sample time (mins)		
		Fasting	60	120
Venous plasma				
FH diab				
No	269	4.2 ± 0.5	7.2 ± 1.7	6.1 ± 1.4
Yes	28	4.6 ± 1.0	7.7 ± 1.7	5.9 ± 1.3
Smoker				
No	88	4.5 ± 0.8	7.7 ± 1.5[a]	6.0 ± 1.4
Yes	38	4.3 ± 0.5	7.7 ± 1.6[b]	5.9 ± 1.2
Parity				
0	145	4.2 ± 0.6	7.3 ± 1.8	6.0 ± 1.4
1	208	4.2 ± 0.6	7.6 ± 1.8	6.4 ± 1.4
Capillary whole blood				
FH diab				
No	162	3.8 ± 0.5	7.2 ± 1.4	5.8 ± 1.1
Yes	11	3.7 ± 0.4	7.0 ± 0.6	5.6 ± 0.8
Smoker				
No	144	3.7 ± 0.5	7.1 ± 1.3	5.7 ± 1.1
Yes	29	4.0 ± 0.4	7.7 ± 1.3	6.1 ± 1.2
Parity				
0	86	3.7 ± 0.4	7.2 ± 1.4	5.7 ± 1.2
1	142	3.8 ± 0.5	7.6 ± 1.4	6.1 ± 1.2

FH diab, Family history of diabetes
[a] $n = 45$.
[b] $n = 21$.

mothers were therefore divided into two groups depending upon whether or not the 2-h blood glucose value reached or exceeded 8 mmol/l. Relatively few did, therefore patients with venous plasma data were combined with those having capillary whole blood levels yielding 79 such mothers and 760 who were normally responsive. Because some centres reported glucose concentrations on both sample types there were more "positive" tests than individuals hence the data which follow were based upon individuals; if a mother had both blood samples assayed but only one reached or exceeded 8 mmol/l she was included.

Family History of Diabetes. There was no preponderance of first-degree relatives having diabetes in those mothers having a high 2-h level.

Smoking Habits. Whether or not the mothers were smokers did not influence the test responses.

Parity. To keep the numbers as large as possible women in their first pregnancy were compared to those in their second or subsequent pregnancy. No parity differences were noted in the high responders.

Maternal Height. There was no difference in the mean height of the two groups.

Gestation at Delivery. Both groups delivered close to term (mean gestation 276±15 d and 274±15 d respectively).

Baby Weight. Both groups delivered babies of comparable weight (3367±508 g and 3366±556 g respectively).

Maternal Age. Age was accurately recorded (i.e. as date of birth) in 58 of those at or above 8 mmol/l; they were significantly older at 29±5.3 years relative to 26±4.6 years ($P<0.001$).

Maternal Weight. Because this increases progressively throughout pregnancy we compared the 290 normal mothers tested during the last trimester with the 35 having raised 2-h levels. The latter group were heavier (74.8±15.9 to 69.8±11.0 kg) and had an increased body mass index (28.3±5.2 to 26.1±3.9; $P<0.02$).

Perinatal Outcome. None of the abortions, stillbirths or the neonatal deaths was associated with a high 2-h blood glucose level.

Other Aspects of the Test Response. Defining impaired glucose tolerance upon a 2-h blood glucose value carries the presumption that previous post-load concentrations were even higher. For IGT the WHO suggested that the 60-min value be 11 mmol/l or higher. In this series the majority of mothers having a 2-h value of 8 mmol/l or more did not have other abnormal values: as discussed above only nine women had a fasting value of 6.9 mmol/l or more and seven came from one centre (Belfast); 13 women had a 60-min level of 11 mmol/l or more but nine of these had a normal fasting value. If only those with two abnormal blood glucose levels be regarded as having IGT or diabetes then of the 79 in the group, two mothers had diabetes and 13 had IGT.

Adopting a 2-h Level of 9 mmol/l as the Cut-off

If, because of the pregnancy effect, a 2-h value of 9 mmol/l was adopted as the cut-off (the 95th centile for 2 h) then 32 mothers in our series would have been detected. The two diabetic women and 10 of the 13 classed as IGT would still have been diagnosed. But inspection of their data again suggests that maternal age and body mass may be influencing the way they handle a glucose load. The mean age of these 32 patients was 30.8±4.7 years relative to 26.4±4.7 years for the remainder ($P<0.001$) while the body mass indices were 29.2±6.2 and 25±4 respectively ($P<0.003$). The lengths of gestation did not differ (273±15 and 276±15 d respectively) nor did birthweight (3422±604 g and 3366±510 g).

Conclusions

If a 75-g OGTT is to be used during pregnancy to screen for diabetes and IGT, allowances must be made for the normal physiological adaptations which occur. We offer the following suggestions.

1. About 10% of pregnant women will reach or exceed a value of 8 mmol/l at 2-h but it is unlikely that 10% of the European population have disordered carbohydrate metabolism.

2. By increasing the 2-h cut-off value to 9 mmol/l or more the number of mothers regarded as at risk would reduce by about half (from 79 to 32 in this series).

3. The 1-h value could be included in any further analysis of the response of the patient. By doing this many fewer women will be regarded as "abnormal"; in this series it reduced the 79 women with a 2-h value >8 mmol/l to 15 who were considered to have carbohydrate intolerance (two with diabetes; 13 with IGT).

4. We would recommend that a 75-g oral glucose load be used and preferably at least two blood samples should be obtained: 60 and 120 min. To diagnose carbohydrate intolerance, venous plasma or capillary whole blood concentration should be 9 mmol/l or more and associated with a 60-min value of 10.5 mmol/l or more (the venous plasma 95th centile). Diabetes should be diagnosed on the existing WHO criteria. The theoretical advantages of using the 95th centile values specific for capillary whole blood and venous plasma are probably outweighed by the practical advantage of using one set of interpretive criteria.

5. From the obstetric viewpoint mothers who "screen positive" do not have bigger babies, they deliver close to term and do not have particular stigmata such as a family history of diabetes, an increased tendency to smoke or an adverse obstetric outcome. However they do tend to be older and heavier.

6. The term "gestational diabetes" should be reserved for those in whom the blood glucose levels are diagnostic of diabetes and not IGT. If the term "impaired glucose tolerance during pregnancy" is too long the abbreviation to "gestational IGT" seems a reasonable alternative.

References

WHO Expert Committee on Diabetes Mellitus (1980) World Health Organization Technical Report Series 646

Diabetes Mellitus Report of a WHO Study Group (1985) World Health Organization Technical Report Series 727

20. Targets in Oral Glucose Tolerance Testing

K. Fuhrmann

Introduction

Accurate estimates of the incidence of abnormal glucose tolerance during pregnancy and of the frequency and the value of gestational diabetes (GDM) risk factors are virtually non-existent. Screening select populations of women with risk factors for the condition, and the non-random, non-population-based nature of most studies, have given rise to wide variations in the reported incidence and significance of risk factors and GDM.

Methods

We examined a randomized population-based group of 2510 pregnant women from Berlin (GDR). All women who came for the first clinic visit during early pregnancy were ascribed serial numbers and the patients with an odd number were asked to take part in the study. In order to ensure representative socioeconomic status of the group, three typical districts of Berlin were chosen. A careful medical history was recorded and subsequently all the laboratory values obtained generally during pregnancy were documented. During the 26th and 36th weeks of pregnancy a 50-g OGTT was performed under standardized conditions. (Capillary whole blood glucose was analysed by an automated glucose oxidase method.) In order to study the reproducibility of the 50-g OGTT during pregnancy, a second test was performed after 14 d in nearly 150 cases. During the GTT insulin and triglyceride levels were estimated.

No treatment was instituted in the intervals between the tests in the reproducibility studies.

Results were considered to be normal when two or three values were equal to or below mean +1 SD. This allowed one value to lie between mean +1 SD and mean +2 SDs.

Carbohydrate Metabolism in Pregnancy and the Newborn IV

Table 20.1. Mean blood glucose values (mmol/l) and standard deviation (SD) of 2510 50-g OGTT during the third trimester of pregnancy in a normal city population

	Mean	Mean + 2 SD gestational diabetes[a]
Fasting	3.89 ± 0.83	≥5.55
60 min	5.99 ± 1.44	≥8.87
120 min	4.66 ± 1.22	≥7.10

[a] See text for criteria.

The rounded criteria for normality in the OGTT are as follows (mean +2 SD of the whole population):

fasting 5.55 mmol/l (100 mg/dl)
1 h 8.88 mmol/l (160 mg/dl),
2 h 7.22 mmol/l (130 mg/dl) (Table 20.1)

Women identified as having two or more abnormal OGTT values (i.e. ≥ mean ± 2 SDs) were designated as having gestational diabetes (GDM).

Women with blood glucose values intermediate between these two categories were classified as having impaired glucose tolerance (IGT).

To study the reproducibility of a 75-g OGTT during pregnancy two tests were performed in 53 healthy pregnant women and in 10 women with GDM.

Results and Discussions

The GDM prevalence in this defined population of 2510 women was 1.1%; 6% had IGT and 92.9% had normal glucose tolerance. Gestational diabetes prevalence increased with the duration of pregnancy as does the IGT prevalence in a more pronounced way (Table 20.2).

There is no significant blood glucose rise during the later stages of pregnancy (Table 20.3). The reproducibility of a 50-g OGTT is good in more than 70% of

Table 20.2. Glucose tolerance depending on gestational age (%)

Week of pregnancy	Normal	IGT	GDM
Mean	92.9	6.0	1.1
≤28th week	94.6	4.4	1.0
29th–32nd week	93.3	5.9	0.8
33rd–36th week	88.9	8.8	2.3
≥37th week	87.7	10.8	1.5

Table 20.3. Blood glucose mean (mmol/l) and SD depending on the weeks of pregnancy

Weeks of pregnancy	0 min	60 min	120 min
≤28th week	3.8 ± 0.8	5.8 ± 1.3	4.5 ± 1.1
29th–32nd week	3.9 ± 0.8	5.9 ± 1.3	4.7 ± 1.1
33rd–36th week	3.9 ± 0.9	6.2 ± 1.4	4.8 ± 1.2
≥37th week	3.9 ± 0.8	6.4 ± 1.3	4.7 ± 1.1

Table 20.4. Mean blood glucose values ± SEM (mmol/l) in the first (I) and second (II) OGTT

	I	II
Normal glucose tolerance (n = 101)		
0 min	4.11 ± 0.87	4.16 ± 0.89
60 min	7.08 ± 1.66	7.38 ± 1.84
120 min	5.21 ± 1.42	5.55 ± 1.70
IGT (n = 41)		
0 min	5.05 ± 1.08	4.45 ± 0.99
60 min	8.24 ± 1.52	7.18 ± 1.58
120 min	6.58 ± 1.08	5.89 ± 1.89
Gestational diabetes (n = 5)		
0 min	6.08 ± 0.92	3.91 ± 0.76
60 min	9.04 ± 1.54	7.97 ± 0.60
120 min	7.16 ± 2.47	5.62 ± 2.15

pregnant women with normal carbohydrate metabolism. In women with IGT or with GDM the reproducibility is worse (Table 20.4 and Figs. 20.1 and 20.4). In the studies of reproducibility represented in Fig. 20.1 it will be seen that, at the second time of testing, there were 106 women found to have normal OGTT results comprising those categorised *in the first test as*: normal (n = 75), IGT (n = 28) and GDM (n = 3).

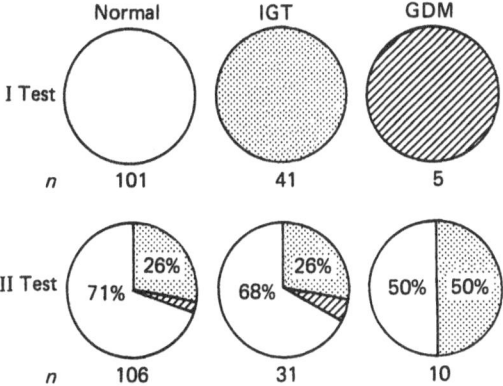

Fig. 20.1. Reproducibility of a 50-g OGTT during pregnancy. Second OGTT after 14 d.

Similarly at the second test, there were 31 women found to have IGT results comprising those classified *in the first test* as: normal ($n = 21$), IGT ($n = 8$) and GDM ($n = 2$). At the second time of testing, 10 women had GDM, none of whom had GDM at the first test, but five had been classified as IGT and five had been normal.

Therefore in an additional study the reproducibility of a 75-g OGTT was tested. The results of these tests are shown in Fig. 20.5.

In normal pregnant women the reproducibility of the 75-g test is similar to that of the 50-g test and in GDM the reproducibility is no better than with the 50-g test. The insulin response after a 50-g OGTT is not significantly different between the normal, impaired and pathological glucose tolerance groups (Fig. 20.2). The increase of glycerol after an OGTT during the first 60 min in the gestational diabetic group (Fig. 20.3) and in addition a significantly reduced insulin glucose index (Table 20.5) indicate a relative lack of circulating insulin. The historical and clinical factors traditionally employed to identify patients who are at high risk for the occurrence of gestational diabetes (risk factors) were determined and evaluated (Table 20.6)

Table 20.5. Δ Insulin/Δ Glucose index after a 50-g OGTT in women with normal glucose tolerance and without risk factors, in gestational diabetes and in pregnant women with different risk factors

Normal glucose tolerance	1.58
Gestational diabetes	0.53
Age $\geqslant$30 years	0.70
Relat. overweight $\geqslant$30%	0.79
Glucosuria	0.82
Family history of diabetes (1st or/and 2nd degree relative)	1.41

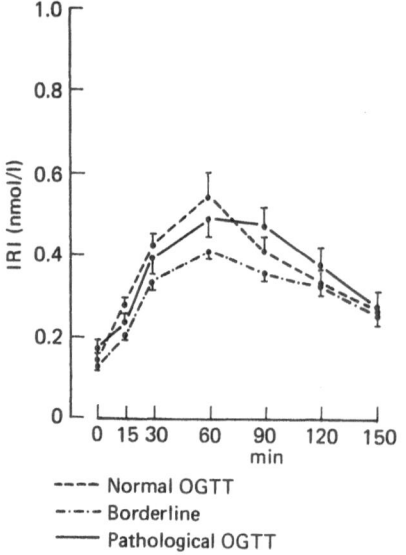

---- Normal OGTT
–·–· Borderline
—— Pathological OGTT

Fig. 20.2. Immunoreactive insulin during a 50-g OGTT in pregnant women with normal, impaired and pathological glucose tolerance.

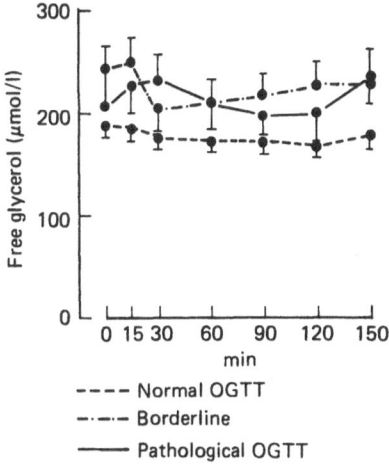

Fig. 20.3. Free glycerol during a 50-g OGTT in pregnant women with normal, impaired and pathological glucose tolerance.

Table 20.6. The frequency of risk factors in 2510 pregnant women of a city population and in gestational diabetic women

Risk factors	n	Frequency % in population	Frequency % in gestational diabetic women
1. Age ≥25 years	740	29.6	65.5
2. Overweight ≥20%	277	11.1	48.3
3. Glucosuria during the first half of pregnancy (24th week)	223	8.9	51.7
4. Birthweight ≥4000 g in the history	79	3.2	13.8
5. Stillbirth in the history	27	1.1	0.0
6. Abortions in the history	259	11.8	24.1
7. Previous deliveries	967	38.7	72.4
8. Blood pressure ≥140/90	598	23.9	34.5
9. Pathological weight gain during pregnancy	1596	63.4	62.0
10. Proteinuria	78	3.12	13.8
11. Diabetes heredity 1st and/or 2nd relative	600	24.0	48.3
12. Absence of risk factors	364	14.5	0.0

Of the whole population, 85.5% had at least one of the presumed risk factors mentioned in the literature. Thus only 14.5% were without risk factors. Most of the risk factors used for GDM screening in the literature really indicate an increased risk of GDM. Only a past history of fetal death and pathological weight gain during pregnancy do not indicate an increased risk of having GDM. There is no specific risk factor for GDM. Therefore it is of importance to determine how often a risk factor occurs in the population. With a single risk factor it is possible to detect from 13% to 72% of all GDM (Table 20.6). When only patients with a combination of two risk factors are tested, a maximum of 31% of those with GDM are detectable; a combination of three risk factors allows the identification of a maximum of 17% of all those with GDM (Table 20.7).

Table 20.7. Combinations of risk factors existing in a city population and in those with GDM

1. Risk factor	2. Risk factor	3. Risk factor	% of population	% of gestational diabetics
Overweight ≥20%	Glucosuria		1.3	31.0
Overweight ≥20%	Family history		4.0	27.6
Overweight ≥20%	Abortions		1.5	6.9
Overweight ≥20%	Glucosuria	Family history	0.56	17.3
Overweight ≥20%	Family history	Abortions	0.70	3.45
Glucosuria	Family history		3.3	27.6
Glucosuria	Abortions		1.3	10.4
Family history 1st°	Abortions		4.3	6.9
Family history 1st°	Pathological weight gain		20.4	24.2

In this study screening based on the presence of any of the risk factors with the exception of pathological weight gain and previous stillbirth, demonstrates that such factors detect a maximum of approximately 70% of all those with GDM. Moreover this is more or less independent of which risk factors are used. The risk factors which are chosen determine the number of OGTTs that will be performed. In our study the risk factors overweight ≥20% or age ≥30 years, or glucosuria, or heredity first degree, or large-for-gestational-age baby ≥4.000 g or three or more deliveries were found in 27% of the whole population. In this group we found 72.4% of all women with gestational diabetes. The risk factors overweight ≥30%, glucosuria, age ≥30 years and heredity first degree were found in 21.2% of the whole population. In this group also 72.4% of all the women with gestational diabetes were present. The risk factors investigated are of differing importance. In women with one risk factor, we found GDM two to twelve times more often than in women without risk factors. In comparison with women without risk factors, in women with two risk factors GDM was found up to 20 times more often. Unfortunately only 1.3% of the population had the combination of the two risk factors (glucosuria and overweight ≥30%) and therefore only 30% of those with GDM could be detected. The risk factors we investigated with the highest GDM prevalence were: glucosuria before the 24th week of pregnancy, overweight ≥30%, age ≥30 years and a history of diabetes in the mother. These four factors were found to be present in 20% of the population and were represented in 70% of all women with GDM. Patients with these risk factors had also a significantly decreased insulin glucose index (Table 20.5).

Screening Using Fasting Blood Glucose Values

We evaluated fasting blood glucose (FBG) and the 1-h and 2-h postglucose challenge values for their suitability in a screening programme for GDM.

Out of 2510 pregnant women 26.8% exceeded an FBG of ≥4.4 mmol/l (70 mg/dl). One hundred per cent of those with GDM had an FBG of ≥4.4 mmol/l.

17.8% of the whole group exceeded 4.72 mmol/l (84 mg/dl) and using this level for screening, 93% of those with GDM could be detected.

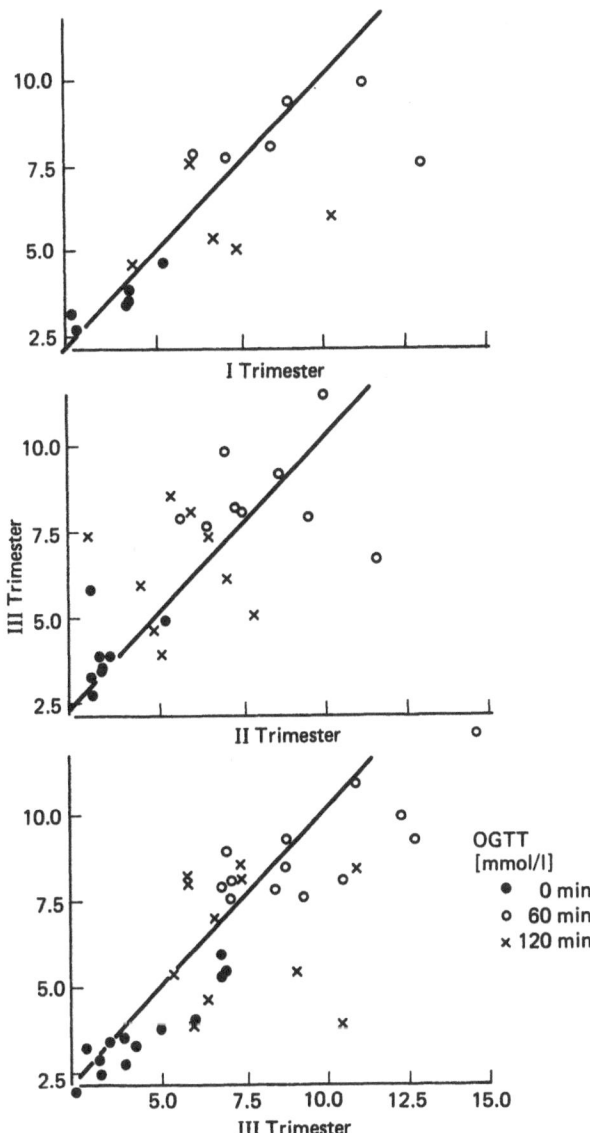

Fig. 20.4. Reproducibility of a 50-g OGTT in women with GDM. (OGTTs of first, second and third trimester are compared to a third-trimester OGTT.)

12.3% of pregnant women exceeded 5.0 mmol/l (90 mg/dl) and this group included 86.4% of the women with GDM.

5.6% of all women exceeded 5.5 mmol/l (98 mg/dl). This group embraced 76% of all women with GDM (Table 20.8).

Gestational diabetes mellitus screening by an FBG has a sensitivity of 100% if the threshold value is 4.4 mmol/l but in 26.8% of all pregnant women an OGTT

Table 20.8. Sensitivity and specificity of fasting and postprandial blood glucose values for a GDM screening. Screening with fasting (FBG) and postprandial blood glucose values

Fasting	≥4.44 mmol/l	≥5.00 mmol/l	≥5.55 mmol/l
Normal OGTT	20.8%	7.4%	3.0%
IGT	80.8%	64.0%	27.8%
Gestational diabetes	100.0%	86.3%	75.9%

60-min postprandial	≥7.22 mmol/l	≥7.77 mmol/l
Normal OGTT	15.0%	6.0%
IGT	74.6%	63.4%
Gestational diabetes	96.6%	96.6%

would be necessary. With an FBG of 5.5 mmol/l the sensitivity is 76% and 5.6% of all pregnant women would need an OGTT.

Screening by Glucose Challenge

Using an oral glucose challenge and measuring the blood glucose value at 60 min for a GDM screening programme, the sensitivity is 96.6% when the borderline value is 7.22 mmol/l (129 mg/dl). 20.6% of all pregnant women exceeded 7.22 mmol/l and would need an OGTT. A threshold value of 7.77 mmol/l (138 mg/dl) included 11% of the population and still detected 96.6% of all GDM women.

Two hours after a 50-g glucose load 207 out of 2510 pregnant women (8.2%) exceeded 6.38 mmol/l (114 mg/dl) and 76.2% of all GDM women were detected. A 2-h "postprandial" BG value of 6.94 mmol/l (124 mg/dl) included only 3.8% of normals, but 76.2% of those with GDM. Fasting and postglucose load blood glucose values are suitable for screening for GDM. The sensitivity and specificity is similar in the three testing conditions. For the detection of about 76% of all GDM women about 4%–6% of all pregnant women would need an OGTT depending on the kind of BG screening used. Screening with risk factors and blood glucose values enables a less expensive diagnosis of GDM to be made. In comparison with the policy of screening by risk factors two-thirds fewer OGTTs are needed to detect the same number of women with GDM.

Screening by blood glucose alone is more sensitive than screening by risk factors, but more expensive. All pregnant women need one blood glucose value and 4%–6% need one OGTT to detect 76% of those with GDM.

For general screening in the GDR we advise the following steps.

First Step. At 24 weeks gestation, documentation should be taken of all women to identify the presence of one or more of the following risk factors (approximately 20% of all pregnant women): glucosuria before the 24th week of pregnancy, overweight ≥30%, age ≥30 years and heredity first degree (especially the mother).

Second Step. The fasting blood glucose value should be measured in the risk group. Women with an FBG ≥4.44 mmol/l require an OGTT.

Third Step. An OGTT.

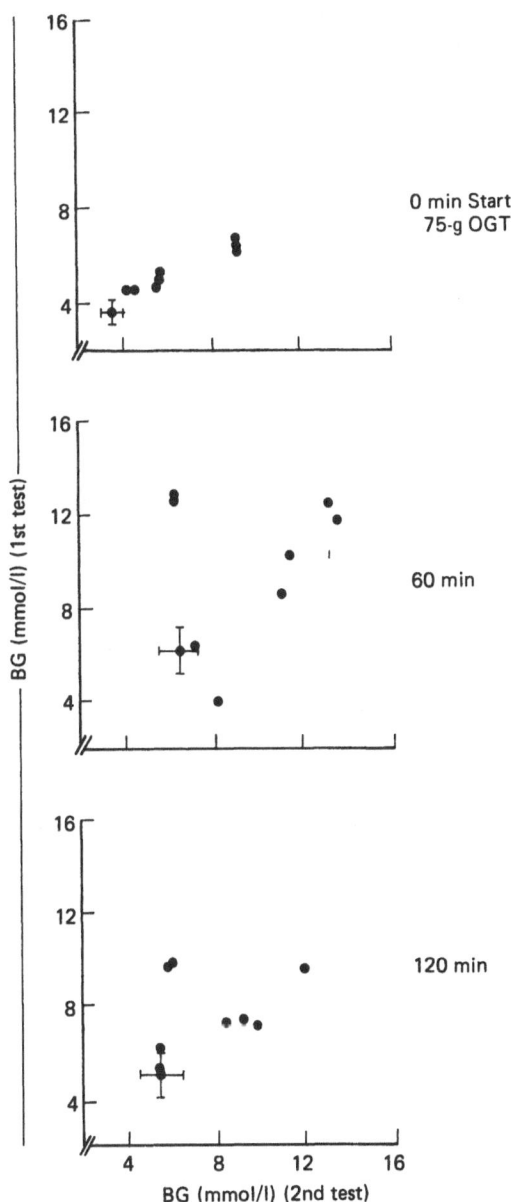

Fig. 20.5. Reproducibility of a 75-g OGTT in women with normal carbohydrate metabolism and in GDM.

Fourth Step. Gestational diabetes mellitus women need a day (night) blood glucose profile to be performed every month. Women with a mean blood glucose (MBG) value of ⩾5.0 mmol/l are transferred to a high-risk pregnancy clinic. We start insulin therapy if the MBG exceeds 5.5 mmol/l.

Follow-up. To evaluate the OGTT criteria we used in our study a follow-up was performed during the 8 years after delivery of all IGT and gestational diabetic women. For our follow-up programme we used the 75-g OGTT according to the WHO recommendations. 75-g OGTTs were performed at 3 months, 6 months, 1 year and 8 years after pregnancy. Applying the WHO criteria, within 8 years 46% of those with GDM became diabetic, mostly with NIDDM (Table 20.9). Only 3% of the IGT group were diabetic after 8 years (Table 20.10). From the risk factors investigated during pregnancy only overweight and age showed significant correlations with diabetes incidence 1 and 8 years after pregnancy.

Table 20.9. Eight year follow-up of glucose tolerance in women with gestational diabetes ($n=50$)

	3 months after pregnancy	6 months after pregnancy	12 months after pregnancy	8 years after pregnancy
Diabetes	4% (2)	4% (2)	18% (9)	46% (23)
IGT	4% (2)	8% (4)	20% (10)	16% (8)
Normal	92% (46)	88% (44)	62% (31)	38% (19)

Table 20.10. Eight-year follow-up of glucose tolerance in women with IGT during pregnancy ($n=29$)

Diabetes mellitus	3% (1)
IGT	28% (8)
Normal	69% (20)

Close correlations were found also between the diabetes incidence 1 and 8 years after pregnancy and both the need for insulin treatment during pregnancy and the occurrence of diabetic fetopathy.

Conclusions

The GDM incidence in a German city population is about 1%. As early as 3 months after delivery, four out of 100 of those who had GDM have overt diabetes.

One year after pregnancy 18% and 8 years after pregnancy 46% of those with GDM had become diabetic, mostly with NIDDM.

The diabetes incidence of borderline cases was only 3% after 8 years (Table 20.10).

The reproducibility of a 50-g OGTT is good only in pregnant women with normal carbohydrate metabolism: a pathological test is poorly reproducible.

The 75-g OGTT has no better reproducibility of a pathological test than has the 50-g test.

Women with one pathological OGTT are at risk and should be followed up during pregnancy and afterwards.

Screening for GDM is possible with blood glucose values in the fasting as well as the postchallenge state. Screening with risk factors and fasting or postchallenge blood glucose values is less expensive.

21. The Spectrum of Glucose Tolerance During Pregnancy

G. Russell, G. Farmer, D. R. Hamilton-Nicol, I. S. Ross and H. W. Sutherland

This chapter is based on data collected in the course of a study of glucose tolerance in 918 non-diabetic women (Farmer et al. 1988), selected randomly from the antenatal clinics at Aberdeen Maternity Hospital and subjected to a 25-g intravenous glucose tolerance test (IVGTT) (Fisher et al. 1974) at about 32 weeks gestation. The results were not made available to the patients or their medical attendants, and no treatment or advice was offered.

Although no prospective attempt was made to ensure that the population studied was representative of the population from which it was drawn, a retrospective comparison of the study population with the entire population of pregnant women attending Aberdeen Maternity Hospital during the study period (Fig. 21.1) showed that the two groups were similar in terms of maternal age, parity and ultimate mode of delivery; the study population contained a slight excess of women in the upper social classes, a finding almost unavoidable in a study demanding patient time and cooperation.

Maternal glucose disposal was assessed using the following indices:

1. *Absolute index* (AI) (disappearance rate of injected glucose).
2. *Increment index* (II) (disappearance rate of injected glucose relative to fasting).
3. *Summed plasma glucose* (SPG) (sum of glucose values including fasting but excluding 4-min value).

The indices of glucose disposal were distributed unimodally with no evidence of a separately identifiable pathological subgroup towards the "diabetic" end of the spectrum (see Fig. 21.2). The interpretation of individual values must therefore be statistical; abnormality cannot be assigned on the criterion of 2 SD beyond the mean because the distributions are skewed, so centile values (e.g. 2.5th) must be used. However, unless clinical problems can be shown to be associated with such arbitrarily defined biochemical abnormality, the use of the terms "normal" and "abnormal", even if mathematically correct, has no clinical relevance and in particular there is no justification for recommending treatment solely on the basis of such results.

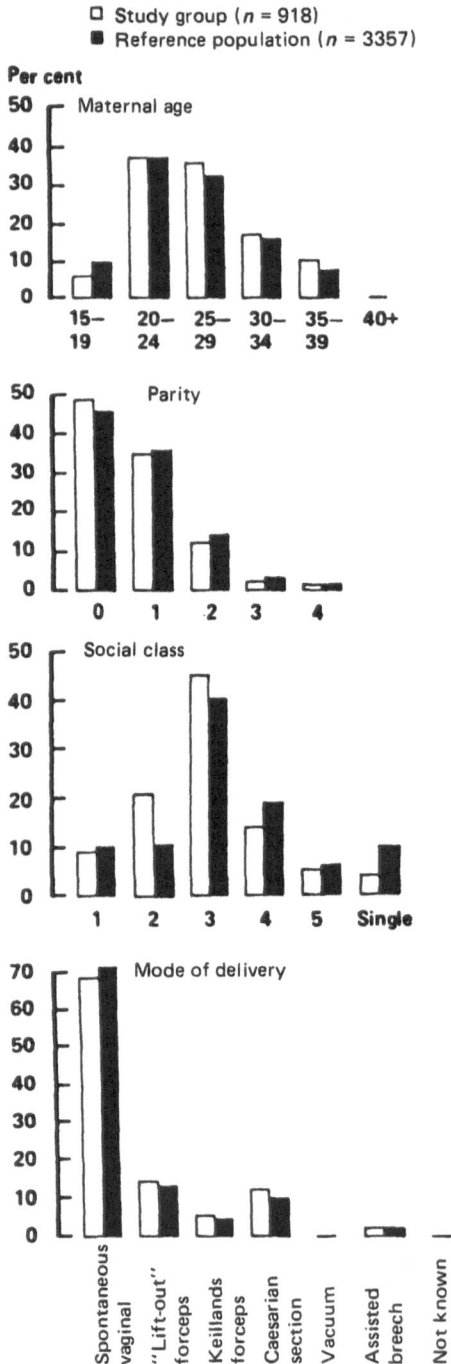

□ Study group (n = 918)
■ Reference population (n = 3357)

Fig. 21.1. Comparison of study population with reference population.

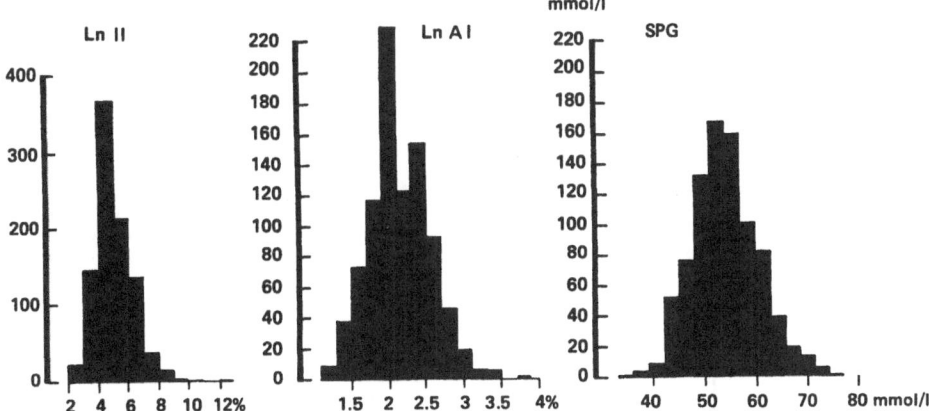

Fig. 21.2. Distributions of increment index (II), absolute index (AI) and summed plasma glucose (SPG).

We have therefore examined the relationships between the indices of maternal glucose tolerance and various aspects of fetal growth and morbidity; details of these relationships have been published elsewhere (Farmer et al. 1988) and will not be repeated here.

When the indices of maternal glucose disposal were correlated with measurements of fetal growth, the relationships were continuous with no evidence of a subgroup in whom a pathological effect might be operating. Nevertheless, although the effects of maternal glucose on fetal growth were slight, they were statistically highly significant; for example the regression coefficient for AI against Infant Birthweight Standard Deviation Score (Altman and Coles 1980) was only −0.2819, but because 917 cases were included in the analysis, the result attained a high degree of statistical significance ($P<0.001$). There is no evidence from our study that these effects on fetal growth are due to a pathological effect of glucose intolerance at one end of the scale (the effect of glucose "supertolerance" in producing light babies is similar to the effects of glucose "intolerance" in producing heavy babies, see Fig. 21.3) or that they pose any danger to the fetus.

Of much greater clinical interest is the relationship between maternal glucose disposal and the presence of neonatal morbidity. In the previous Colloquium (Farmer and Russell 1984) we published a preliminary analysis of the relationship between SPG and congenital malformation; this relationship is presented in Fig. 21.4 which illustrates clearly that abnormalities of all grades are more frequent in the offspring of mothers with higher SPG values, but that this relationship is not the result of the malign influence of glucose tolerance impaired beyond a certain cut-off point at one end of the spectrum. Grouping of the data by centiles, deciles and quartiles fails to demonstrate a cut-off point, which emerges only when the distribution is divided into halves.

The relationship between maternal SPG and other indices of neonatal morbidity is illustrated in Fig. 21.5 in which it can be seen that at gestational ages beyond 40 weeks perinatal asphyxia, admission to the Special Care Baby Unit (SCBU), transient tachypnoea of the newborn and suspected sepsis (which probably reflects perinatal asphyxia) were associated with significantly increased

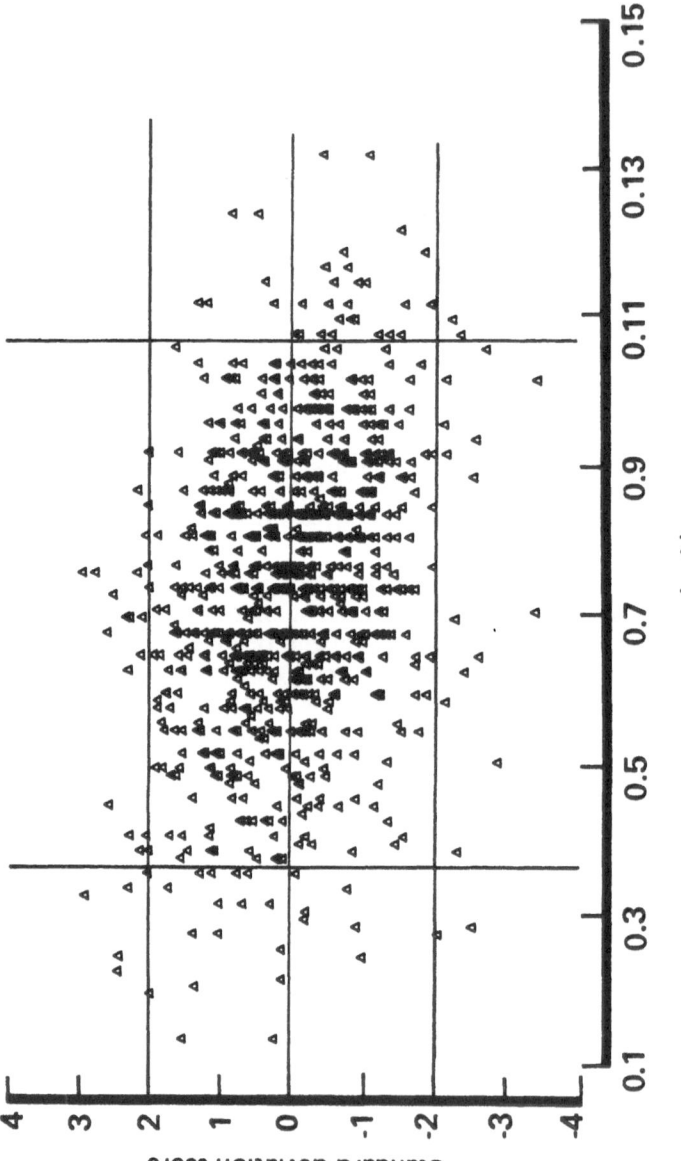

Fig. 21.3. Scattergram of relationship between absolute index (AI) (logged) and birthweight standard deviation score. The *horizontal lines* divide the infants into those whose birthweights lie more than 2 SD above or below the mean for gestational age, and the *vertical lines* divide the AI values at the 3rd and 97th centiles.

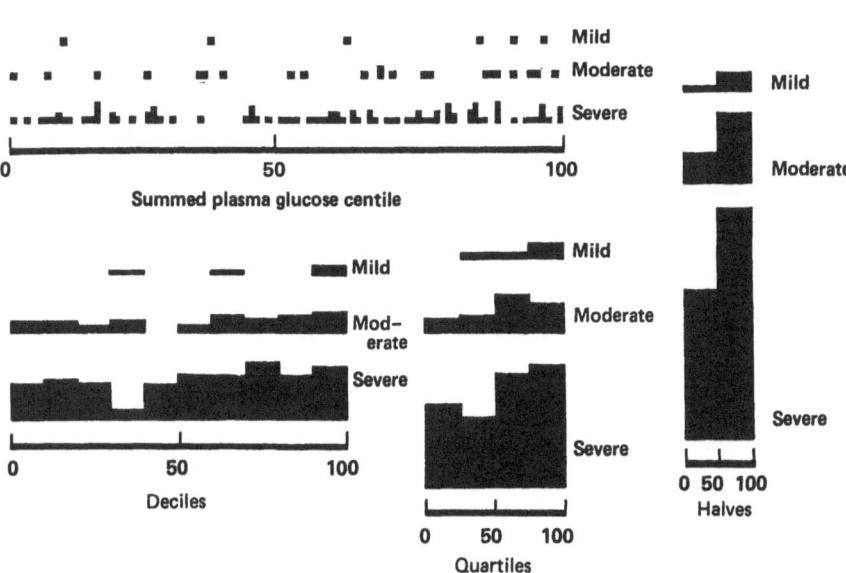

Fig. 21.4. Incidence of congenital malformations at different levels of maternal summed plasma glucose (SPG), grouped in centiles, deciles, quartiles and halves.

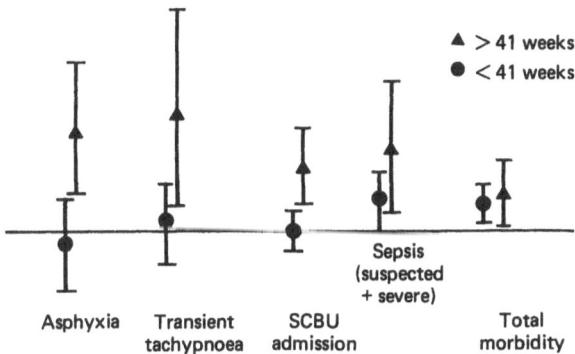

Fig. 21.5. 95% confidence limits for mean maternal summed plasma glucose associated with various types of neonatal morbidity; the *horizontal line* indicates the mean for mothers of babies who did not suffer that particular type of morbidity.

maternal SPG. These associations were either absent or much less strong at gestational ages of less than 41 weeks.

There is therefore good reason to suggest that glucose tolerance as assessed by the IVGTT in non-diabetic mothers has an effect on the occurrence of various types of neonatal morbidity, particularly congenital malformations and asphyxia in post-term infants. This in turn raises interesting therapeutic possibilities; if the mothers in the "diabetic" centiles could be transferred to the "normal" centiles, then perhaps the prognosis for the infant might be improved; there is certainly good reason to imagine so. There would seem to be little point in trying to identify a small "pathological" group of mothers using the IVGTT; our data suggest that the adverse effects of maternal glucose intolerance are graded throughout the range of normal values, and that there is no cut-off point at one end of the distribution beyond which the well-being of the fetus is predictably compromised, nor a point at the other end beyond which fetal wellbeing is secure. Instead of searching for ever milder forms of gestational diabetes, treatment should be universal, should start before pregnancy is embarked upon and should focus on simple dietary recommendations of the type already widely applied in the management of diabetes (American Diabetes Association 1979; British Diabetic Association 1982), with advice to consume a diet high in fibre and low in refined carbohydrate.

References

Altman DG, Coles EC (1980) Assessing birth-weight-for-dates on a continuous scale. Ann Hum Biol 33:717–720

American Diabetes Association (1979) Principles of nutrition and dietary recommendations for individuals with diabetes mellitus. Diabetes 28:1027–1030

British Diabetic Association (1982) Dietary recommendations for diabetics in the 1980s. Hum Nutr Appl Nutr 36A:1027–1030

Farmer G, Russell G (1984) Indices of fetal growth and neonatal morbidity in relation to glucose tolerance during pregnancy. In: Sutherland HW, Stowers JM (eds) Carbohydrate metabolism in pregnancy and the newborn. Churchill Livingstone, Edinburgh, pp 190–194

Farmer G, Russell G, Hamilton-Nicol DR et al. (1988) The influence of maternal glucose metabolism on fetal growth, development and morbidity in 917 singleton pregnancies in nondiabetic women. Diabetologia 31:134–141

Fisher PM, Hamilton PM, Sutherland HW, Stowers JM (1974) The effect of pregnancy on intravenous glucose tolerance. J Obstet Gynaecol Br Commonw 81:285–290

22. Further Observations in Lean and Obese Women with Gestational Diabetes During a 400-Kilocalorie Meal Tolerance Test

Dorothy R. Hollingsworth, D. Ney, V. Fujimoto, M. Milewski and H. Murphy

Glucose loading tests have provided useful criteria for the diagnosis of gestational diabetes (GDM) (O'Sullivan and Mahan 1964; Gillmer et al. 1980; Barden and Knowles 1981; Carpenter and Coustan 1982). Clinical observations during a 400-kilocalorie meal tolerance test in lean and obese women with GDM have demonstrated heterogeneity in the disorder (Cheney et al. 1985; Hollingsworth et al. 1985), and Freinkel et al. (1986) have described both phenotypic and genotypic heterogeneity in the syndrome.

A diagnosis of GDM may have adverse long-term implications for both mothers and infants. Is it possible to utilize a brief, practical, physiological test to provide a better metabolic definition of women with this problem? Since 1980 we have administered a 400-kilocalorie breakfast meal tolerance test (MTT) to all pregnant diabetic women (IDDM, NIDDM, GDM) who served as research subjects at the University of California, San Diego Medical Center. This report describes our experience with the MTT in 83 lean and obese women with GDM and 27 normal pregnant women of comparable weights. The purpose of the study was to assess the degree of glucose intolerance following an isocaloric breakfast meal and possible metabolic differences to this physiological challenge in lean and obese women with GDM. A second objective was to compare the neonatal problems and size of infants of mothers with quantitatively defined metabolic profiles.

Methods

Patients

Normal pregnant women and those with gestational diabetes were recruited from the obstetric clinics at the University of California, San Diego Medical Center.

Four groups of subjects participated in the study: lean women with GDM (BMI ≤27, $n = 45$); obese women with GDM (BMI >27, $n = 38$); lean normal women (BMI ≤24, $n = 22$) and obese normal women (BMI >27, $n = 10$). Women with gestational diabetes had no previous history of glucose intolerance and met the criteria of O'Sullivan and Mahan (1964) for the diagnosis of gestational diabetes. Patients with a previous diagnosis of diabetes, a history of therapy with oral hypoglycaemic medications or HbA1 ≥8% (normal: 5%–8%) before 20 weeks gestation were excluded from the diagnosis of gestational diabetes because they had evidence of impaired glucose tolerance when not pregnant. Women with an abnormal 75-g oral glucose tolerance test (WHO criteria, 1980) at or after 6 weeks postpartum were also excluded from the data analysis and reclassified as having diabetes or impaired glucose tolerance when not pregnant.

Anthropometric and skinfold measurements for normal newborn infants (values at sea level) were obtained for 199 Mexican–American and Caucasian baby boys and girls. Buccal, triceps and subscapular skinfolds were measured with Harpenden skinfold callipers (Brans et al. 1974) on the first day of life along with weight, length, head circumference, hip and waist circumferences and crown–rump length. Informed consent for the meal tolerance study was obtained from each patient and from all mothers of newborn infants in the anthropometric study.

Treatment of Gestational Diabetes

Diet (Algert et al. 1985)

Patients with GDM were individually instructed in the American Diabetes Association diet (1979). Obese women with GDM were prescribed a total daily caloric intake of approximately 1700–1800 kcal (not less than 25 kcal/kg ideal body weight) and lean women with GDM were prescribed a daily caloric intake of 2000–3000 kcal (not less than 36 kcal/kg). Record keeping included a daily tally of food intake using an exchange list. Control subjects were given dietary instruction on the recommended diet for pregnancy (National Research Council 1980).

Insulin

All GDM patients were seen in the Diabetes in Pregnancy clinic each week where a 2-h postbreakfast blood glucose level was obtained using an Accuchek II meter. Women who had more than one value greater than 120 mg/dl (6.7 mmol/l) were treated with small doses of regular insulin before each meal based on glucose meter readings performed in the clinic and at home.

400-Kilocalorie Meal Tolerance Test (MTT)

This procedure was performed by the staff at the Clinical Research Center (CRC) and has been described previously (Cheney et al. 1985). Tables 22.1a and 22.1b describe the meal and results ± standard deviation in 23 normal lean and 10 obese pregnant women in the third trimester. Each patient fasted for 12 h before the test. Fasting blood samples were drawn at 8:00 a.m. for measurement of glycosylated haemoglobin A_1, plasma total triglyceride, total cholesterol, glucose, insulin, C-peptide, glucagon and human chorionic somatomammotropin (hCS). Measurements of glucose and hormone responses to the test meal were obtained at 30, 60 and 120 min. The 400-kcal breakfast was eaten in 10 min. Timing of the test began with the first bite of food.

Table 22.1a. 400-kilocalorie mixed breakfast test meal

Exchange	Food	Amount	Carbohydrate (g)	Protein (g)	Fat (g)	Kilocalories	Dietary fibre (g)
1 Fruit	Grape juice	3 oz	15.8	0.4	—	65	—
1 Bread	White bread	25 g	11.9	2.2	0.8	64	0.68
1 Meat	1 Egg (large)	50 g	0.35	6.4	5.8	79	—
1 Fat	Margarine	4 g	—	—	4.0	36	—
1 Milk	Whole milk	8 oz	11.0	8.0	9.0	157	—
Total			39.1	17	19.6	401	0.68
Per cent (energy)			39	17	44	100	NS (0.1)

Table 22.1b. Breakfast meal tolerance test in 23 lean and 10 obese normal pregnant women

Time (min)	Glucose mg/dl (mmol/l)	Insulin μU/ml	C-peptide ng/ml	Glucagon pg/ml	hCS μg/dl	CHOL ng/dl	TG ng/dl
L	75 ± 7 (4.2)	17 ± 9	2.3 ± 1	158 ± 67	4.6 ± 1.4	259 ± 46	244 ± 82
O	80 ± 6 (4.4)	26 ± 19	5.1 ± 3	179 ± 80	4.9 ± 1.4	256 ± 24	229 ± 72
30							
L	111 ± 13 (6.2)	102 ± 45	6.5 ± 4	161 ± 73	4.4 ± 1.1	—	—
O	112 ± 8 (6.2)	123 ± 63	10.5 ± 6	188 ± 77	4.5 ± 1.7	—	—
60							
L	106 ± 12 (5.9)	90 ± 42	6.7 ± 4	152 ± 58	4.7 ± 1.4	—	—
O	108 ± 15 (6.0)	109 ± 45	11.0 ± 4	187 ± 74	4.3 ± 1.6	—	—
120							
L	84 ± 8 (4.7)	51 ± 36	6.1 ± 4	170 ± 79	4.8 ± 1.6	—	—
O	92 ± 6 (5.1)	56 ± 20	9.5 ± 5	187 ± 72	4.8 ± 1.6	—	—

All values are presented as mean ± standard deviation.
hCS, human chorionic somatomammotropin (hPL, human placental lactogen); CHOL, cholesterol; TG, triglyceride; L, lean (BMI ⩽24); n=22); O, obese (BMI >27; n=10).

Plasma glucose was measured by a glucose oxidase method and glycosylated haemoglobin by the Isolab fast haemoglobin test system (Cousins et al. 1984). Determinations of immunoreactive insulin and C-peptide were by the methods of Kuzuya et al. (1977). Plasma immunoreactive glucagon was measured by the method of Harris et al. (1978) and hCS by a modification of the Moser and Hollingsworth method (1973).

The data from the four groups of patients were compared using t-tests and linear correlation and regression analysis. Unless otherwise indicated, random variation is given as standard deviation of the mean.

Results

Patients

In our clinic the majority of women with GDM are Mexican–American (Table 22.2); the higher number of Caucasian normals in the comparison groups reflects the recruitment process for experimental subjects. As a group obese women with GDM were appreciably heavier (P 0.0) and taller ($P<0.02$) with a higher body mass index (P 0.0) than lean women with GDM. They gained less weight during pregnancy (PNS), they had larger placentas (PNS) and heavier infants (PNS).

Table 22.2. Characteristics of lean and obese women with gestational diabetes

Group	Age (years)	Weight (kg)	BMI (kg/m²)	Weight gain in pregnancy (kg)	Hb$_{A1}$ (at term) (%)	Placental weight (g)	Infant birth weight (g)	Gestational age (weeks)
Gestational diabetes								
Lean (38)	31 ± 7	56 ± 7	23 ± 3 (36)	14 ± 6 (32)	6.4 ± 0.8	530 ± 100 (34)	3574 ± 570	40 ± 1
Obese (45)	31 ± 5	93 ± 17	36 ± 5 (34)	14 ± 10 (34)	6.9 ± 1	570 ± 105 (32)	3812 ± 535	40 ± 1
P	NS	0.0	0.0	NS	0.02	NS	NS	NS
Normal								
Lean (23)	26 ± 4	57 ± 8	22 ± 3	16 ± 5 (10)	5.8 ± 0.5 (16)	542 ± 114 (10)	3368 ± 60 (199)	40 ± 0.1
Obese (17)	28 ± 6	93 ± 18	35 ± 5	11 ± 5 (12)	6.0 ± 0.9 (9)	611 ± 164 (13)	3813 ± 588 (16)	40 ± 1
P	NS	0.0	0.0	0.02	NS	NS	0.0	NS

All values are presented as mean ± standard deviation.
( ) = Number of subjects.

Diagnosis of Gestational Diabetes

Table 22.3 shows mean plasma glucose values during screening tests for gestational diabetes performed at 24–28 weeks gestation. Our somewhat lower plasma glucose levels during these tests compared with those in the North

Table 22.3. Plasma glucose values during 1 h (50 g glucose) and 3 h (100 g glucose) screening tests in lean and obese women with gestational diabetes

Test	Time (min)			
	0	60	120	180
1 h Glucola (50 g glucose)				
Lean		198 ± 45 (11)		
Obese		184 ± 29 (10.2)		
P		NS		
3 h Glucola (100 g glucose)				
Lean	98 ± 19 (5.4)	219 ± 33 (12.2)	202 ± 35 (11.2)	148 ± 43 (8.2)
Obese	111 ± 20 (6.2)	218 ± 29 (12.1)	192 ± 40 (10.7)	135 ± 39 (7.5)
P	0.02	NS	NS	NS

( ) = mmol/l.

American literature reflect the elimination of women with NIDDM (type II diabetes) which is a different clinical and metabolic entity during pregnancy than GDM. Women with NIDDM were detected by (a) early screening at the first prenatal visit if risk factors for gestational diabetes were present or (b) by later confirmation at the 6 weeks postpartum visit when they received a 2-h 75-g glucose loading test. World Health Organization criteria were used postpartum to distinguish normal women from those with impaired glucose tolerance or diabetes.

Aside from higher fasting plasma glucose levels in obese women with GDM (111 ± SD 20 mg/dl vs 98 ± SD 19 mg/dl; $P<0.02$), during the 3-h confirmatory OGTT with 100 g of glucose, there were no significant differences in the tests between lean and obese women with GDM.

Treatment

All subjects received individualized dietary therapy as described in the methods section. Insulin was prescribed for 21 (47%) obese women and 10 (26%) lean women with GDM.

Metabolic Observations

Glucose

Mean plasma glucose levels at each time period during the 2-h test were significantly higher in obese women with GDM ($P<0.01$; Fig. 22.1). This

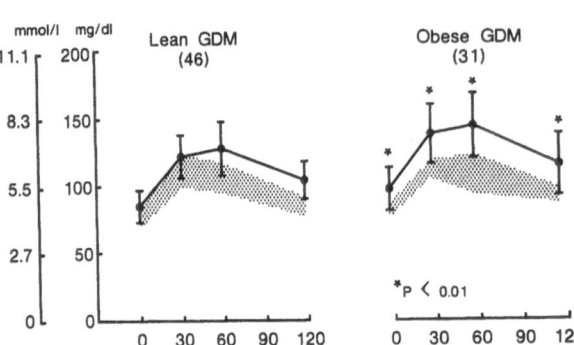

Fig. 22.1. Plasma glucose levels during a 2-h 400-kcal breakfast meal tolerance test during the third trimester in lean and obese women with gestational diabetes (GDM). The *stippled areas* indicate mean ± standard deviation of glucose values in 23 lean and 10 obese normal pregnant women. Obese women with GDM had significantly higher glucose values at each test period.

observation was also confirmed by higher mean integrated glucose units under the 2-h curve (obese: 15 374 ± SD 2218; lean: 13 805 ± 1745, $P<0.01$).

Insulin and C-Peptide

Normal obese pregnant women had higher fasting and meal-stimulated plasma insulin values than lean normal subjects throughout the breakfast test as shown on Fig. 22.2 (PNS). The peak rise in insulin levels in both lean and obese normals occurred at 30 min.

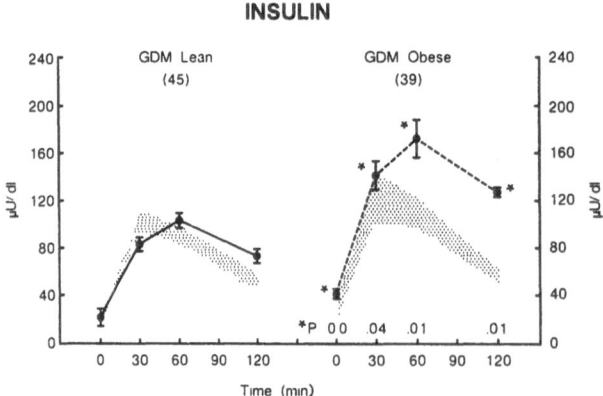

Fig. 22.2. Plasma insulin levels ± standard error of the mean (SEM) during a 2-h 400-kcal meal tolerance test in 45 lean women with GDM and 39 obese women with GDM. The *stippled areas* in Figs. 22.2, 22.3 and 22.4 represent the mean ± SEM in normal comparison groups. Obese women with GDM had significantly higher insulin levels at each time period than women in any other group.

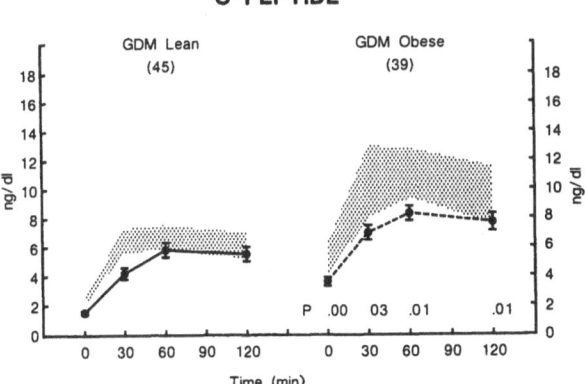

Fig. 22.3. Plasma C-peptide levels ± SEM at fasting and over 2 h following breakfast meal stimulation.

In obese women with GDM, mean plasma insulin values were higher than those of any other comparison group at all time periods (Fig. 22.2). Both lean and obese women with GDM had a delay in peak insulin levels to 60 min after starting the breakfast meal. There was no difference in mean integrated insulin units (IIU) under the 2-h curve between lean normal and lean GDM subjects (9167 ± SD 4155 vs 9692 ± SD 3549 IIU; PNS).

In contrast, obese women with GDM exhibited hyperinsulinaemia with respect to both normal and lean women with GDM ($P<0.001$) and obese normals (obese NL: 10 637 ± SD 4183 IIU vs obese women with GDM 16 535 ± SD 814; $P=<0.03$). These findings suggest greater gestational insulin resistance in pregnant obese women with GDM.

Integrated C-P units (IC-PU) under the 2-h test curve were significantly higher in obese compared with lean normal women ($P<0.03$; Fig. 22.3). This was also true when obese women with GDM were compared with lean women with GDM (833 ± SD 315 vs 571 ± SD 309 IC-PU units; $P<0.01$). However, in contrast to insulin measurements in obese subjects, C-P values were significantly lower in obese women with GDM than obese normals (833 ± SD 15 IC-PU vs 1171 ± SD IC-PU; $P<0.04$).

Glucagon

In normal pregnant lean and obese women there were no significant differences in plasma glucagon levels at any point during the meal stimulation test. In lean and obese patients with GDM fasting and meal-stimulating glucagon values were higher in obese women throughout the test (Fig. 22.4). These values were significant when obese women with GDM were compared with obese normal women and lean women with GDM ($P<0.01$).

Human Chorionic Somatomammotropin (hCS)

Measurements of hCS levels did not differ among the four patient groups at any point in the meal tolerance test or in integrated areas under the 2-h curve. Hourly

GLUCAGON

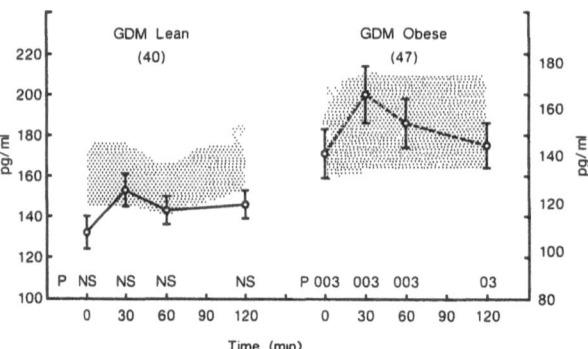

Fig. 22.4. Plasma glucagon levels ± SEM during a 2-h breakfast meal test in lean and obese normal women compared with women with GDM. Lean women with GDM had lower values at fasting and during all postprandial test periods.

hCS determinations around the 24-h metabolic clock did not vary among groups or during 8-h periods of the day or night. There was no correlation of hCS levels with those of glucose, insulin or glucagon. In addition, fasting and meal-stimulated hCS values were not correlated with infant birthweight.

Lipids

In this study we were unable to demonstrate significant differences in fasting levels of total cholesterol or triglyceride between lean or obese normal women or those with GDM.

Taken together, these data indicate that obese women with GDM can be distinguished metabolically from lean women with GDM by their higher glucose, insulin, C-peptide and glucagon responses to a small breakfast.

Infants of Mothers with Gestational Diabetes

Table 22.4 describes the complications in the babies of the two groups of mothers with GDM. More problems are associated with pregnancies in obese women with GDM. Thirty-eight per cent of these mothers had Caesarean sections (vs 26% in lean GDM); five had shoulder dystocia (10% vs 0% in lean) and two had birth injuries (4% vs 0% in lean). The most striking difference, considering the excellent diabetic control and Hb$_{A1}$ values within the normal range in both groups, was the higher number of macrosomic babies and greater frequency of hypoglycaemia, hyperbilirubinaemia, infections and polycythaemia in the infants of obese mothers. The only fetal loss was in an obese woman with GDM.

Table 22.4. Complications in infants of lean and obese diabetic mothers

Group (n)	Fetal distress n (%)	Caesarean section n (%)	Birth injury n (%)	Still-born n (%)	Macro-somia n (%)	Hypogly-caemia n (%)	Hyperbili-rubinaemia n (%)	Poly-cythaemia n (%)	Infec-tion n (%)
Lean (38)	4 (11)	10 (26)	0 (0)	0	7 (18)	2 (5)	0	0	0
Obese (45)	3 (7)	17 (38)	2 (4)	1 (2)	15 (33)	11 (24)	4 (9)	3 (7)	7 (16)

Complications were not mutually exclusive.

Anthropometric Measurements

Table 22.5 presents a summary of measurements in infants of the four groups of women. Infants of 12 normal obese mothers were larger in all dimensions except the buccal skinfold when compared with babies of 199 normal lean mothers.

Table 22.5. Anthropometric measurements in infants of lean and obese diabetic and normal mothers

Infants	Mothers					
	Normal lean (199)	Normal obese (12)	P	GDM lean (32)	GDM obese (38)	P
IBW (g)	3368 ± 60	3813 ± 588	0.04	3574 ± 570	3812 ± 535	NS
IBL (cm)	50 ± 0.5	52 ± 2	0.04	51 ± 2 $P<0.01^a$	52 ± 2	0.04
BMI (kg/m³)	26 ± 0.2	27 ± 3^a	NS	26 ± 2 $P<0.001^b$	30 ± 4^a	0.04
HC (cm)	35 ± 0.5	36 ± 1^b	0.0	35 ± 1 $P<0.02^c$	35 ± 1^b	NS
CR (cm)	34 ± 0.3	36 ± 2^c	0.04	34 ± 1	35 ± 1^c	NS
Waist (cm)	32 ± 0.3	34 ± 2	0.03	32 ± 2	33 ± 2	0.03
Hip (cm)	28 ± 0.08	30 ± 2	0.04	28 ± 2	30 ± 2	0.03
W/H × 100	112 ± 0.01	111 ± 2	0.0	114 ± 2	113 ± 4	NS
Skinfold measurements						
Buccal (mm)	4.8 ± 1	5.0 ± 1	NS	4.6 ± 1	5.5 ± 1	0.01
Triceps (mm)	3.8 ± 0.2	4.5 ± 1	0	4.1 ± 0.6 $P<0.04^d$	4.5 ± 1	NS
Subscap (mm)	3.9 ± 0.2	4.8 ± 1^d	0	4.4 ± 0.9	5.5 ± 1^d	0.01
TSF (mm)	13.1 ± 2	14.4 ± 2	0	13.1 ± 2	15 ± 3	0.03

All values represent means ± SD.
IBW, infant birthweight; *IBL*, infant birth length; *BMI*, body mass index; *HC*, head circumference; *CR*, crown–rump; *W/H*, waist/hip ratio; *Subscap*, subscapular; *TSF*, total skin fold measurement. Small letters a, b, c and d refer to figures compared and related P values.

The most interesting observations were in the babies of normal and obese GDM mothers. Although mean birthweights were not different in the two groups, infants of obese women with GDM clearly had a different distribution of body fat. Their body mass index (BMI) was higher ($30 ± 4$ vs $27 ± 3$; $P<0.01$) and they had an increased truncal deposition of fat manifested by high subscapular skinfold measurements (5.5 mm $\pm$ 1 vs 4.8 mm $\pm$ 1 in infants of normal obese mothers; $P<0.04$). When compared with infants of lean women with GDM, buccal ($P<0.01$), subscapular ($P<0.01$) and total skinfold measurements ($P<0.03$) were all significantly higher. There was no difference in triceps skinfold measurements in babies of women with GDM but the babies of lean women with GDM had increased triceps skinfolds compared with those of babies of lean normal women (lean women with GDM: 4.4 $\pm$ 0.9; lean normal 3.8 $\pm$ 0.2, $P=0$).

Discussion

The pathophysiology of GDM is unknown; the disorder represents a complex interrelationship and interaction of the genetics of susceptibility to various types of diabetes and the normal metabolic and hormonal alterations of pregnancy.

Glucose loading tests in pregnant women exaggerate glucose intolerance and permit detection of gestational diabetes. These tests are highly unphysiological and bear little resemblance to carbohydrate tolerance as it affects individuals from day to day (Lefèbre and Luyckx 1976; Owens et al. 1979). In addition, they may cause nausea and vomiting and are generally unpleasant.

Once the diagnosis of GDM is made, we have found it helpful to examine glucose and hormonal responses to a more physiological mixed meal challenge (Cheney et al. 1985). Coustan et al. (1987) have suggested that a breakfast tolerance test rather than a glucose loading test might be employed as a threshold screening test for GDM. Fitch and King (1987) have utilized 500-kcal moderate and high protein breakfast test meals to measure the responses of plasma glucose, insulin and amino acids in normal women and two with GDM. They found that pregnant women had higher insulin responses to both test meals and smaller rises of arginine, ornithine and branched-chain amino acids. The importance of these observations on fetal outcome in normal and diabetic pregnancies remains to be determined.

The heterogeneity of pregnant women with impaired glucose tolerance (GDM) is similar to that of non-pregnant individuals. Our ability to predict subsequent deterioration to frank diabetes is limited (Keen et al. 1982). Ward et al. (1985) have observed that women with histories of GDM who are predisposed to NIDDM have impairments both of insulin secretion and insulin action before the development of hyperglycaemia. Thus, it seemed reasonable to us to devise a test of short duration (2 h) that would provide a metabolic profile of lean and obese women with GDM. The National Diabetes Data Group (1979) also defines NIDDM in these to categories.

The fetus represents a bioassay of the genetic and in utero metabolic environment. Thus, we also examined the perinatal outcome and anthropometric measurements of infants of lean and obese women with GDM and normal mothers. The GDM mothers had similar degrees of glucose intolerance at diagnosis as assessed by the 50-g and 100-g glucose loading tests and Hb_{A1} concentrations at baseline (6.9 $\pm$ 1% in obese women with GDM and 6.8 $\pm$ 0.2 in lean women with GDM; normal: 5%–8%). Our more rigorous screening procedures for GDM eliminate the dilution of the study groups with women who have more severe, but not previously diagnosed, asymptomatic NIDDM (type II diabetes) or slow onset IDDM. The major difference between lean and obese groups of women with GDM was the significant obesity in the heavier women and their stronger family histories of diabetes.

This study expands our observations on the breakfast meal challenge test described in earlier reports (Cheney et al. 1985; Hollingsworth et al. 1985). In this larger group of women with GDM, the physiological stimulation of a breakfast meal resulted in significantly higher plasma levels of glucose, insulin, C-peptide and glucagon in obese women with GDM.

Although Hb$_{A1}$ concentrations were virtually identical in lean and obese women with GDM at diagnosis, lean women with GDM had significantly lower values before delivery (6.4% vs 6.9%; $P<0.02$). This difference was observed despite the lower dietary prescriptions given to obese women with GDM and the greater percentage who received insulin therapy.

We were unable to demonstrate differences in fasting plasma levels of cholesterol or total triglyceride in lean versus obese women with GDM. Moreover, their lipid values did not differ from those of normal pregnant women of comparable weights. This may have reflected the mildness of the glucose intolerance in GDM. Golay et al. (1986) have reported normal free fatty acid (FFA) levels in seven obese non-pregnant individuals with impaired glucose tolerance, higher postprandial glucose levels and elevated ambient insulin values. These findings were in contrast to the significantly increased FFA concentrations and grossly abnormal FFA metabolism they observed in seven obese subjects with NIDDM.

Perhaps the most interesting aspects of our study were the differences in the infants of obese GDM mothers. They were more likely to be born by Caesarean section following maternal dystocia and to have more neonatal metabolic complications. The only fetal loss during the study occurred in the fetus of an obese woman with GDM. Anthropometric studies showed that infants of obese women with GDM (but not obese normal women) had a greater truncal accumulation of fat that was characterized by increased subscapular skinfold measurements. This central adiposity was apparent in all macrosomic and some normal weight babies of obese women with GDM. This finding is of interest because it is analogous to the upper segment obesity described in older individuals with NIDDM.

In neither lean nor obese women with GDM were we able to correlate maternal plasma glucose or insulin levels during the meal test or areas under the curve with the birthweights of their infants. The complex interactions of variable concentrations of maternal nutrients, the metabolic functions of the placenta, transport of the umbilical diet to the fetus and the role of fetal endocrine and paracrine growth factors remain an unexplained and puzzling area of human physiology.

In summary, in the absence of genetic markers for all types of diabetes, we suggest the possibility that gestational diabetes may provoke an early genetic and environmental interaction which can unmask *susceptibility* to diabetes. For the present, a physiological breakfast meal tolerance test provides a better metabolic description of individual patients or groups of women with GDM than a glucose loading test with measurements limited to changes in plasma concentrations of glucose.

References

Algert S, Shragg P, Hollingsworth DR (1985) Moderate caloric restriction in obese women with gestational diabetes. Obstet Gynecol 65:487–491

American Diabetes Association (1979) Principles of nutrition and dietary recommendations for individuals with diabetes mellitus: 1979. Diabetes 28:1027–1030

Barden TP, Knowles HC (1981) Diagnosis of diabetes in pregnancy. Obstet Gynecol 24:3–19

Brans YW, Summers JE, Dweck HS, Cassady G (1974) A non invasive approach to body composition in the neonate. Dynamic skin fold measurement. Pediatr Res 8:215–222

Carpenter JW, Coustan DR (1982) Criteria for screening tests for gestational diabetes. Am J Obstet Gynecol 144:768–773

Cheney C, Shragg P, Hollingsworth DR (1985) Demonstration of heterogeneity in gestational diabetes by a 400-kcal breakfast meal tolerance test. Obstet Gynecol 65:17–23

Cousins L, Dattel BJ, Hollingsworth DR, Zettner A (1984) Glycosylated hemoglobin as a screening test for carbohydrate intolerance in pregnancy. Am J Obstet Gynecol 150:455–460

Coustan DR, Widness JA, Carpenter MW, Rotondo L, Pratt DH (1987) The "breakfast tolerance test": screening for gestational diabetes with a standardized mixed nutrient meal. Am J Obstet Gynecol 157:1113–1117

Fitch WL, King JC (1987) Plasma amino acid, glucose, and insulin responses to moderate-protein and high-protein test meals in pregnant, nonpregnant, and gestational diabetic women. Am J Clin Nutr 46:243–249

Freinkel N, Metzger BE, Phelps RL et al. (1986) Gestational diabetes mellitus: a syndrome with phenotypic and genotypic heterogeneity. Horm Metab Res 18:427–430

Gillmer MDG, Oakley NW, Beard RW, Nithyananthan R, Cawston M (1980) Screening for diabetes during pregnancy. Br J Obstet Gynaecol 87:377–382

Golay A, Chen Y-DI, Reaven GM (1986) Effect of differences in glucose tolerance on insulin's ability to regulate carbohydrate and free fatty acid metabolism in obese individuals. J Clin Endocrinol Metab 62:1081–1088

Harris V, Faloona GR, Unger R (1978) Glucagon methods of hormone radioimmunoassay, 2nd ed, Academic Press, New York, pp 643–656

Hollingsworth DR, Ney D, Stubblefield N, Fell T (1985) Heterogeneity of lean and obese women with gestational diabetes. Metabolic assessment with isocaloric meal tolerance tests. Diabetes 34 (Suppl 2):81–87

Keen H, Jarrett RJ, McCartney P (1982) The ten-year follow-up of the Bedford Survey (1962–1972): glucose tolerance and diabetes. Diabetologia 22:73–78

Kuzuya H, Blix P, Horwitz D, Steiner DF, Rubenstein AH (1977) Determination of free and total insulin and C-peptide in insulin treated diabetics. Diabetes 26:22–29

Lefèbre PJ, Luyckx AS (1976) One breakfast tolerance test: return to physiology. Diabet Metab 2:15–19

Moser RJ, Hollingsworth DR (1973) Radioimmunoassay of human chorionic somatomammotropin (HCS) in serum, amniotic fluid and urine. Clin Chem 119: 602–605

National Diabetes Data Group (1979) Classification and diagnosis of diabetes mellitus and other categories of glucose intolerance. Diabetes 28:1039–1057

National Research Council Committee on Dietary Allowances, Food and Nutrition Board (1980) Recommended dietary allowances, 9th edn. National Academy of Sciences, US Government Printing Office, Washington DC

O'Sullivan JB, Mahan CB (1964) Criteria for the oral glucose tolerance test in pregnancy. Diabetes 13:278–285

Owens DR, Wragg KG, Briggs PI, Luzio G, Kimber G, Davies C (1979) Comparison of the metabolic response to a glucose tolerance test and and standardized test meal and the response to serial test meals in normal healthy subjects. Diabetes Care 2:409–412

Ward WK, Johnston CLW, Beard JC, Benedetti J, Halter JB, Porte D (1985) Insulin resistance and impaired insulin secretion in subjects with histories of gestational diabetes mellitus. Diabetes 34:861–869

World Health Organization Expert Committee on Diabetes Mellitus (1980) Second report. Tech Rep Ser WHO, no. 646

23. Standardized Test Meal in Human Pregnancy

Doris M. Campbell, H. W. Sutherland and S. Tuttle

Introduction

There is much dissatisfaction with both oral and intravenous glucose tolerance testing in pregnancy, resulting in different groups striving to find alternatives such as the 24-h glucose profile (Gillmer et al. 1975), the measurement of random plasma glucose at an antenatal clinic at a known interval after food (Lind and MacDougall 1981), the use of glucose polymer (Court et al. 1984) and more recently "a breakfast tolerance test" (Paris-Bockel et al. 1983; Coustan et al. 1987). Both latter groups of workers have found that the breakfast tolerance test could possibly be used as an alternative to oral glucose tolerance testing in pregnancy either for screening or diagnosis. Neither group, however, gives any indication as to the reproducibility of their breakfast tolerance tests or indicated whether any variation in the response to their "standard" meal at different stages of pregnancy was found. The breakfast meal provided by both the American and French workers consisted of foods commonly eaten at this time of day and was of approximate nutrient content rather than a standard meal of fixed nutrient intake.

Our studies have been carried out to look at the reproducibility and variability of the blood glucose response to a standardized prepacked test meal (constituents are listed in Appendix) under standard conditions in the same woman, to examine the changes in response according to the time of day the test was undertaken and level of activity undertaken by individuals and to see whether there are any changes in the blood glucose after the meal in the same women studied serially throughout pregnancy.

Methodology

Study A

Twenty healthy women with no predisposition to diabetes, i.e. with no risk features for gestational diabetes (Sutherland et al. 1979), were recruited at 30–32 weeks gestation. There were 10 primigravidae and 10 multipara. Standardized test meals were given as breakfast tolerance tests after the subjects fasted overnight on two occasions, 7 d apart. Ear-prick capillary samples of blood were taken for plasma glucose analysis in the fasting state, at 4, 10, 15, 20, 30, 40, 50, 60, 90 and 120 min after completion of the meal.

Study B

Ten healthy women were recruited at 30–34 weeks gestation. There were five primigravidae and five multipara, two of whom smoked. 75-g oral glucose tolerance tests were performed 7 d apart. The subjects fasted overnight. Earlobe capillary samples were taken for plasma glucose measurement in the fasting state and at 4, 10, 20, 30, 40, 60, 90 and 120 min.

Study C

Ten healthy women with no predisposition to diabetes were recruited at 30–32 weeks gestation. There were five primigravidae (two smokers) and five multipara (one smoker). The plasma glucose response to the standardized glucose test meal was measured once after consumption of the meal at breakfast time and once after consumption at lunchtime, with no preliminary fast, within the same week of gestation. The time of the first test was randomly allocated. The protocol followed was as in study A.

Study D

Ten normal healthy women with no predisposition to diabetes were recruited at 30–32 weeks gestation. There were three primigravidae (one smoker) and seven multipara (two smokers). Five women ate the standardized test meal twice at breakfast time and five twice at lunch time; on one occasion the women were resting in the clinical research unit (CRU), and on the other occasion the meal was eaten in their own home, and the women instructed to make their own way to the hospital following consumption of the meal. The order of the tests was randomly allocated. On the occasions that the women ate the test meal at home, plasma glucose was analysed at 60, 90, 120 and 150 min after eating their meal. The protocol otherwise was as for study A.

Study E

Eighteen normal healthy primigravidae were recruited at booking at the antenatal clinic. Standardized test meals with the measurement of earlobe capillary plasma glucose in the fasting state and at 30, 60, 90 and 120 min following the completion of the meal were carried out three times during the pregnancy, i.e. at 16, 26 and 36 weeks gestation. All of these women have since delivered normal healthy infants.

Results

The results for study A are given in Table 23.1a. Paired t-tests have been performed on the matched samples from individual women. It should be noted that the mean difference between test 1 and test 2 is small at all time intervals studied, the largest being 0.24 mmol/l difference in plasma glucose at 10 min (statistically significant). Table 23.1b confirms that there is no difference in the summed plasma glucose between test 1 and test 2 or in the maximum plasma glucose reached. The median time to maximum plasma glucose on both occasions was 30 min with no significant difference between the first and second test time to maximum level.

Table 23.1a. Standardized test meal reproducibility (20 women, two tests 7 d apart)

Time (min)	Mean plasma glucose (mmol/l)			
	Test 1	Test 2	Difference	"t"
0 (fasting)	4.43 (0.38)	4.35 (0.36)	0.08	1.62
4	4.82 (0.54)	4.84 (0.51)	−0.02	−0.02
10	5.18 (0.62)	5.42 (0.66)	−0.24	−2.55*
15	5.80 (0.93)	5.85 (0.75)	−0.06	−0.41
20	6.16 (0.86)	6.26 (0.83)	−0.10	−0.78
30	6.48 (0.87)	6.54 (0.80)	−0.06	−0.51
40	6.27 (0.87)	6.34 (0.78)	−0.07	−0.46
50	5.95 (0.71)	5.99 (0.63)	−0.04	−0.27
60	5.78 (0.69)	5.77 (0.66)	0.01	0.07
90	5.39 (0.50)	5.50 (0.66)	−0.11	−0.86
120	5.18 (0.48)	5.15 (0.62)	−0.03	0.23

Numbers in brackets are SDs
*$P=0.05$

Table 23.1b. Standardized test meal reproducibility (20 women, two tests 7 d apart)

	Test 1	Test 2	Difference	"t"
Mean summed plasma glucose (mmol/l)	57.01 (5.46)	57.66 (5.30)	−0.66	−1.045
Mean maximum plasma glucose (mmol/l)	6.80 (0.73)	6.74 (0.71)	0.06	0.69
Median time to maximum plasma glucose (min)	30	30	Mann Whitney $U = 184.5$ NS	

Numbers in brackets are SDs

Similar results for the 75-g oral glucose tolerance test (study B) are presented in Tables 23.2a and 23.2b. It is to be noted that the mean differences between tests at the majority of time intervals studied are larger than for the test meal but paired t-testing reveals no statistically significant difference between them. Table

Table 23.2a. 75-g oral glucose tolerance test reproducibility (10 women, two tests 7 d apart)

Time (min)	Mean plasma glucose (mmol/l)			
	Test 1	Test 2	Difference	"t"
0 (fasting)	4.48 (0.18)	4.59 (0.35)	−0.11	−1.24
4	4.94 (0.65)	4.86 (0.46)	−0.08	−0.66
10	6.04 (0.93)	5.90 (0.62)	0.14	0.51
20	7.57 (1.14)	7.19 (1.31)	0.38	0.94
30	8.57 (1.17)	8.02 (1.63)	0.55	1.64
40	8.97 (1.54)	8.50 (1.79)	0.47	1.29
50	8.53 (1.52)	8.83 (1.81)	−0.31	−0.87
60	8.04 (1.76)	8.43 (1.84)	−0.38	−0.90
90	6.76 (1.68)	7.56 (2.18)	−0.80	−2.09
120	6.49 (1.41)	7.27 (1.90)	−0.78	−1.58

Numbers in brackets are SDs

Table 23.2b. 75-g oral glucose tolerance test reproducibility (10 women, two tests 7 d apart)

	Test 1	Test 2	Difference	"t"
Mean summed plasma glucose (mmol/l)	65.92 (9.93)	66.56 (10.19)	−0.64	−0.31
Mean maximum plasma glucose (mmol/l)	9.13 (1.40)	9.40 (1.42)	−0.27	−0.83
Median time to maximum plasma glucose (min)	40	50	Mann Whitney $U = 22$ $P<0.025$	

Numbers in brackets are SDs

23.2b confirms that, as expected, the mean maximum plasma glucose is higher following an oral glucose load than a meal and likewise the summed plasma glucose is higher, but there are no significant differences between the two tests 1 week apart. There was a statistically significant difference however in time to maximum plasma glucose, the median in the first test being 40 min and in the second test 50 min (Table 23.2b). On examining the mean difference between the two oral glucose tolerance tests it is to be noted that in the early part of the tests, i.e. 10–40 min, the mean plasma glucose levels were higher on the first occasion than on the second occasion, whereas from 50 min through to 120 min, levels were lower on the first occasion than on the second occasion. This is in keeping with the later time to peak in test 2. Such a pattern is not apparent following test meals (Table 23.1a). Because plasma glucose levels are higher in the first glucose tolerance test in the early part of the test and lower in the later part of the test, the differences cancel each other out and there is no difference in the summed glucose values. Ignoring whether the differences were higher or lower in the first and second test, the average difference over 10 time intervals for the standardized test meals was 0.08 mmol/l (SD 0.07) whereas for the oral glucose tolerance test, the average difference was 0.40 mmol/l (SD 0.26). This is statistically significant (t = 3.86; $P<0.01$).

Table 23.3a compares the glucose response to the test meal at breakfast and at lunch. In general, the lunchtime glucose values were lower than those of the morning test but there is only one statistically significant difference between the two tests performed at breakfast and at lunch time, i.e. the 90-min glucose value was lower at lunchtime. There were no differences noted in the summed plasma

Table 23.3a. Standardized test meal: Breakfast/lunch comparison (10 women, tests 4–7 d apart)

Time (min)	Mean plasma glucose (mmol/l)			
	At breakfast	At lunch	Difference	"t"
0 (fasting)	4.48 (0.46)	4.72 (0.77)	−0.25	−1.03
4	4.91 (0.53)	5.18 (0.96)	−0.27	−0.89
10	5.86 (0.63)	5.67 (0.97)	−0.08	−0.33
15	6.09 (0.63)	6.13 (0.86)	−0.04	−0.22
20	6.57 (0.69)	6.41 (0.71)	0.16	0.90
30	6.91 (0.73)	6.78 (0.69)	0.13	0.65
40	6.72 (0.87)	6.60 (0.70)	0.13	0.65
50	6.52 (1.08)	6.29 (0.64)	0.23	0.83
60	6.15 (1.05)	5.85 (0.60)	0.30	1.13
90	5.85 (0.63)	5.39 (0.65)	0.45	3.13*
120	5.28 (0.69)	5.21 (0.70)	0.08	0.39
150	4.63 (0.44)	4.75 (0.46)	−0.12	−0.83

Numbers in brackets are SDs
*$P<0.02$

Table 23.3b. Standardized test meal: breakfast/lunch comparison (10 women, tests 4–7 d apart)

	At breakfast	At lunch	Difference	"t"
Mean summed plasma glucose (mmol/l)	65.21 (6.54)	64.25 (6.47)	0.96	0.62
Mean maximum plasma glucose (mmol/l)	7.11 (0.73)	6.91 (0.68)	0.20	1.46
Median time to maximum plasma glucose (min)	35	30	Mann Whitney $U = 45.50$ NS	

Table 23.4. Standardized test meal: effect of activity (10 women, tests 5–7 d apart)

Time (min)	Mean plasma glucose (mmol/l)			
	"Resting – CRU"	"Active – home"	Difference	"t"
60	5.73 (0.59)	5.51 (0.71)	0.22	1.14
90	5.23 (0.51)	5.27 (0.47)	−0.03	−0.20
120	5.11 (0.51)	4.85 (0.52)	0.26	2.07
150	4.75 (0.39)	4.53 (0.41)	0.22	2.00

Numbers in brackets are SDs

glucose, the maximum plasma glucose reached or the time to maximum plasma glucose at lunchtime as compared with breakfast time (Table 23.3b).

As expected, when the women undertook some activity following the test meal, the mean capillary plasma glucose levels were slightly lower although not significantly so, than when the test was performed under standard resting conditions (Table 23.4).

Table 23.5a gives the results of the plasma glucose response following the standardized test meal at three separate occasions during pregnancy. Analyses of variance are carried out to determine differences by the interval at testing. As has been documented before, fasting plasma glucose declined significantly as gestation advanced. However, following consumption of the test meal, the mean plasma glucose levels at 30, 60, 90 and 120 min were virtually identical at all gestations tested. Likewise the summed plasma glucose and maximum plasma glucose following the test meal and the median time to maximum were similar at the three gestations, 16, 26 and 36 weeks (Table 23.5b).

Table 23.5a. Standardized test meal: serial study in pregnancy (18 women)

Time (min)	Mean fasting plasma glucose (mmol/l)			
	16 weeks	26 weeks	36 weeks	Analysis of variance F
0 (fasting)	4.42 (0.37)	4.23 (0.41)	4.03 (0.46)	3.97*
30	6.20 (0.80)	6.37 (0.62)	6.26 (0.65)	0.29
60	5.54 (0.58)	5.54 (0.58)	5.70 (0.70)	0.40
90	5.24 (0.47)	5.24 (0.53)	5.18 (0.67)	0.11
120	4.84 (0.31)	4.91 (0.41)	4.90 (0.34)	0.16

Numbers in brackets are SDs
*$P<0.025$

Table 23.5b. Standardized test meal: serial study in pregnancy (18 women)

	16 weeks	26 weeks	36 weeks	Analysis of variance F
Mean summed plasma glucose (mmol/l)	21.81 (1.32)	22.06 (1.53)	22.02 (1.77)	0.12
Maximum plasma glucose (mmol/l)	6.31 (0.70)	6.37 (0.63)	6.32 (0.65)	0.04
Median time to maximum (min)	30	30	30	

Numbers in brackets are SDs

Discussion

Our studies have indicated that the glucose response following the standardized test meal is highly reproducible and compares favourably with the 75-g oral glucose tolerance test (OGTT). The differences between two consecutive tests in the same women are greater for an OGTT under similar conditions than for the test meal. This agrees with the work of Lind et al. (1968) who commented that the OGTT response varied "almost as much between successive tests in the same patient as between patients".

In contrast to both oral glucose tolerance which is known to deteriorate throughout the day (Jarrett et al. 1972) and the diminishing carbohydrate tolerance after a standardized test meal during the day in the non-pregnant (Owens et al. 1979) there was little difference in the glucose response when the meal was eaten at lunchtime as compared with breakfast time. Rather surprisingly, the plasma glucose values following consumption at lunchtime were slightly lower. As expected (Lipman et al. 1972) the levels when the woman ate the meal in her own home and then journeyed to the hospital for blood sampling were lower than those when the entire test was carried out with the woman seated at rest. However, the differences were very small.

In contrast to both oral glucose tolerance (Lind et al. 1973) and intravenous glucose tolerance (Fisher et al. 1974), both of which tend to "worsen" during the course of gestation, no such trend is apparent following the test meal. It is known that glucose absorption from an oral glucose load may be delayed when compared with a starch meal (Lind and Hytten 1969). Following an intravenous glucose load, gut absorption and the response of gut hormones to food is bypassed and it is only the insulin response that is tested. It can be concluded from our results that the gut may exert a major influence in controlling the level of blood glucose achieved following food, both by changes in relative roles of absorption of different dietary constituents and by the interaction between gastrointestinal hormones such as gastrin and cholecystokinin with the pancreatic hormones insulin and glucagon. Hornnes et al. (1979, 1981) have examined some of the endocrine interaction following oral glucose or a protein-rich meal and concluded that there is considerable adaptation and change in pregnancy of gastro-entero-pancreatic endocrinology.

Our results are in keeping with those of Gillmer et al. (1975) who studied glucose profiles in nine normal women in early and late pregnancy and found no major differences in glucose values by gestation.

In conclusion, we have found that in pregnancy the plasma glucose response following a standard prepacked test meal is highly reproducible, does not vary significantly with the time of day or level of activity of the individual, is acceptable to pregnant women although a few found difficulty in eating it all in early pregnancy and it does not change at all with the stage of pregnancy. In all of these respects, therefore, a test meal is superior to a glucose tolerance test and it is more physiological. Provided that it can be shown to be of clinical value in detecting pathological pregnancies, it could be used in place of glucose tolerance tests for the diagnosis of gestational diabetes.

Appendix

Aberdeen Mixed Nutrient Meal (Supplied by Boots Co. PLC)

I. Biscuits
  Ingredients by Order of Weight

1. Oats
2. Brown sugar
3. Bran
4. Sultanas
5. Vegetable fat
6. Hazelnuts
7. Soya kernels
8. Skimmed milk powder
9. Honey

10. Malt extract
11. Guar gum
12. Dicalcium phosphate
13. Salt
14. Emulsifier
15. Vitamin C
16. Niacin
17. Reduced iron
18. Riboflavin

19. Thiamin
20. Vitamin A
21. Folic acid
22. Potassium iodide
23. Vitamin D
24. Vitamin B$_{12}$

Dietary Analysis	*Per 100 g*	*Per serving* *2 biscuits (50 g)*
Protein	9.2 g	4.6 g
Fat	18.0 g	9.0 g
Carbohydrate	62.5 g	31.3 g
Energy	1926 kJ	963 kJ
	460 calories	230 calories
Vitamin A	500 μg	250 μg
Vitamin B_1	0.8 mg	0.4 mg
Vitamin B_2	1.1 mg	0.55 mg
Niacin	12 mg	6 mg
Vitamin B_{12}	1.4 μg	0.7 μg
Folic acid	200 μg	100 μg
Vitamin C	20 mg	10 mg
Vitamin D	7 μg	3.5 μg
Calcium	334 mg	167 mg
Iodine	95 μg	47.5 μg
Iron	8 mg	4 mg
Dietary fibre	10.2 g	5.1 g

II. Milk Drink
Ingredients by Order of Weight

1. Skimmed milk powder
2. Dextrose
3. Vegetable fat with anti-oxidant
4. Modified starch
5. Dried malt extract
6. Sodium chloride
7. Emulsifiers
8. Ferrous sulphate
9. Emulsifiers
10. Niacin
11. Riboflavin
12. Thiamin
13. Vitamin A
14. Folic acid
15. Potassium iodide
16. Vitamin D
17. Vitamin B_{12}

Dietary Analysis	*Per 100 g*	*Per serving (50 g)*
Protein	19.6 g	9.8 g
Fat	16.9 g	8.5 g
Carbohydrate	54.7 g	27.4 g
Energy	1862 kJ	931 kJ
	445 calories	223 calories
Vitamin A	260 μg	130 μg
Vitamin B_1	0.45 mg	0.23 mg
Vitamin B_2	0.55 mg	0.28 mg
Niacin	6.3 mg	3.2 mg
Vitamin B_{12}	0.7 μg	0.35 μg
Folic acid	105 μg	52.5 μg
Vitamin C	12 mg	6 mg
Vitamin D	3.4 μg	1.7 μg
Calcium	600 mg	300 mg
Iodine	50 μg	25 μg
Iron	7 mg	3.5 mg

III. Total Product Dietary Analysis	Per meal
Protein	14.4 g
Fat	17.5 g
Carbohydrate	58.7 g
Energy	1694 kJ
	453 calories
Vitamin A	380 μg
Vitamin B_1	0.63 mg
Vitamin B_2	0.83 mg
Niacin	9.2 mg
Vitamin B_{12}	1.05 μg
Folic acid	152.5 μg
Vitamin C	16 mg
Vitamin D	5.2 μg
Calcium	467 mg
Iodine	72.5 μg
Iron	7.5 mg
Dietary fibre	5.1 g

References

Court DJ, Stone R, Killip M (1984) Comparison of glucose and a glucose polymer for testing oral carbohydrate tolerance in pregnancy. Obstet Gynecol 64:251–255

Coustan DR, Widness JA, Carpenter MW, Rotondo L, Pratt DC (1987) The "breakfast tolerance test". Screening for gestational diabetes with a standardized mixed nutrient meal. Am J Obstet Gynecol 157:1113–1117

Fisher PM, Hamilton PM, Sutherland HW, Stowers JM (1974) The effect of pregnancy on intravenous glucose tolerance. J Obstet Gynaecol Br Commonw 81:285–290

Gillmer MDG, Beard RW, Brooke FM, Oakley NW (1975) Carbohydrate metabolism in pregnancy, part I. Diurnal plasma glucose profile in normal and diabetic women. Br Med J 3:399–404

Hornnes PJ, Kuhl C, Lauritsen KP (1979) Diminished gastric inhibitory polypeptide response to oral glucose in late human pregnancy. J Clin Endocrinol Metab 48:506–508

Hornnes PJ, Kuhl C, Lauritsen KP (1981) Gastro-entero-pancreatic hormones in normal pregnancy: response to a protein-rich meal. Eur J Clin Invest 11:345–349

Jarrett RJ, Baker IA, Keen H, Oakley NW (1972) Diurnal variation in oral glucose tolerance: blood sugar and plasma insulin levels morning, afternoon and evening. Br Med J 1:199–201

Lind T, Hytten FE (1969) Blood glucose following oral loads of glucose, maltose and starch during pregnancy. Proc Nutr Soc 28:64A

Lind T, MacDougall AN (1981) Antenatal screening for diabetes mellitus by random blood glucose sampling. Br J Obstet Gynaecol 88:346–351

Lind T, Cheyne GA, Billewicz WZ, Fairweather DVT (1968) Observations on the oral glucose tolerance test in pregnancy. J Obstet Gynaecol Br Commonw 75:540–545

Lind T, Billewicz WZ, Brown C (1973) A serial study of changes occurring in the oral glucose tolerance test during pregnancy. J Obstet Gynaecol Br Commonw 80:1033–1039

Lipman RL, Raskin P, Love T, Triebwasser J, Lecocq FR, Schnure JJ (1972) Glucose intolerance during decreased physical activity in man. Diabetes 21:101–107

Owens DR, Wragg KG, Briggs PI, Luzio S, Kimler C, Davies C (1979) Comparison of the metabolic response to a glucose tolerance test and a standardized test meal and the response to serial test meals in normal healthy subjects. Diabetes Care 2:409–413

Paris-Bockel D, Comte F. Jeanmougin P, Keller B, Schlienger JL (1983) The breakfast tolerance test: application to the diagnosis of gestational diabetes (in French) Sem Hop Paris 59 (31):2167–2172

Sutherland HW, Stowers JM, Fisher PM (1979) Detection of chemical gestational diabetes. In: Sutherland HW, Stowers JM (eds) Carbohydrate metabolism in pregnancy and the newborn. Springer-Verlag, Berlin Heidelberg New York, pp 436–461.

24. Breakfast Tolerance Test in Pregnancy

H. W. Sutherland, D. W. M. Pearson,
M. E. J. Lean and D. M. Campbell

There are many reservations about the use of the OGTT in pregnancy (Sutherland et al. 1979; Court et al. 1985).

At present, gestational diabetes mellitus (GDM) is diagnosed by the use of the oral glucose tolerance test (OGTT) applied in pregnancy (Freinkel 1985). The World Health Organization (WHO) recommends that 75 g glucose is given and it is "often sufficient to measure the blood glucose values only after fasting and at two hours" although it is also stated that "for the asymptomatic patient, at least one additional test result with a value in the diabetic range is desirable, either from a random sample or from the OGTT" (WHO 1985). The WHO criteria for impaired glucose tolerance (IGT) are for *fasting*: whole blood (venous or capillary) <6.7 mmol/l and plasma (venous or capillary) <7.8 mmol/l. The *2-h* criteria for IGT also depend particularly on the type of sample: whole blood (venous) 6.7–10 mmol/l; whole blood (capillary) and plasma (venous) 7.8–11.1 mmol/l; and plasma (capillary) 8.9–12.2 mmol/l. These procedures and criteria for the diagnosis of IGT have been translated to pregnant women for the purpose of diagnosis of GDM.

At a practical level, in our experience many pregnant women in the fasting state find the solution unpalatable. Nausea, fainting and headache are symptoms which may lead to vomiting (Hatem et al. 1988). This occurrence makes interpretation of the blood glucose values unsatisfactory. In our clinic, after such side-effects have occurred there is a high default rate at appointments for re-testing. It has been suggested that the high osmotic pressure of the 75-g glucose drink delays gastric emptying and absorption from the small bowel (Court et al. 1985) which would explain the abdominal bloatedness experienced by pregnant women during OGTT. Moreover, the reproducibility is poor in pregnancy (Lind et al. 1968) even in compliant test subjects and this may be underestimated because those who have experienced these unpleasant symptoms in the first test are unlikely to attend again to provide data for inclusion.

At a theoretical level there is concern about the use of non-pregnant criteria for the OGTT in pregnant women in whom it is well established that the fasting blood sugar level is lower (Sutherland et al. 1987), the plasma volume is expanded (Campbell and MacGillivray 1977) and the renal threshold for glucose excretion is lower but widely variable even on a day-to-day basis (Lind and Hytten 1972).

Gestational diabetes mellitus is a defect of mixed fuel handling and not a disorder of glucose homeostasis alone (Freinkel and Metzger 1979), and several studies have demonstrated clearly that diet affects glucose homeostasis in women with impaired glucose tolerance during pregnancy. In the successful management of GDM, maternal dietary re-adjustment is the first step and frequently the only measure required (Persson et al. 1985). Increasing the dietary fibre has a lowering effect on maternal glycaemia (Fraser 1983; Fraser et al. 1983). Significantly improved glucose tolerance has been observed following the introduction of a low fat, high unrefined carbohydrate diet for a period of as few as 4 d in a randomized cross-over study of women with GDM (Nolan 1984). In insulin-treated pregnant women (10 type 1 and 10 type II diabetics) decreased insulin requirement resulted from adoption of a high carbohydrate, high-fibre, low fat diet (Ney et al. 1982). Evaluation of insulin sensitivity in the third trimester of pregnancy in relation to dietary fibre intake has led to the suggestion that the loss of insulin sensitivity at this time in Western women may be a diet-induced artefact (Fraser et al. 1988). Our own data suggest that dietary adjustment alone could possibly reduce the fetal complications associated with maternal impaired metabolism (Farmer et al. 1988). Pregnant women can raise their blood sugar levels nearly to the WHO GDM diagnostic range by simply consuming a high-energy meal. The next day, they can show normal blood sugar values following a standardized mixed formula test meal (Sutherland et al. 1987). Such data lend support to the view that it may be more appropriate to evaluate maternal handling of food rather than handling of a glucose challenge to detect disordered maternal metabolism which might affect the fetus adversely.

It is possible that the fetal endocrine pancreas might be hyperstimulated as a result of an inappropriate maternal diet composition. Alternatively, if maternal diet is normal, then a pathogenic nutrient mix may reach the fetus if the mother has the disordered metabolism which forms the essence of GDM based on fetal pathological considerations.

What specifically should concern clinicians caring for pregnant women is whether, from an everyday diet, the nutrient mix reaching the fetus is pathogenic or physiological – qualitatively or quantitatively.

The view that the OGTT is adequate to diagnose significantly disordered maternal metabolism is undermined by the increasing use of blood glucose profiles in pregnancy to determine the need for insulin therapy.

Following the workshop on GDM at the last Colloquium in 1983, we concluded that in the context of contemporary knowledge it would be appropriate to study the glycaemic response in pregnancy to a standardized mixed formula test meal. There was little encouragement in the English language literature that such an approach would be an optimal discriminant tool in pregnancy, but a study of non-pregnant subjects showed enhanced insulin responses with a meal compared with oral glucose (Turner et al. 1977). Turner et al. interpreted their finding as a failure of the test meal rather than the alternative view that it was a more effective challenge to insulin synthesis and release. The same Oxford study found that mild diabetic subjects with an abnormal OGTT may have normal or near-normal glucose responses to a standardized breakfast (520 kcal). Also compared to the OGTT, a poorer correlation between the fasting plasma glucose level and incremental area was observed after the breakfast tolerance test (BTT). This allayed our fears that postprandial glycaemia after a modest meal might simply reflect fasting homeostasis rather than define a stimulated glycaemic response.

Another comparative study (Owens et al. 1979) of the OGTT (50 g) and a standardized mixed formula test meal (515 kcal) in non-pregnant, normal, healthy subjects showed that both the amplitude of glycaemic excursion and between-subject variation were less with a test meal. The authors emphasized that the prime function of the OGTT was amplifying any glucose intolerance present and thus aiding diagnosis of diabetes, rather than the alternative view that the meal response gave a "more clinically relevant metabolic status". Paris-Bockel et al. (1983) compared the OGTT (100 g), IVGTT and breakfast tolerance test (BTT) glycaemic responses in 26 pregnant women. The BTT contained 690 kcal (approximately one-third average daily energy intake – 84 g carbohydrates, 22.6 g protein, 9.4 g fat) and lasted 3 h. They suggested that the BTT could be as sensitive as the OGTT for detecting glucose intolerance and stated that the BTT "could be proposed as an easy and economic measure for diagnosing gestational diabetes".

Aberdeen Study of the Breakfast Tolerance Test (BTT) and the Oral Glucose Tolerance Test (OGTT) in Pregnancy

Having reviewed the amount and content of an average UK meal, quality-controlled standardized mixed formula test meals were obtained from Boots Co. PLC in accordance with our specifications which were made with a view to use of the formula both as a breakfast and at other times of the day (Table 24.1). After an overnight fast the glycaemic responses to the tests were compared in 101 pregnant women (primigravida $n=49$), none of whom was known to have diabetes or to have used corticosteroids, at as near to the 26th week for the OGTT and the 27th week for the BTT as was convenient. Earlobe capillary plasma glucose (CPG) was measured by a specific enzymatic method (Beckman glucose analyser) with the subjects sitting at rest. The timing of blood sampling related to the completion of ingestion of the challenges. The study protocol is shown in Table 24.2 and some demographic characteristics of the 101 women who completed the protocol are shown in Table 24.3. Parity is shown in two groups of previous pregnancies (PP), namely those continuing after (PP>28 weeks) and terminating before (PP<28 weeks) 28 completed weeks of pregnancy. Birth-weight percentile ("Percentile" in Table 24.3) was calculated using the appropriate data (Altman and Coles 1980). Body mass index (BMI) was calculated according to the formula weight (kg)/height (m^2). The waist–hip ratio refers to circumferential measurements made at the umbilicus and anterior superior iliac spines respectively. The family history of diabetes mellitus score was derived from allocating points, namely 3 for sibling, 2 for parent and 1 for grandparent for the 19 women for whom this was applicable. The mean score was 2.5 ± 0.8 for those 19 women.

Comparing the total group who completed the protocol ($n=101$) with those who refused to participate in the research ($n=75$) the study group was similar in most respects except for being of higher parity. Also the newborn in the study group had a higher mean percentile birthweight (44.9 vs 36.1) and higher Apgar scores than the defaulters.

Table 24.1. Comparison of nutrients in the Aberdeen test meal and a typical meal (% by weight)

Nutrient	Aberdeen test meal	Typical meal[a]
Protein	15.6	15.7
Fat	17.8	22.9
Carbohydrate	61.3	57.1
Fibre	5.3	4.3
Energy (kcal)	453	743

[a] 1980 UK National Food Survey.

Table 24.2. Study protocol

In pregnancy	
1st antenatal clinic visit, <20 weeks	Height, weight, ultrasound fetal assessment
26 weeks	Weight, 75-g OGTT
27 weeks	453 kcal BTT
After delivery	
Early, 10 d	Obstetric and neonatal notes abstracted
Late, 17–43 weeks	Weight, waist and hips measured

Table 24.3. Characteristics of 101 women and their newborn

Maternal		Newborn		Maternal postnatal[a]	
Age (years)	26.7 ± 3.7	Gestation	39.5 ± 1.9	Weight (kg)	66.88 ± 11.37
Height (m)	161.7 ± 6.1	Birthweight (g)	3355.8 ± 44.9	BMI	23.55 ± 3.96
		percentile	44.9	Waist (cm)	86.78 ± 11.24
26-week	67.8 ± 10.5	Apgar 1 min	8.2 ± 1.4	Hips (cm)	93.98 ± 9.98
weight (kg)					
PP <28 weeks	0.53 ± 0.8	Apgar 5 min	9.1 ± 1.1	Waist–hip ratio	92.24 ± 5.42
PP >28 weeks	0.30 ± 0.6	Mortality	0		

Mean and SD where appropriate.
[a] Interval between delivery and follow-up 29.6 ± 5 weeks.

The relationships of these maternal and fetal characteristics with the OGTT and BTT blood glucose values are shown in Table 24.4. Maternal age (range 19–37 years) was noted to correlate significantly with plasma glucose throughout the OGTT response but only with the 60- and 90-min blood glucose during the BTT. Height (range 147–178 cm) showed an inverse correlation with the BTT and none with the OGTT values. Percentile birthweight and maternal indices of weight correlated with the BTT but not with the OGTT responses. The 2-h CPG after the BTT was the only value to correlate with the family history score of diabetes mellitus ($r=0.404$, $n = 19$, $P=0.043$).

Re-examination of glucose values during the OGTT response, controlling for maternal age, showed significant partial correlations with the waist/hip ratio at 60 and 90 min.

Controlling for height in the BTT, glycaemic response showed partial correlations with observed birthweight but not the birthweight percentile whose derivation has already taken account of maternal height inter alia. Maternal

Table 24.4. All significant Pearson correlation coefficients (r) between maternal and newborn characteristics (n=101) (probabilities appear in parentheses)

Minutes	Glucose tolerance test		Breakfast tolerance test							
	Age	WHR	Age	Height	Weight FU	P-bweight	BMIFU	Waist	Hips	WHR
30	0.199 (0.023)					0.164 (0.05)				
60	0.238 (0.014)	0.185 (0.032)	0.292 (0.014)							
90	0.261 (0.014)		0.189 (0.03)		0.169 (0.046)		0.236 (0.009)		0.170 (0.045)	
120	0.172 (0.043)			−0.278 (0.002)		0.202 (0.022)	0.237 (0.008)			
30+60+90+120	0.272 (0.003)			−0.240 (0.008)		0.215 (0.015)	0.254 (0.015)	0.215 (0.015)	0.197 (0.024)	
30+60	0.224 (0.007)			−0.187 (0.03)		0.186 (0.031)	0.166 (0.049)	0.20 (0.023)		0.199 (0.023)
90+120	0.25 (0.006)			−0.25 (0.006)			0.26 (0.004)		0.181 (0.035)	

WHR, waist/hip ratio; Weight FU and BMIFU refer to maternal data obtained after pregnancy (29.5 ± 5 weeks); P-bweight, percentile birthweight

Table 24.5. Pearson correlation coefficients (r) of capillary plasma glucose concentrations (mmol/l) between BTT and OGTT

Minutes	BTT					
	0	30	60	90	120	B SUM
OGTT						
0	0.7796	0.2728	0.1116	0.3167	0.3109	0.3626
	P=0.000	P=0.003	P=0.133	P=0.001	P=0.001	P=0.000
30	0.1429	0.2671	0.1142	0.2563	0.1324	0.2924
	P=0.077	P=0.003	P=0.128	P=0.005	P=0.093	P=0.002
60	0.1830	0.3064	0.3226	0.3479	0.2055	0.4505
	P=0.034	P=0.001	P=0.001	P=0.000	P=0.020	P=0.000
90	0.1247	0.1272	0.2083	0.2849	0.1879	0.2904
	P=0.107	P=0.102	P=0.018	P=0.002	P=0.030	P=0.002
120	0.1598	0.0062	0.1971	0.3824	0.3724	0.3084
	P=0.055	P=0.476	P=0.024	P=0.000	P=0.000	P=0.001
G SUM	0.1884	0.2342	0.2672	0.3881	0.2654	0.4204
	P=0.030	P=0.009	P=0.003	P=0.000	P=0.004	P=0.000

Table 24.6. Capillary plasma glucose 50th and 97th percentile mmol/l reference values and responses of three women whose babies had clinical suspicion of diabetogenic fetopathy

	Minutes				
	0	30	60	90	120
OGTT 50th	4.4	8.1	7.6	7.0	6.55
BTT 50th	4.4	6.4	5.9	5.4	5.0
OGTT 97th	5.1	10.6	11.0	9.4	8.2
BTT 97th	5.1	7.8	7.3	6.4	6.1
Case					
(a) OGTT	5.16[a]	8.61	9.72	9.0	6.61
BTT	5.1[a]	7.9[a]	7.11	6.0	5.56
(b) OGTT	4.17	12.22[a]	9.0	6.28	7.61
BTT	4.67	7.89[a]	6.22	5.67	5.56
(c) OGTT	5.0	8.56	9.28	5.17	6.89
BTT	4.83	7.17	6.61	6.55[a]	5.78

[a] ≥97th percentile.

weight during pregnancy correlated with the 90- and 120-min BTT CPG values and waist/hip ratio correlated with the 30-min CPG in the BTT.

There are correlations between the fasting CPG levels and 26-week pregnant weight ($r=0.23$, $P=0.01$), and weight ($r=0.296$, $P=0.001$), BMI ($r=0.296$, $P=0.001$), waist ($r=0.258$, $P=0.005$) and hips ($r=0.30$, $P=0.001$) measured approximately 30 weeks postpartum. Controlling for fasting CPG, the effects of age on the OGTT and height on the BTT persisted, but all significant correlations between indices of maternal weight and BTT response were lost. Nevertheless, the relationship of plasma glucose during the BTT with percentile birthweight remained, independent of fasting CPG.

Table 24.5 shows the correlation between the CPG values following the oral glucose and breakfast challenges at 26 and 27 weeks respectively. While as expected the fasting values are similar it will be seen that of the stimulated glucose values, summed postchallenge glucose values (GSUM and BSUM), which could be regarded as glucose area under the curves, had the highest correlation, followed by the 2-h and 1-h values respectively. The 50th percentile glucose peak for both tests was observed at 30 min (Table 24.6).

Clinical Outcome

As expected in 101 unselected women, there was little morbidity. There was one intrauterine death (immediately following repeated amniocentesis for rhesus incompatability) and no neonatal deaths. The mother of the baby whose birthweight was above the 99th percentile had normal blood glucose values during both tests.

Because CPG concentrations were asymmetrically distributed, percentile values were used in relating tolerance test responses to clinical features associated with GDM. Since GDM is regarded as having an incidence of 3% (Merkatz et al. 1980) the pregnancies associated with observed glucose values ≥97th percentile were studied as cases which might be considered as being associated with significantly impaired maternal carbohydrate metabolism.

Amongst the 101 women, values for plasma glucose were ≥97th percentile fasting in four cases, during the OGTT at 14 points in nine women and during the BTT at 9 points in eight women. The 97th percentile CPG values for the two tolerance tests are shown in Table 24.6 with the CPG values of the mothers of the only three babies who were suspected of showing clinical features of diabetogenic fetopathy. Only one had high fasting CPG, and none had an abnormal value at 120 min in the OGTT by the WHO criteria. All three had an abnormal plasma glucose during their BTT.

Three other women with high fasting blood glucose levels had uncomplicated deliveries and no morbidity in the newborn, all of whom had average birthweight percentiles. Of the four women with proteinuric pre-eclampsia, two were included in the ≥97th percentile OGTT group, and none had abnormal BTT: two of the 10 with gestational hypertension were in the ≥97th percentile OGTT group.

In addition to case (b) shown in Table 24.6, only two women also had ≥97th percentile values in both the OGTT and BTT; one had fasting glycosuria (Sutherland et al. 1970) (and a parent with IDDM) and the other delivered a growth-retarded baby who had prolonged neonatal hypoglycaemia and jaundice. The remaining two women in the ≥97th centile OGTT group had unremarkable pregnancies and healthy babies.

Three women with CPG values ≥97th percentile at the BTT remain to be described: the first had a maternal grandmother with type II diabetes and she herself had recurrent troublesome vaginal candidiasis throughout the pregnancy; the second had recently delivered a child with a suspected cranial malformation; the third had a BTT glycaemic response worthy of detailed description, namely: 0 min 4.44, 30 min 6.72, 60 min 6.33, 90 min 6.39 and 120 min 6.28 mmol/l. The 2-h value was the highest in the series of 101 women and yet the OGTT CPG concentrations at 30 min (8.89), 60 min (7.33), 90 min (6.22) and 120 min (6.39 mmol/l) were well within the normal ranges. The baby had a birthweight percentile of 65 and little (jaundice) or no morbidity in the first few days of life.

Conclusions

There is mounting evidence to justify a radical re-appraisal of the approaches to evaluating maternal metabolism in human pregnancy. Our data suggest that the OGTT result may be oversensitive to the effects of maternal age and, more importantly, the 2-h OGTT value failed to identify any of the three women with possible diabetogenic fetopathy. On the other hand, if a BTT is to be used to assess maternal metabolism, maternal height may have to be taken into consideration.

In the context of the potential pathogenic hyperstimulation of the fetal islets, which is the focus of the immediate obstetric view, our data suggest that the glycaemic response to a standardized BTT not only differs from that to the currently recommended OGTT but may well be more associated with the occurrence of diabetogenic fetopathies.

Whether or not a relative impairment in mixed fuel handling, signalled by the BTT, forecasts the later onset of type II diabetes awaits follow-up studies but the correlations between the BTT response and maternal BMI and fat distribution in this study are suggestive that this may be so.

It is our conclusion that the BTT has a valuable place in the standardized assessment of maternal metabolism and merits fuller investigation and more extensive application to clarify its place as a routine investigative procedure.

Acknowledgements. Grateful acknowledgement is made to Boots Co. PLC for their preparation and supply of the test meals. We thank Professor A. A. Templeton and are grateful for the valued help of his staff, Miss Fiona MacGregor, Mrs Margaret Fraser, Mrs. Elaine Stirton and not least, Mrs. Sheila Mearns who typed the manuscript. The Grampian Health Board is due our thanks for financial assistance.

References

Altman DG, Coles EC (1980) Assessing birth weight-for-dates on a continuous scale. Ann Hum Biol 7:35–44

Campbell DM, MacGillivray IM (1977) Maternal physiological responses and birthweight in singleton and twin pregnancies by parity. Europ J Obstet Gynecol Reprod Biol 7:17–24

Court DJ, Mann SL, Stone PR, Goldsbury SM, Dixon-McIvor D, Baker JR (1985) Comparison of glucose polymer and glucose for screening and tolerance tests in pregnancy. Obstet Gynecol 66:491–499

Farmer G, Russell G, Hamilton-Nicol DR et al. (1988) The influence of maternal glucose metabolism on fetal growth, development and morbidity in 917 singleton pregnancies in non-diabetic women. Diabetologia 31:134–141

Fraser RB (1983) High fibre diets in pregnancy. In: Campbell DM, Gillmer MDG (eds) Nutrition in pregnancy. RCOG, London, pp 269–277

Fraser RB, Ford FA, Milner RDG (1983) A controlled trial of a high dietary fibre intake in pregnancy – effects on plasma glucose and insulin levels. Diabetologia 25:238–241

Fraser RB, Ford FA, Lawrence GF (1988) Insulin sensitivity in the third trimester of pregnancy. A randomized study of dietary effects. Br J Obstet Gynaecol 95:223–229

Freinkel N (1985) Summary and recommendations of the Second International Workshop-Conference on Gestational Diabetes Mellitus. Diabetes 34 [Suppl 2]:123–126

Freinkel N, Metzger BE (1979) Pregnancy as a tissue culture experience: the critical implications of maternal metabolism for fetal development. In: Pregnancy metabolism diabetes and the fetus. CIBA Foundation Symposium, No 63, Excerpta Medica, Amsterdam, pp 3–23

Hatem M, Anthony F, Hogston P, Rose DJF, Dennis KJ (1988) Reference values for 75 g oral glucose tolerance test in pregnancy. Br Med J 296:676–678

Lind T, Cheyne GA, Billewicz WZ, Fairweather DVI (1968) Observations on the oral glucose tolerance test in pregnancy. Br J Obstet Gynaecol 75:540–545

Lind T, Hytten FE (1972) The excretion of glucose during normal pregnancy. J Obstet Gynaecol Br Commonwealth 79:961–965

Merkatz IE, Duchon MA, Yamashita TS, Houser HB (1980) A pilot community based screening program for gestational diabetes. Diabetes Care 3:453–457

Ney D, Hollingsworth DR, Cousins L (1982) Decreased insulin requirement and improved control of diabetes in pregnant women given a high carbohydrate, high-fibre, low-fat diet. Diabetes Care 5:529–533

Nolan CJ (1984) Improved glucose tolerance in gestational diabetic women on a low fat high unrefined carbohydrate diet. Aust NZ J Obstet Gynaecol 24:174–177

Owens DR, Wragg KG, Briggs PI, Luzio S, Kimber G, Davies C (1979) Comparison of the metabolic response to a glucose tolerance test and a standardized test meal and the response to serial test meals in normal healthy subjects. Diabetes Care 2:409–413

Paris-Bockel D, Comte F, Jeanmougin P, Keller B, Schlienger JL (1983) The breakfast tolerance test: application to the diagnosis of gestational diabetes (in French). Sem Hop Paris 59:2167–2172

Persson B, Stangenberg M, Hansson U, Norlander E (1985) Gestational diabetes mellitus (GDM). Comparative evaluation of two treatment regimens, diet versus insulin and diet. Diabetes 34 [Suppl 2]:101–105

Sutherland HW, Stowers JM, McKenzie C (1970) Simplifying the clinical problem of glycosuria in pregnancy. Lancet I:1071–1074

Sutherland HW, Stowers JM, Fisher PM (1979) Detection of chemical gestational diabetes. In: Sutherland HW, Stowers JM (eds), Carbohydrate metabolism in pregnancy and the newborn 1978. Springer-Verlag, Berlin Heidelberg New York, pp 436–461

Sutherland HW, Pearson DWM, Kerridge DF, Russell G, Farmer G (1987) Screening for gestational diabetes. In: Duran Garcia (ed) Proceedings of the International symposia 'Diabetes in pregnancy'. Servicio de publicaciones, Universidad de Sevilla, pp 65–86

Turner RC, Mann JI, Simpson RD, Harris E, Maxwell R (1977) Fasting hyperglycaemia and relatively unimpaired meal responses in mild diabetes. Clin Endocrinol 6:253–264

World Health Organization Technical Report Series, 727 (1985) Diabetes mellitus: report of a WHO study group. World Health Organization, Geneva

25. Diabetes Diagnosed During Pregnancy: Follow-up Studies

L. Mølsted-Pedersen, P. Damm and K. Buschard

Introduction

Diabetes diagnosed during pregnancy is clinically represented by several categories of patients. Thus, according to the latest recommendation gestational diabetes mellitus is defined as carbohydrate intolerance of variable severity with onset or first recognition during the present pregnancy (Gabbe 1986a). This definition, which was unanimously approved by the participants of the Second International Workshop Conference on Gestational Diabetes Mellitus, is now widely accepted by clinicians involved in this field. The definition applies irrespective of whether or not insulin is used for treatment or the condition persists after pregnancy. It does not exclude the possibility that the glucose intolerance may have antedated the pregnancy.

Gestational diabetes not only is a risk factor during the index pregnancy but also clearly may be a signal of abnormal glucose metabolism in later life (O'Sullivan 1984).

In the present study the women with gestational diabetes in a previous pregnancy were divided into three groups according to the severity of the maternal diabetes in the index pregnancy. The aim of the study was to present the preliminary results of the glucose tolerance at follow-up in the three different groups, and to study factors which might be of prognostic influence and therefore could help in the planning of adequate patient control.

Materials and Methods

Selection of Patients and Classification

The Rigshospital has no general diabetes clinic, although it has a centre for referred pregnant diabetic women at the Obstetric Department. Therefore the source of population for this study included patients visiting the general out-patient clinic of the obstetric department as well as pregnant women referred from other hospitals with diabetes diagnosed during pregnancy. The screening procedure used was that described by Guttorm (1975), in which pregnant women designated as potential diabetics and/or glucosurics had their fasting blood glucose determined twice. If the fasting blood glucose (capillary whole blood) is above 4.1 mmol/l twice an oral glucose tolerance test (OGTT) is performed at least once after week 28. The 3-h 50-g OGTT has been used. The control population comprised 46 normal, non-pregnant women. These controls were non-potential diabetic women (Pedersen 1977) who had normal OGTT when they were pregnant 2–3 years before the present investigation. During pregnancy, the controls had not shown glucosuria, and their infants had been of normal birthweight. The mean glucose values of the non-pregnant controls were calculated together with the mean glucose curve plus 2 and 3 SD. At least two glucose values should exceed the mean plus 3 SD curve of the non-pregnant controls to be designated diabetic (Kühl 1975). The designation "borderline" means that two points or more are above the mean plus 2 SD curve.

According to the treatment during pregnancy the patients were divided into three groups: A, treated with diet alone (White 1965), A⁺, treated with diet + anti-diabetic compounds and (A)B, treated with diet + insulin (Table 25.1). Women with diabetes diagnosed before pregnancy were not included in this study.

Table 25.1. Diabetes diagnosed in pregnancy. Classification according to treatment

Group	Treatment
A	Diet
A⁺	Diet and oral anti-diabetic compounds
(A)B	Diet and insulin

Principles of Treatment

The fundamental treatment has been a restricted diet of 5.000–7.500 kJ daily depending on the weight of the pregnant woman. Additional therapy with oral drugs or insulin was instituted according to the blood glucose level (capillary whole blood). If the fasting blood glucose at admission was above 8.0 mmol/l insulin treatment was started immediately. All of the overweight were given a 5.000 kJ diet. If the 24-h blood glucose level as estimated by six blood glucose measurements per 24 h surpassed 6.0 mmol/l, oral compounds were given in addition to diet. This treatment has only been initiated after the 20th week of gestation. Normal weight women have had tolbutamide (maximum 500 mg three times daily) and overweight women have been given metformin (maximum 500 mg three times daily) which may be replaced by insulin if the criteria cannot be fulfilled within 3 to 4 d. The start of trials with oral compounds took place in the ward, whereas some patients began treatment with diet as out-patients. The treatment with oral compounds was stopped at the end of 1984 and replaced by treatment with insulin. Therapy with insulin and oral compounds was normally discontinued after delivery depending on the blood glucose level. Those who were on dietary therapy only were given a full diet after delivery and the blood glucose levels were followed.

Follow-up Studies

Since 1978 all women with diabetes diagnosed during pregnancy have been offered an OGTT 2 months postpartum and again once a year thereafter. From 1981 the offer has been given by a yearly letter sent from the hospital and since then nearly 80% of the patients have accepted the offer. When the OGTT is diabetic or the fasting blood glucose is excessively increased at the follow-up examination the patient is referred to a diabetes hospital or department in most cases. In the case of no reply from these women during the last 2 years the diabetes department or the general practitioner have been contacted.

The study period covered the two decades from 1965 to 1984 and for each of the three groups (A, A$^+$, (A)B) shorter periods were selected for the follow-up investigation.

Results

Data from the Index Pregnancy

In the 20-year period 1965 to 1984 a total of 769 women with diabetes diagnosed during pregnancy had been treated at the diabetes centre (Table 25.2). Nine per cent were treated with oral compounds while another 10% developed insulin-dependent diabetes during pregnancy and insulin treatment was initiated. A two- to threefold increase in the number of patients was seen from period I to period II, most marked in class A (Table 25.2). In Table 25.3 the perinatal mortality from the two 10-year periods is given for each class and for comparison the figures from White's class B from the same period are shown.

A significant decrease in perinatal mortality from period I to period II is seen in all the classes, but is most pronounced in class A.

Congenital malformations (CM) from the same period and the same group plus a control group are shown in Table 25.4. In infants of mothers who had their diabetes diagnosed for the first time during the actual pregnancy the frequency of CM was not different from a control group, irrespective of the treatment during pregnancy. In contrast the frequency of congenital malformations was significantly increased in White's class B patients compared to the control group.

As previously mentioned some of the women with diabetes diagnosed in pregnancy were referred from other hospitals and others were found by screening among the patients visiting the out-patient obstetric clinic. In women treated with diet only (class A) 72% were found by screening while among women treated with oral compounds or insulin the percentages were 48 and 27 respectively (Table 25.5).

Table 25.2. Diabetes diagnosed in pregnancy, Rigshospital series 1965–1984

Period	A	A$^+$	(A)B	Total
I 1965–1974	138	27	25	190
II 1975–1984	485	42	52	579
Total	623 (81%)	69 (9%)	77 (10%)	769

Table 25.3. Diabetes diagnosed in pregnancy. Perinatal mortality in two periods, Rigshospital series 1965–1984

Period	Class A		Class A$^+$		Class (A)B		Class B	
	Total no.	Perinatal mortality (%)	Total no.	Perinatal mortality (%)	Total no.	Perinatal mortality (%)	Total no.	Perinatal mortality (%)
1965–1974	138	3.6	27	7.4	25	8.0	120	6.6
1975–1984	485	0.8	42	2.4	52	3.8	143	2.8

Table 25.4. Congenital malformations in newborn infants of mothers with diabetes diagnosed in pregnancy, Rigshospital series 1965–1984

White class	Total no. of infants	Infants with congenital malformations	
		No.	Per cent
A	623	17	2.7
A+	69	2	2.9
(A)B	77	2	2.6
B	263	16	6.1
Non-diabetic control group	1715	48	2.8

A, A+, (A)B bracketed together: 2.7

Table 25.5. Origin of the women with diabetes diagnosed during pregnancy

White class	Found by screening (%)	Referred from other hospitals (%)
A	72	28
A$^+$	48	52
(A)B	27	73

In the follow-up investigation of the class A diabetics the period 1981 to 1985 was selected for the present study since the percentage of women who responded to our yearly recall for OGTT was high in that time period. Two hundred and thirty-seven women were treated with diet alone and 182 (77%) had an OGTT performed at least 12 months after delivery (Table 25.6).

In the decade 1975 to 1984 a total of 60 women were treated with oral compounds for shorter or longer periods during pregnancy but 18 (30%) had to be changed to insulin therapy later in pregnancy. Of the remaining 42 women, 37

Table 25.6. Follow-up studies of women with diabetes diagnosed during pregnancy, I

White class	Period	Average follow-up period (months)		No. diagnosed in pregnancy	No. at follow-up
		Mean	Range		
A	1981–1985	33.2	12–82	237	182 (77%)
A⁺	1975–1984	92.0	48–156	42	37 (88%)
(A)B	1966–1980	96.0	50–204	63	60 (95%)

(88%) participated in the follow-up studies for an average of 7.6 years after the index pregnancy (Table 25.6). Twenty-nine were treated with sulphonylurea and 13 with metformin.

Some data from the patients who were insulin dependent during pregnancy have been published already (Buschard et al. 1987). At the time of diagnosis the average fasting blood glucose level was 15.6 mmol/l and 81% of the women had ketonuria. Only nine of the 63 patients (14%) had to continue with insulin after delivery without interruption until the follow-up investigation on average 8 years later. Sixty (95%) took part in the follow-up investigation (Table 25.6).

In Table 25.7 the data at onset of diabetes in the index pregnancy in each group are given. There was no significant difference in parity or maternal age between the three groups. The gestational week at onset of diabetes tended to be higher in the diet-treated group but the difference was not significant. The percentage of overweight women was significantly lower among the insulin-dependent diabetics ((A)B) than in the two other groups.

Table 25.7. Follow-up studies of women with diabetes diagnosed during pregnancy, II. Clinical details

White class	Gestational week at onset of diabetes		Parity	Maternal age (years)		Overweight ≥20% (%)
	Mean	Range		Mean	Range	
A	33	12–42	1.9	29.0	16–43	32
A⁺	28	26–37	2.3	30.5	17–47	31
(A)B	27	2–37	2.0	27.1	18–43	14

State of Glucose Tolerance at Follow-up

At the follow-up examination on average 33 months after delivery 45 (25%) of the women with diet-treated diabetes during pregnancy had a diabetic OGTT and were again treated with diet. Another four were treated with diet and oral compounds while three were on insulin. Fifty (28%) had borderline OGTT which leaves only 80 (44%) with a normal OGTT (Table 25.8).

Table 25.8. Follow-up studies of women with diabetes diagnosed during pregnancy. State of glucose tolerance at follow-up

White class	Borderline OGTT		Diabetic						Normal OGTT	
			Diet		Diet plus oral anti-diabetic		Diet plus insulin			
	No.	Per cent	No.	Per cent	No.	Per cent	No.	Per cent	No.	Per cent
A	50	27.5	45	24.7	4	2.2	3	1.6	80	44.0
A$^+$	3	8.3	8	22.2	6	16.2	13	36.0	6	16.7
(A)B	0	0	8	13.3	6	10.0	46	76.7	0	0

Of those given oral compounds during the index pregnancy only six (16.2%) had a normal OGTT at follow-up, while 35% were insulin dependent, 16.2% were taking oral anti-diabetics, 24.3% were on diet and 8.3% showed a borderline OGTT and were untreated. There was no difference in the length of follow-up period between the groups currently on treatment with insulin, oral compounds, diet or no treatment at all (Table 25.8).

Of the patients with insulin-dependent diabetes in the index pregnancy 60 participated in the follow-up examination and 46 were currently insulin treated, nine of these without interruptions from time of onset of the disease. Thirty-seven had stopped taking insulin during the remission period (average 8.5 months), beginning on average 9 d after delivery. Fourteen patients were not insulin treated at follow-up, but all of the 11 examined displayed abnormal carbohydrate metabolism, seven with fasting blood glucose values above 14 mmol/l, and four with markedly pathological glucose tolerance tests. Six were treated with diet and oral compounds while eight were treated with diet alone. These non-insulin-treated patients were seen 4.5 years after delivery (range 3.2–13.0 years), whereas the average interval between delivery and follow-up in the insulin-treated patients was 8.1 years (range 1.6–16.3 years).

Patients currently taking insulin were significantly younger than those not currently taking insulin; this applies also to those who started with insulin in the index pregnancy and to those who were treated with oral compounds (Table 25.9). Also patients not currently taking insulin had significantly higher prepregnancy weights than the insulin-treated group. When grouped by weight (Natvig 1956) around 80% of the currently insulin-treated patients were normal or underweight, whereas 64% of those not currently taking insulin were more than 10% overweight; this applies also to those who started with insulin and to those who started with oral compounds. The women who currently were insulin treated tended to have a lower parity than those not currently insulin treated, but the difference was not significant (Table 25.9).

In White's class A patients no difference in maternal age, weight and parity could be found between those with diabetic, borderline or normal OGTTs at the follow-up examination. The perinatal mortality in White's class (A)B deserves further comment as the intrauterine deaths in all four pregnancies could be directly related to severe, acute derangement in carbohydrate metabolism in women previously not known to be diabetic. Antenatal care had taken place in other obstetrical departments within our referral area. It is noteworthy that even though indicators of gestational diabetes were present weeks to months before

Table 25.9. Clinical data from the index pregnancy correlated to the follow-up results

	Treatment with insulin in pregnancy			Treatment with oral compounds in pregnancy		
	All patients ($n=63$)	Currently insulin-treated patients ($n=46$)	Not currently insulin-treated patients ($n=14$)	All patients ($n=42$)	Currently insulin-treated patients ($n=13$)	Not currently insulin-treated patients ($n=24$)
Age (years)	27	26*	30*	30	26***	32***
Parity	2.0	1.8	2.5	2.2	1.5	2.5
Weight (kg)	62	59**	74**	73	67***	78****
Height (cm)	164	165	162	165	165	165

*$P<0.05$, **$P<0.001$, ***$P<0.005$, ****$P<0.05$

Table 25.10. Perinatal mortality in White's class (A)B, 4 of 63 = 6.3%. All referred from other hospitals at the time of diagnosis

Indicators of gestational diabetes	Gestational age at delivery (weeks)	Birthweight (g)	Maternal state at admission
1. ++ glucosuria in 22nd and 30th week of gestation	31	Stillborn 1950	Precoma (hydramnios)
2. Delivery of a stillborn baby of 4650 g 3 years previously	35	Stillborn 3650	Severe acidosis
3. ++ glucosuria in 21st and 22nd week of gestation	33	Stillborn 2200	Precoma
4. ++ glucosuria in 36th week of gestation	37	Stillborn 3700	Precoma

the acute episodes of severe acidosis or precoma arose, no steps were taken to diagnose gestational diabetes (Table 25.10).

Discussion

Gestational diabetes mellitus is a heterogeneous disorder which complicates 2%–3% of all pregnancies in the Western world (Gabbe 1986b). The treatment of and clinical research in diabetes complicating pregnancy in the east of Denmark has for many years been centralized at the Diabetes Centre at the Obstetrical Department, Rigshospitalet, Copehagen. The present study underlines the profound heterogeneity which characterizes a series of women with diabetes diagnosed during pregnancy in our centre, which takes care of almost unselected case material.

The number of pregnancies in which diabetes is diagnosed for the first time has increased considerably during the last decade (Table 25.2). This can be explained by an intensified screening procedure for diabetes in pregnancy; furthermore there has been a sharp rise in referrals from other hospitals. The duration of treatment in pregnancy was extremely variable and generally short, as diabetes was detected in the last trimester in 80% of our patients.

During the last investigation period, 1975–1984, the perinatal mortality in White's class A patients was not different from that found in the general population (0.8%). In the groups treated with oral compounds or insulin the perinatal mortality was increased three- to fourfold compared to the non-diabetic population, and was of the same magnitude as seen in women with IDDM of short duration diagnosed before pregnancy.

The possible adverse effects on the fetus, similar to those found in pregnancies with IDDM established before pregnancy, might be operative in the last part of gestation.

On the other hand, a malformation rate similar to that seen in the non-diabetic population favours a normal carbohydrate metabolism at conception and in the first trimester (Fuhrmann et al. 1983).

In a 10-year period 60 patients had a trial with oral compounds in the Copenhagen Centre. Eighteen (30%) of the patients were "drug failures" requiring insulin to decrease blood glucose levels. This is in accordance with the results from the first Copenhagen series (Pedersen and Mølsted-Pedersen 1975) and other studies (Coetzee and Jackson 1979). We are not proposing the use of oral compounds in pregnancy but have been studying their use. The case for a limited place for oral drugs may perhaps be established or when ongoing follow-up studies of the offspring have been completed.

Since our trial with oral compounds finished at the end of 1984, 149 women with diabetes diagnosed during pregnancy have been treated at the Diabetes Centre. Nineteen per cent required treatment with insulin in accordance with our established criteria, and this figure makes it probable that those women who previously had a trial with oral agents are now treated directly with insulin. The group of women with gestational diabetes who will benefit from insulin therapy was of the same magnitude in the study of Persson et al. (1985).

Although the follow-up period for class A diabetic women was as short as 33 months on average, already 28% of the women have turned out to be clinically diabetic or to have a definitely diabetic oral glucose tolerance test. The high incidence of clinical diabetes in classes A[+] and (A)B is less surprising because the derangement of carbohydrate metabolism in the index pregnancy was more profound. A recent follow-up study also covering a wide spectrum of glucose intolerance in pregnancy gives a comparably high incidence of abnormal postpartum glucose intolerance (Metzger et al. 1985). Also the most extensive and only controlled follow-up study of gestational diabetes (O'Sullivan 1984) has shown that women with diabetes diagnosed during pregnancy are at high risk for future diabetes.

The distribution of tissue types among the class (A)B patients has shown a high proportion with HLA-DR3,4 (Møller-Jensen et al. 1987), which is a similar picture to that seen in non-pregnant women with IDDM but very definitely "skewed" in relation to the normal background population. Since gestational diabetic women (Rubinstein et al. 1981) as well as patients with NIDDM (Rimoin and Rotter 1984) have a tissue-type distribution which does not differ from that of the normal population, the "skewed" distribution among the class (A)B patients gives evidence that their diabetes was true IDDM.

At follow-up the women currently treated with insulin were significantly younger in age, had a lighter prepregnancy weight and their parity tended to be lower than those not currently insulin treated; this applies to both class (A)B and class A$^+$. For several years it has been emphasized that women acquiring diabetes in pregnancy comprise two main categories: the young, thin and the older more or less obese women, respectively, with a stronger tendency to acquire clinical diabetes after a short period of time in the young, lean group (Pedersen 1977). The present results provide further evidence for this.

Conclusions

1. On the basis of follow-up studies it is recommended that women with gestational diabetes should be subjected to an oral glucose tolerance test approximately 2 months after delivery to evaluate whether they are still glucose intolerant. Even if the postpartum OGTT is normal, yearly control OGTTs should be arranged since gestational diabetic subjects have a considerably increased risk of developing manifest diabetes later in life.

2. Women with diabetes diagnosed during pregnancy constitute a hetero-geneous group of which around 20% need insulin during pregnancy. Most of those requiring insulin during pregnancy have true IDDM. Of those who are treated with insulin or oral compounds in pregnancy the young and lean women have the highest risk of developing manifest diabetes after a short period of time.

3. Screening for diabetes in pregnancy is important since proper treatment of the mother seems to improve the prognosis for the fetus.

References

Buschard K, Buch I, Mølsted-Pedersen L, Hougaard P, Kühl C (1987) Increased incidence of true type I diabetes acquired during pregnancy. Br Med J 294:275–279

Coetzee EJ, Jackson WPU (1979) Metformin in management of pregnant insulin-independent diabetics. Diabetologia 16:241–245

Fuhrmann K, Reiher H, Semmler K, Fisher F, Fisher M, Glöckner E (1983) Prevention of congenital malformations in infants of insulin-dependent diabetic mothers. Diabetes Care 6:219–224

Gabbe SG (1986a) Definition, detection and management of gestational diabetes. Obstet Gynecol 67:121–125

Gabbe SG (1986b) Gestational diabetes mellitus. N Engl J Med 315:1025–1026

Guttorm E (1975) Practical screening for diabetes mellitus in pregnant women. In: Sutherland HW, Stowers JM (eds) Carbohydrate metabolism in pregnancy and the newborn. Churchill Livingstone, Edinburgh, pp 142–152

Kühl C (1975) Glucose metabolism during and after pregnancy in normal and gestational diabetic women. Acta Endocrinol (Copenh) 79:709–710

Metzger BE, Bybee DE, Freinkel N, Phelps RL, Radvany RM Vaisrub N (1985) Gestational diabetes mellitus. Correlations between phenotypic and genotypic characteristics of the mother and abnormal glucose tolerance during the first year post partum. Diabetes 34 [Suppl 2]:111–115

Møller-Jensen B, Buschard K, Buch I et al. (1987) HLA associations in insulin-dependent diabetes
    mellitus diagnosed during pregnancy. Acta Endocrinol (Copenh) 116:387–389
Natvig H (1956) Nye høyde-vekttabeller for norske kvinner og menn. Landsforeningen for kosthold
    og helse. Universitetsforlaget, Oslo
O'Sullivan JB (1984) Subsequent morbidity among gestational diabetic women. In: Sutherland HW,
    Stowers JM (eds) Carbohydrate metabolism in pregnancy and the newborn. Churchill Liv-
    ingstone, Edinburgh, pp 174–180
Pedersen J (1977) The pregnant diabetic and her newborn. Munksgaard, Copenhagen
Pedersen J, Mølsted-Pedersen L (1975) Oral antidiabetic compounds in pregnancy. In: Camerini-
    Davalos RA, Cole HS (eds) Early diabetes in early life. Academic Press, New York, pp 487–494
Persson B, Stangenberg M, Hansson U, Nordlander E (1985) Gestational diabetes mellitus (GDM).
    Comparative evaluation of two treatment regimens, diet versus insulin and diet. Diabetes 34
    [Suppl 2]:101–105
Rimoin DL, Rotter JI (1984) The genetics of diabetes mellitus. In: Adreani D, Di Mario U, Federlin
    KF, Heding LG (eds) Immunology in diabetes. Kimpton Medical Publications, London, pp 45–62
Rubinstein P, Walter M, Krassner J et al. (1981) HLA antigens and islet cell antibodies in gestational
    diabetes. Hum Immunol 3:271–275
White P (1965) Pregnancy and diabetes. Medical aspects. Med Clin North Am 49:1015–1024

26. The Boston Gestational Diabetes Studies: Review and Perspectives

J. B. O'Sullivan

The major conclusions for two controlled intervention trials conducted in Boston City and Boston Lying-In Hospitals have been presented at previous Aberdeen Colloquiums. At the first Aberdeen Colloquium, the study design, its rationale and pregnancy outcomes were described (O'Sullivan 1975). On the occasion of the second Colloquium, the subsequent development of diabetes mellitus and predictor variables were explored (O'Sullivan 1979). Finally, at the third Colloquium, the experience with both morbidity and mortality in our study subjects was described (O'Sullivan 1984).

In general, a significantly higher perinatal mortality was found among those women with gestational diabetes (GDM) than among randomly selected control patients whose only requirement was to exhibit a normal 3-h oral glucose tolerance test (OGTT). Insulin treatment was found to reduce the higher incidence of large-baby births to the rate of the negative controls but did not reduce the perinatal mortality rate (O'Sullivan and Mahan 1980). Consequently, a second study, using the current OGTT criteria, was initiated. These criteria for GDM were shown to select patients closer to the development of diabetes in later years than did the diagnostic standards employed in the earlier study. The second study showed, in a more convincing manner, a significantly higher perinatal loss rate among gestational diabetics than in controls. Although the rate was impressively lower among GDMs randomized into an insulin-treatment category than among the GDM controls, it did not achieve statistical significance by the time the study had prematurely closed.

When the data from these two studies were combined, then a significant beneficial effect on perinatal mortality for the insulin-treated group was found. This joining of two studies, however, required redefining the selection criteria for the first study and restrictions concerning the duration of insulin therapy for both investigations. Such retrospective analyses dictate that the conclusions be used for hypothesis setting only. I am unaware of any subsequent studies proving this apparently beneficial effect of insulin treatment on perinatal mortality rates in those with GDMs. Subsequent improvement in perinatal salvage across the whole sprectrum of diabetes, and particularly so for the woman with GDM, renders the question, as originally posed, moot. It is now a matter of defining the indications for the commencement of insulin in the individual case rather than deciding whether all those with GDM would benefit from its universal use.

Similarly, insulin managment of the gestational diabetic in the Boston studies appeared to have no effect on the progression to diabetes in subsequent years. Here again some unanswered questions remain. For example, insulin management was found to reduce the incidence rates for diabetes when clinical criteria (large-baby birth; family history of diabetes) were used to describe subsets of gestational diabetics (O'Sullivan and Mahan 1980). As before, these results involved redefining retrospectively the baseline data and consequently are limited to hypothesis setting.

The morbidity and mortality findings on follow-up indicated a greater frequency of hypertension, hyperlipidaemia and abnormal resting and stress electrocardiograms among former gestational diabetics than among the negative control patients and a significantly lower mortality rate for the gestational diabetics who had received insulin treatment in their index pregnancies. The number of morbid endpoints were too few for multivariate analyses and the deaths too few for exploring mortality by cause. It is hoped that the study can be re-opened, if not for re-testing, then for a mortality follow-up.

Having briefly outlined the salient findings of the Boston Gestational Diabetes Studies, those achieving statistical significance and those needing confirmation, data that have relevance to the continuing need for identifying the gestational diabetic will be reviewed. Questions have also been raised concerning the absence of maternal age and weight analyses in the Boston studies and, indeed, concerning the whole concept of gestational diabetes (Jarrett 1981). One example of Jarrett's concern about the existing evidence for a relationship between glucose levels and perinatal mortality is the study of Hadden (1980). Hadden's perinatal mortality rate for the years 1966 to 1977 in the major Northern Ireland hospital was only marginally higher among women with an abnormal GTT than in the general prenatal population. Any generalization of these results, however, must consider the fact that the whole prenatal population did not receive glucose tolerance tests to separate out those with GDM. Our experience with screening suggests that a substantial number of those with GDM would have been missed by the screening procedures in use throughout that time period in Belfast. Inclusions of gestational diabetics in the general pregnant, rather than in the GDM study population, would have had little impact on the perinatal mortality rates of the former given its large denominator, but a potentially significant effect on increasing the rates from the latter due to the smaller numbers (denominator) of gestational diabetics.

Analyses from the second study of gestational diabetics at Boston City Hospital, confining the data to the untreated gestational diabetics and negative controls, are shown in Table 26.1. These data explore the significantly higher perinatal losses of the gestational diabetics in that study by subgrouping on maternal age and body weight. The data indicate that all of the losses among those with GDM are confined to women aged 25 years and over. Table 26.2 provides the mean venous whole blood glucose values obtained from the gestational OGTT results for the four GDM subsets in Table 26.1. No difference was found among the four groups with respect to blood glucose levels. In addition, the 1-h GTT values, averaging 174 mg/dl, were within 1 mg/dl of each other. It would appear from these analyses, then, that gestational hyperglycaemia in this study could be tolerated by the younger age group without adverse effects on the outcome of their pregnancies. Whether such excellent results among gestational diabetics under age 25 years could be replicated in settings without expertly focused care is a major question that must be answered before age-limiting gestational screening for obstetric purposes can be recommended.

Table 26.1. Perinatal mortality (PM) in gestational diabetic and negative controls by age and body weight

Age	Weight	Negative controls		Gestational diabetics	
		No.	PM (%)	No.	PM (%)
<25	Normal	138	1.4	40	0.0
	Obese[a]	33	3.0	13	0.0
>25	Normal	54	0.0	54	7.4[b]
	Obese	34	2.9	80	10.1[b]

[a] Overweight: 120% or more.
[b] PM rate significantly higher in those with GDM ($P<0.05$).

Table 26.2. Mean glucose tolerance in those with GDM by age and body weight

Age	Weight	No.	Glucose Tolerance Test[a]	
			Fasting	2-h
<25	Normal	40	84	157
	Obese[b]	13	94	163
>25	Normal	54	86	160
	Obese	80	90	160

[a] Venous whole blood glucose means (mg/dl).
[b] Overweight: 120% or more.

Given the current high quality of care and excellence of results in specialized centres, a prime target for investigation is the study of perinatal mortality by age in a community that does not have access to such expertise. Now that the World Health Organization Expert Committee on Diabetes Mellitus (WHO 1980) has recommended that impaired glucose tolerance (WHO–IGT) criteria be employed to characterize glucose intolerance in pregnancy this task is more complex. It should be noted that the WHO Expert Committee recommended that its management should be the same as for diabetes, i.e. WHO–IGT is their equivalent of gestational diabetes. One cannot readily answer a question raised by one study by employing different diagnostic criteria. The WHO–IGT criteria necessitate a 75-g oral glucose challenge and a 2-h blood glucose sample. The diagnosis is defined as being "intermediate between normal and diabetic" with a fasting venous whole blood value below 120 mg/dl and a 2-h post challenge between 120 and 180 mg/dl. Strict adherence to these guidelines, however, will leave unclassified persons with glucose levels of 180 mg/dl or higher who fail to meet the WHO diagnostic standards for diabetes, which requires confirmation either by the presence of diabetic symptoms or by an additional elevated blood glucose value.

Table 26.3 provides fasting and 2-h venous whole blood glucose distributions for 752 unselected pregnancies at Boston City Hospital. These data can be used to count the number of women meeting the individual WHO–IGT glucose criteria. One adjustment must first be made in order to compensate for using the 100-g

Table 26.3. Distribution of OGTT values in 752 unselected pregnancies

Venous whole blood (mg/dl)	Fasting no.	2-h no.
<50	12	13
50–59	80	21
60–69	323	82
70–79	253	138
80–89	68	148
90–99	12	122
100–109	1	92
110–119	1	53
120–129	0	27
130–139	1	30
140–149	0	11
150–159	0	8
160–169	0	2
170–179	0	0
180+	1	5
Totals	752	752

instead of the 75-g glucose challenge recommended by the WHO Expert Committee. Castro et al. (1970) compared the 75-g and 100-g tests and found that the 2-h values averaged 4 mg higher following the larger challenge. Rather than adjusting the 2-h valves in Table 26.3 down by 4 mg/dl, the same effect is achieved by increasing the WHO diagnostic standard from 120 mg/dl to 124 mg/dl. Table 26.3 provides data by 10 mg intervals only, so the WHO 120 mg/dl criterion was overadjusted to 130 mg/dl instead of 124 mg/dl. With this adjustment, a total of 56 women are found to meet or exceed this criterion level, two of whom would be excluded by having a fasting level in excess of 120 mg/dl. The resulting prevalence of gestational diabetes by WHO–IGT criteria is 7.2% or close to three times the rate calculated using the criteria currently recommended in the US. Using an exact adjustment to 124 mg/dl would have resulted in a higher prevalence rate. Indeed, the data presented earlier in this volume by Lind were based on patients diagnosed by WHO standards and can be used to calculate the frequency of GDM by those criteria. The GDM prevalence in his collaborative study estimates 8.2%, not inconsistent with the foregoing data from our unselected pregnancies. Consequently, when these findings are related to the results obtained in the Boston studies which effectively reduced the prevalence of gestational diabetes to 2.3%, the use of the WHO diagnostic criteria in pregnancy would appear to be undesirable for the research purposes suggested.

The final section of this review will focus on the incidence of diabetes mellitus in women originally identified as having GDM. Three diagnostic criteria for diabetes mellitus are presented. The first has been applied from the outset of our studies, namely the United States Public Health Service (USPHS) criteria which require the fasting and 3-h combination, or three or more values at or above the following venous whole blood levels: fasting 110 mg/dl; 1-h 170 mg/dl; 2-h 120 mg/dl; 3-h 110 mg/dl. Early in the study, when the course of diabetes diagnosed by the USPHS criteria revealed many remissions, there was a question whether this finding reflected a problem with the criteria or truly reflected a remittent course for diabetes. The need to differentiate the results with levels of hyperglycaemia that would leave no doubt about the presence of diabetes was met by employing a second and arbitrary set of "decompensation" standards. These criteria required two or more of the following venous whole blood values: fasting 120 mg/dl; postprandial 180 mg/dl; postglucose 300 mg/dl. Thirdly, the WHO Diabetes criteria (WHO–DM 1985), which require a random venous whole blood glucose of 180 mg/dl and symptoms of diabetes, or in the absence of symptoms, one additional test either from a random sample (180 mg/dl or higher) or from the OGTT (fasting 120 mg/dl or 2-h 180 mg/dl or higher), were employed. The 2-h value was adjusted 5 mg/dl upwards (to 185 mg/dl) in order to allow a better comparison with the results from the Boston studies. In addition, the diagnoses were made without regard to the presence or absence of symptoms which, in the opinion of the author, hamper interstudy comparisons inasmuch as investigators will differ in the significance they attach to varying degrees of symptoms and patients can either exaggerate or deny their presence.

Table 26.4 provides the 22- to 28-year incidences of diabetes by all three criteria. The rate obtained when the WHO–DM criteria were applied to the data can be seen to be intermediate between those obtained with the USPHS and decompensation criteria. Adjustment for the effects of the 100-g challenge was explored further by re-applying the WHO criteria using a 10 mg/dl instead of a 5 mg/dl modification of the 2-h criterion value (i.e. 190 mg/dl instead of 185 mg/dl). The resulting WHO–DM incidence rate was 1% for former gestational diabetics and remained unchanged for the negative controls. This surprisingly small change in the incidence of diabetes resulted from the fact that most of these subjects had substantial hyperglycaemia, often in the 300–600 mg/dl range.

Table 26.4. Incidence (22–28 years) of diabetes in gestational diabetics and controls by three diagnostic criteria

Category	No.	Subsequent diabetes (%)		
		Total USPHS	Decompensation	WHO–DM
Negative controls	328	7.0	3.4	5.5
Former gestational diabetics	615	49.9	24.7	36.4

The incidence of diabetes mellitus can also be examined by confining the figures to women who exhibited a non-diagnostic postpartum glucose tolerance test, in each instance employing the respective criteria for the diagnosis of diabetes mellitus. The resulting incidence rates are provided in Table 26.5 and being designed by subtracting from both the numerator and denominator women who had a diagnostic test postpartum, they are, as expected, lower. In the Boston studies the difference is relatively small because only a small number (2.1%) failed to exhibit a non-diagnostic OGTT postpartum. The broad definition of gestational diabetes in current use can, however, include persons with overt diabetes. Consequently, expressing incidence rates for subsequent diabetes mellitus based only on the gestational, and not the postpartum status, will be less valuable and will create problems when comparisons between rates from different studies are attempted. The wide range of such rates is shown in Table 25.6, and others have been presented in this volume. In general, the rates vary from 2% to 86% per year. With these incidence rates, the difference in frequency

Table 26.5. Incidence (22–28 years) of diabetes in gestational diabetics with non-diagnostic OGTTs postpartum

Diagnostic criteria	No.	Subsequent diabetes (%)
USPHS	602	48.8
Decompensation	603	23.2
WHO–DM	603	35.2

Table 26.6. Follow-up studies of gestational diabetics

Authors	Gestational diabetics	Follow-up[a] (years)	Diabetics (%)
Hagbard and Svanborg (1960)	37 transient diabetics	7	27.0
Konradi and Matveeva (1974)	43 abnormal GTT	6	42.2
Mestman (1980)	181 abnormal GTT	5	45.3
Pettitt et al. (1980)	233 abnormal GTT	8	4.5–45.5
Metzger et al. (1985)	Abnormal GTT:	1	
	61 FPG <105		23.0
	30 FPG 105<130		43.0
	22 FPG >130		86.0
Stowers (1984)	72 abnormal IVGTT	Av.10	2%/yr
O'Sullivan (1984)	615 abnormal GTT	28	49.9

[a] Maximum duration of follow-up, except as noted.

of diabetes over several years can be so large that it becomes obvious that the baseline criteria, their application or other factors, resulted from selecting very different populations of glucose-intolerant pregnant women.

The study of Hagbard and Svanborg is included in Table 26.6 because it provides an excellent example of the degree to which remissions can occur and because it raises questions relating to current definitions of gestational diabetes. There seems little doubt that these patients would qualify as gestational diabetics by the current definition namely "carbohydrate intolerance of variable severity with onset or first recognition during the present pregnancy" (Second International Workshop Conference on Gestational Diabetes Mellitus 1985). In this fascinating study, 71 prenatal patients presented for the first time with symptoms of diabetes and fasting capillary glucose values exceeding 200 mg/dl at some large hospitals in Sweden between 1948 and 1954. Ketosis of varying degrees was present in 40% of the cases, including eight patients with incipient coma. The diabetes proved transitory in 52% ($n=37$) of the cases, all evidence of diabetes having disappeared and blood glucose values having returned to normal when retested after delivery and lactation. Of the eight cases in coma or incipient coma four had only transient diabetes. Follow-up revealed that 27% of the transitory cases had insulin-requiring diabetes. This incidence rate is almost certainly grossly understated because it was based on questionnaire information without additional testing.

Because these patients qualify as gestational diabetics they point to the necessity for the addition of an exclusion statement to the description of the current diagnostic standard. The Boston gestational diabetes studies had a requirement to exclude symptomatic diabetics, even if diagnosed in the current pregnancy. The criterion used for this purpose was the presence of classic diabetic symptoms and an abnormal OGTT or, in the absence of symptoms, confirmed hyperglycaemia of 300 mg/dl or higher. Symptoms are used for exclusion of cases and their use for this purpose is defended on the basis that subjects were randomized into defined study categories for a future endpoint, the outcome of pregnancy. Such exclusions may account, in part, for the high percentage of normal OGTTs in our studies.

It should be noted that all of the incidence rates in Table 26.6 are for different spans of time. In addition, they relate to varying lengths of follow-up for the participants within each study. The effect of this latter consideration can be shown in data from the Boston study where a life table projection of the results based on estimates assuming that all patients had been observed for a full 24 years showed an incidence rate of 73% (SE 2.8 years) for those with GDM and 11.2% (SE 2.4 years) for the negative controls.

Definition of the population's baseline status and consideration of the effects of varying periods of follow-up are fundamental to all observational studies. Other factors can then be explored, such as the influence on incidence rates of varying degrees of gestational hyperglycaemia, of maternal age and weight and other variables, either by cross-classification tables or, more fully, by multifactor analyses. These analyses have been carried to varying degrees by the listed studies. More fundamental explorations with aetiological possibilities have also been pursued, such as the islet cell antibody analysis of Stowers et al. (1985) and additional factors related to the authors' genetic hypothesis by Metzger et al. (1985).

Despite the fundamental problems that arise when attempting to compare diabetes incidence rates, there is broad general agreement on the predictive nature of gestational glucose levels. Hyperglycaemia, in addition to indicating at risk pregnancies, also identifies those women who are at risk for future diabetes. The gestational diabetic provides an outstanding opportunity for the practice of preventive medicine. In addition to focusing on events relating to pregnancy, it is worth emphasizing opportunities for the prevention or amelioration of both subsequent diabetes and cardiovascular disease. Nutritional and behavioural education to achieve continuing weight control should serve to counter the tendency to both obesity and diabetes; advice should also be given concerning the restriction of dietary cholesterol and saturated fat, the promotion of exercise, the cessation of smoking and regarding intermittent blood tests and blood pressure control. The peripregnancy period allows patient contact for up to 9 months and thus provides an excellent opportunity to expand the routine care of these patients to include cardiovascular risk assessment and education aimed at the postpregnancy years. Such a programme has the potential of making a significant contribution to reducing the high risk of morbid events that characterize the years subsequent to the diagnosis of gestational diabetes.

References

Castro A, Scott JP, Grettie DP, MacFarlane D, Bailey RE (1970) Plasma insulin and glucose responses of healthy subjects and of varying glucose loads during 3-hour glucose tolerance tests. Diabetes 19:842–851

Hadden DR (1980) Screening for abnormalities of carbohydrate metabolism in pregnancy 1966–77: the Belfast experience. Diabetes Care 3:440–446

Hagbard L, Svanborg A (1960) Prognosis of diabetes mellitus with onset during pregnancy. Diabetes 9:296–302

Jarrett RJ (1981) Reflections on gestational diabetes mellitus. Lancet II:1220–1222

Konradi LI, Matveeva OF (1974) Prognostic value of disorders of glucose tolerance in pregnant women. Probl Endokrinol (Mosk) 20(2):10–13

Mestman JH (1980) Outcome of diabetes screening in pregnancy and perinatal morbidity in infants of mothers with mild impairment in glucose tolerance. Diabetes Care 3:447–452

Metzger BE, Bybee DE, Freinkel N, Phelps RL, Radvany RM, Vaisrub N (1985) Gestational diabetes mellitus: correlations between the phenotypic and genotypic characteristics of the mother and abnormal glucose tolerance during the first year postpartum. Diabetes 34:111–115

O'Sullivan JB (1975) Prospective study of gestational diabetes and its treatment. In: Sutherland HW, Stowers JM (eds) Carbohydrate metabolism in pregnancy and the newborn. Churchill Livingstone, Edinburgh, pp 195–204

O'Sullivan JB (1979) Gestational diabetes: factors influencing the rates of subsequent diabetes. In: Sutherland HW, Stowers JM (eds) Carbohydrate metabolism in pregnancy and the newborn. Springer, New York, pp 425–435

O'Sullivan JB (1984) Subsequent morbidity among gestational diabetic women. In: Sutherland HW, Stowers JM (eds) Carbohydrate metabolism in pregnancy and the newborn. Churchill Livingstone, Edinburgh, pp 174–180

O'Sullivan JB, Mahan CM (1980) Insulin treatment and high risk groups. Diabetes Care 3:482–485

Pettitt DJ, Knowler WC, Baird HR, Bennett PH (1980) Gestational diabetes: infant and maternal complications of pregnancy in relation to third-trimester glucose tolerance in the Pima Indians. Diabetes Care 3:458–464

Report of a World Health Organisation Study Group (1985) Diabetes mellitus. Technical Report Series 727. World Health Organisation, Geneva

Stowers JM (1984) Follow-up of gestational diabetic mothers treated thereafter. In: Sutherland HW, Stowers JM (eds) Carbohydrate metabolism in pregnancy and the newborn. Churchill Livingstone, Edinburgh, pp 181–183

Stowers JM, Sutherland HW, Kerridge DF (1985) Long range implications for the mother. The Aberdeen experience. Diabetes 34 (Suppl):106–110

World Health Organization (1980) Expert Committee on Diabetes Mellitus: 2nd Report. Technical Report Series 646. World Health Organization, Geneva

27. The Obstetrician's Role in the Management of Diabetic Pregnancy: The Aberdeen Approach

H. W. Sutherland and N. C. Smith

Introduction

The purpose of this chapter is to describe the obstetrician's role in the management of pregnancy in women with insulin-dependent diabetes mellitus (IDDM) and gestational diabetes mellitus (GDM) and it should be read in conjunction with Chap. 14.

The Nature of the Maternity Service

Optimal obstetric care for women with diabetes comprises attention to care prepregnancy, prenatal, intrapartum and in the puerperium by a specialist with particular knowledge and interest in the reproductive hazards associated with compromised maternal carbohydrate metabolism. The care setting should be equipped with the facilities of a tertiary maternity care centre (Traub et al. 1986), and optimally the obstetrician should be an integral part of the care team comprising, additionally, a diabetologist, a paediatrician, a midwife and a dietitian, and when required, an ophthalmologist, an anaesthetist and a medical social worker with a special commitment to the problems of diabetes. Interdisciplinary communication is important. Individualized patient care is highly desirable. In Aberdeen we aim to achieve a partnership between the health care team and the patient, and where possible her partner, before and throughout the pregnancy, by emphasizing that we share in the common objective of a successful pregnancy because we believe that without the patient's cooperation, avoidable complications are more likely to occur.

Information about the availability and desirability of prepregnancy care is widely broadcast in the area and diabetic women in the reproductive age group are especially targeted. We aim to establish good rapport as soon as possible with each diabetic woman seeking a successful pregnancy, preferably at the Prepregnancy Clinic visits which have a large educational component. Since 1962, there has been a weekly joint antenatal diabetic clinic operating in Aberdeen Maternity Hospital at which in the same clinic room the obstetrician, diabetologist and midwife give each diabetic woman a joint consultation. Since the inception of this joint clinic it has been the aim to admit diabetic women into hospital as infrequently as possible and discharge them from hospital as quickly as possible. Since the mid-1970s prepregnant women have also attended this clinic and a dietitian has been at hand. Since 1977 when we introduced glucose self-monitoring to our clinic only two of 197 pregnancies in women with IDDM and with a normally formed fetus have had a therapeutic abortion for medical reasons, but this approach may be necessary more frequently, e.g. eight of 223 pregnancies in a 53-month period from 1981 in Copenhagen were so terminated (Mølsted-Pedersen and Kuhl 1986).

Prepregnancy Care

The obstetrician's responsibility is to ensure that the diabetic woman enters pregnancy in optimal health and with a sense of realistic optimism about its outcome and confidence in herself and in the health care team. Her past menstrual, contraceptive, fertility, social and reproductive history is reviewed in detail and appropriate investigations are made, e.g. rubella and thyroid status, haematology and bacteriology of the urinary and genital tracts. The use of mechanical contraception, preferably condoms, is advised for the 3 months prior to attempting conception and during this interval plasma progesterone is measured to assess ovulatory function. Induction of ovulation may rarely be required (see Chap. 7). Rubella immunization is sometimes indicated which may prolong the period of planned effective contraception. Advice is given about cigarette smoking and alcohol intake. An assessment is made of the amount of exercise taken by the diabetic woman and her diet reviewed and appropriate counsel given.

Pre(Ante)-natal Care

As soon as pregnancy is suspected serum beta subunit human chorionic gonadotrophin is measured and an ultrasound scan of the uterus is made (Chap. 9). Except where indicated by vaginal discharge or bleeding, pelvic examination is not performed in early pregnancy. All are booked for delivery in the tertiary maternity centre. A regular (minimal) programme of clinic attendance is instituted (see Fig. 27.1). The frequency of visits shown has been determined over our 25-year experience in the combined diabetic prenatal clinic.

Following the diagnosis of GDM women attend the combined clinic and the following week enter the protocol of care as for IDDM women but also have an initial assessment of renal and thyroid function. Obese older type II diabetic women also have an electrocardiagram (Chap. 14).

Ward Admission

Ward admission for obstetric reasons is uncommon but short stays are required for genital tract bleeding (threatened or incomplete abortion) and missed

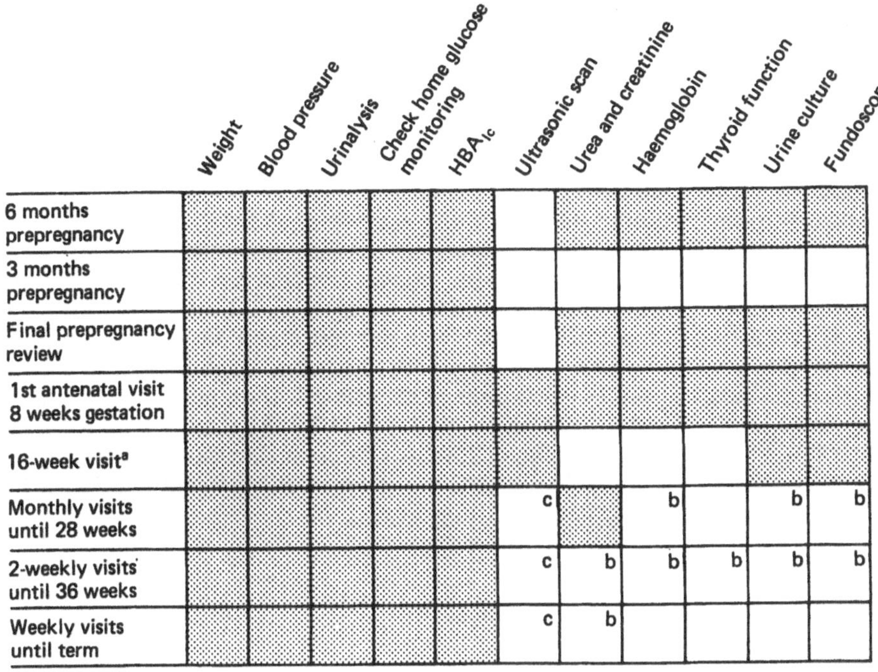

	Weight	Blood pressure	Urinalysis	Check home glucose monitoring	HBA$_{1c}$	Ultrasonic scan	Urea and creatinine	Haemoglobin	Thyroid function	Urine culture	Fundoscopy
6 months prepregnancy											
3 months prepregnancy											
Final prepregnancy review											
1st antenatal visit 8 weeks gestation											
16-week visit[a]											
Monthly visits until 28 weeks						c		b		b	b
2-weekly visits until 36 weeks						c	b	b	b	b	b
Weekly visits until term						c	b				

[a] Also measure C-peptide and α-fetoprotein.
[b] Required at one of these visits only.
[c] See text.

Fig. 27.1. Assessments made (*shaded boxes*) before and during pregnancy at the Aberdeen Combined Antenatal Diabetic Clinic.

abortion and more prolonged admissions may be required on account of hyperemesis gravidarum (Chap. 14), pyelonephritis and pregnancy-induced hypertension or antepartum haemorrhage. In the absence of pyrexia, vomiting, excessive uterine contractions or concomitant genital tract bleeding, women with lower urinary tract infections are treated with appropriate antibiotics as outpatients. In late pregnancy admission to hospital may be the most convenient way to effect the dual purposes of fetal monitoring and improving or maintaining metabolic control. Some units routinely admit women with IDDM for 2–6 weeks prior to term but this has never been Aberdeen policy. Nonetheless we concur with the view that it is safer to admit too many rather than too few (Skyler and O'Sullivan 1986).

Exercise

Most of our patients are well aware of the effect of exercise on their metabolic control before pregnancy is contemplated. As mentioned above, the educational messages are rehearsed at the Prepregnancy Clinic. The women who develop IDDM in pregnancy for the first time or who are new to the clinic for other reasons are counselled about the possibility of exercise-induced hypoglycaemia, the effect of more rapid insulin absorption from injected exercising limbs and the need to increase the intake of food before exercise and possibly the need for additional carbohydrate intake after strenuous exercise. In some women with (long-) established IDDM, exercise-induced hypoglycaemia may be problematic in pregnancy because of failure to raise their catecholamine levels in response to exercise as normal women can in pregnancy (Artal et al. 1981). Finally the question of participation in sport may be raised. We take the view and share it with the patient that the pregnancy is precious and short in duration in the context of her life, and the younger the diabetic woman is when she has her family the better. Moreover, we point out that even if a potential complication of pregnancy such as miscarriage or preterm labour was not the direct result of a sporting activity, the patient herself may engender lingering doubts that it was a contributory factor to the development of the complication and for this reason alone, very moderate participation in sport would be the maximum advisable. This counsel in our experience has allowed satisfactory accommodation of the pregnancy within an acceptable lifestyle, e.g. swimmers have continued to swim throughout pregnancy, but gently.

Assessment of the Fetoplacental Unit

Biochemical Techniques. Following extensive experience, several studies of our own and review of those of others (Lavin et al. 1983; Sutherland 1986), we have abandoned the assessment of fetoplacental function by measurement of placental steroids and proteins because it was generally unhelpful in the management of the individual case and had a low cost/benefit ratio compared with biophysical techniques.

Ultrasound Scan. In contrast, throughout pregnancy serial ultrasound scans are invaluable in the management of diabetic women. Apart from the detection of plural pregnancy, missed abortion, hydatidiform mole and continuing intrauterine pregnancy in the first trimester they allow assessment of the development of the fetoplacental unit and its function beyond the limits of clinical manual evaluation. Accurate assessment of the gestational age has been discussed in the context of initial growth delay in Chap. 9. Accuracy of gestational age assessement early in pregnancy is essential in the correct management of diabetic pregnancy and may become a critical issue if at a later stage early delivery of the infant is contemplated, e.g. for maternal reasons such as advancing retinopathy.

In early second trimester, evidence of fetal malformation should be actively sought in diabetic women. The serum alphafetoprotein is often lower in women with IDDM (Wald et al. 1979), but the reason for this is unknown (Powrie et al. 1987). Therefore, detailed ultrasonic fetal examination by an appropriately experienced practitioner is the method of choice. The clinical suspicion of excessive amniotic fluid can be further evaluated with ultrasound and if found to be present, detailed sonar examination of the fetus may demonstrate malformation. Otherwise, in our experience the explanation is usually unsuspected suboptimal maternal metabolic control. The serial measurement of maximum depth of amniotic fluid pools allows progressive monitoring of the favourable effect of tightening of metabolic control. In our practice, our patients routinely have fetal growth ultrasound scans at 20, 24 and 28 weeks and full fetal assessment scans at 32, 36, 38 and 40 weeks. The measurements made in the fetal growth scans include the biparietal diameter, femoral length, abdominal circumference and greatest amniotic pool depth. Full fetal assessment scans in addition to the above-mentioned growth indices also include head/abdominal circumference ratio, comment on fetal presentation, placental site, calcification and thickness, the fetal "breathing" and limb movements and estimated fetal weight. If this weight is greater than 4000 g at 38 weeks and the presentation is cephalic, it is recommended that the chest–biparietal diameter difference is estimated to evaluate the potential risk of shoulder girdle dystocia at vaginal delivery. If this value is greater than 1.4 cm (Elliot et al. 1982) Caesarean section is indicated in primigravidae and may be advisable also in multigravidae depending on the past obstetric history. Following review of the obstetric history in multigravidae, if vaginal delivery is contemplated, an expert obstetric practitioner should attend the second stage of labour. We are fortunate to have a magnetic resonance imaging facility (Chap. 10) with which abdominal fat can be quantified and also shoulder width and pelvic dimensions may be measured. Onset of IDDM in a girl before age 13 is associated with a significantly shorter transverse diameter of the pelvic inlet (Mølsted-Pedersen 1974).

Fetal Heart Rate Monitoring. The evidence that stress testing is superior to non-stress testing is unconvincing. Non-stress cardiotocography (CTG) is useful in selected cases and we have found it unnecessary to use this technique routinely except in those who also have thyroid dysfunction and who are receiving treatment. We believe that routine CTG monitoring is stressful to our diabetic women. Therefore it is used only in the last weeks of pregnancy when delivery before term is contemplated, when there is reason to believe the fetus is comprised, e.g. following genital tract bleeding; where pre-eclampsia has developed; if there is evidence of retarded fetal growth; if there is evidence of macrosomia; or if maternal metabolic control has been poor. Under such circumstances, and with prolonged pregnancy, CTG monitoring is done frequently, i.e. daily or more often, as indicated clinically. It is also used to evaluate the significance of reported fewer fetal movements at any time in the third trimester. Following such a report, when the CTG is found to be normal, a kick chart of the count-to-ten type is given to the patient with instructions on how to carry out daily plotting of clock time when 10 movements have been felt and how to act on her own responsibility should no movements be felt over a period of 6 h, namely make immediate arrangements for inpatient evaluation by CTG. Otherwise these charts are reviewed weekly at the combined clinic. A mildly abnormal CTG is repeated within a few hours. A seriously abnormal CTG usually calls for immediate delivery by Caesarean section.

Umbilical Artery Velocity Wave Forms (UAVW). The employment of this technique using continuous Doppler ultrasound to measure the velocity of erythrocytes in the umbilical artery has demonstrated a significant relationship between maternal metabolic control and abnormal placental vascular resistance indicated by the systolic/diastolic ratio in diabetic pregnancy (Bracero et al. 1986). More work is required to show that this technique is helpful in identifying fetuses who should be rescued by delivery rather than by improving maternal metabolic control.

Amniocentesis. The use of this technique in later pregnancy is discussed in extenso in Chap. 12. Our views coincide in every respect with those expressed by the authors. Since changing our policy in 1980 to allow diabetic pregnancy to continue to term, amniocentesis has been rarely performed except in early second trimester for cytogenetic reasons, e.g. the age-related risk of Down's syndrome in women older than 38 years, or later for the evaluation of potential haemolytic disease of the newborn. In situations where it is not possible to achieve good metabolic control, an early delivery for fetal reasons may be the preferable course of action and under such circumstances a shake test or measurement of the phosphatidylglycerol in the amniotic fluid following amniocentesis would be a satisfactory approach (vide infra).

Preterm Labour

This complication is particularly serious in diabetic women because the infant is apparently functionally less mature than the infant of the non-diabetic mother of similar gestational age. Moreover, both beta sympathomimetic and steroid drugs used in the management of the extreme preterm labour have marked hyperglycaemic effects which may lead quickly to ketoacidosis in the mother and these drugs are to be used with utmost caution and never without an insulin infusion and regular, very frequent, at least hourly, monitoring of maternal blood sugar, ketones, electrolytes and cardiopulmonary function. Avoidance (prevention) of extreme preterm labour is the best approach, thus predisposing factors such as a previous history of premature fetal expulsion, polyhydramnios (vide supra) or urinary tract and genital tract infections should be given serious consideration, and where abnormality is found, prompt treatment should be instituted if possible. Contractions of the pregnant uterus induced by nipple stimulation are readily demonstrable by cardiotocography and in women with a history of preterm labour, sexual stimulation is probably best avoided. Preterm labour has been found to be twice as common in diabetic as compared with non-diabetic pregnancies (Lufkin et al. 1984) but this is controversial (Zabut et al. 1985). The real importance of preterm labour lies in the serious prognostic significance for the prematurely expelled infant of the diabetic mother (IDM) (Chap. 31).

Placental Abruption

This complication is very dangerous for the fetus and requires immediate certain diagnosis and prompt delivery by Caesarean section with full intensive care regime for the mother, e.g. central venous pressure line, blood replacement transfusion etc. and the services of the skilled anaesthetist and expert paediatrician. Sometimes small and perhaps frequent slightly painful or pain-free warning haemorrhages occur allowing more consideration and some choice in timing and of mode of delivery guided by biophysical monitoring of the fetal condition. Under such circumstances, haematology measurements with particular reference to haemoglobin, platelet count and rhesus factor should be made to evaluate the maternal condition and whether or not an injection of prophylactic anti-D is required. Elsewhere in our practice we have found that massive abruption can occur in women with IDDM even lying at rest in hospital in reasonably good metabolic control. These retroplacental haemorrhages have occurred without any warning and even on detailed retrospective review no predisposing suspicious warning factor including diminution of perceived fetal movements could be identified.

Infections

Because of the adverse effects of infection on maternal metabolic control and the separate and additional risk of preterm labour, maternal bacterial infection should be diagnosed and treated promptly by parenteral antibiotics in the first instance in pregnant women with IDDM.

Pyelonephritis, one of Pedersen's bad prognostic signs (Pedersen and Pedersen 1965), should be treated by urgent hospital admission, intravenous infusion of fluids, intravenous or intramuscular antibiotics and analgesia. We have noted that a marked increase in urinary glucose excretion may be indicative of pyelonephritis and now culture the urine in this event.

Fungal vulvo-vaginitis can apparently be acute and extensive without causing upset in metabolic control. Nonetheless, frequently such infections may become mixed bacterial and fungal infections and should be treated promptly. Enquiry about vaginal blood loss, discharge or irritation should be specifically made at regular intervals during antenatal care. Respiratory tract and dental or subcutaneous abscesses should be treated aggressively and promptly in hospital.

Pregnancy-Induced Hypertension: Pre-eclampsia

Pre-eclampsia is another of the prognostically bad signs identified by Pedersen (Pedersen and Pedersen 1965), the validity of which has been verified in contemporary practice (Diamond et al. 1987). Blood pressure, body weight (lightly robed) and urine analysis for protein (Chap. 16) are estimated at every antenatal visit. When estimating blood pressure in obese women it is important to use a large sphygmomanometer cuff. Young (<20 years) and older (>35 years) primigravidae are more likely to develop pre-eclampsia. The very young "neglector" (Pedersen and Pedersen 1965) who defaults from clinic attendance in later pregnancy is always a source of concern in this context in addition to metabolic control considerations. High maternal weight gain >0.6 kg per week between 20 and 30 weeks in such patients is a particularly ominous sign and arrangements must be made for regular, daily if necessary, measurement of the urine for proteinuria. The development of proteinuria signals the requirement to confirm its presence in a clean catch midstream specimen of urine which should then be evaluated for pyuria and cultured. The development of true non-pyogenic proteinuria requires immediate hospital admission for further evaluation. In all diabetic women serum urate, urea and creatinine are measured routinely prepregnancy on one or more occasions, and subsequently early in pregnancy and again at 20, 32 and 38 weeks gestation to monitor renal function.

Duration of Pregnancy

With the careful evaluation of the date of conception in women with IDDM and serial scanning in pregnancy, in practice we have found that pregnancy prolonged 5 d beyond the expected date of delivery is rarely a problem. In contrast, women with GDM do have a problem with prolonged pregnancy, but this may be unreal because reliable information establishing gestational age with accuracy in early pregnancy is frequently absent. Immediately before or on the expected date of delivery, examination per vaginam to assess suitability for induction of labour is made in both groups of women because there is convincing evidence that neonatal asphyxia is associated with prolonged pregnancy in the presence of even mild abnormalities of maternal glucose tolerance (Farmer et al. 1988).

In practice over the years we rarely found assessment of amniotic fluid indices of fetal pulmonary maturity provided information useful in deciding when delivery was indicated, only when it was not indicated. Given the choice of incubator for the fetus of the metabolically well-controlled mother with IDDM or GDM, we much prefer the uterus and our policy has been to await the physiological fetomaternal signal of maturity, namely the spontaneous onset of labour. This approach has been rewarded with a higher vaginal delivery rate and more importantly a substantial reduction in neonatal morbidity which confirms the achievements of the Dublin group (Drury 1986). However, we concede that in centres where this approach is inappropriate because of poor maternal metabolic control arising from suboptimal facilities or poor patient cooperation, early delivery after day 260 following the demonstration of a reassuring amniotic fluid phosphatidylglycerol concentration is possibly the optimal choice of management of women with poorly controlled IDDM. The cost of this approach is probably morbidity extending far beyond the neonatal period (Chap. 31) and higher rates of Caesarean section. When elective Caesarean section is planned, e.g. for contracted pelvis, a date 3–5 d before the reported date of delivery is chosen for surgery and the choice of regional or general anaesthesia discussed in advance with the patient and her partner.

Plural Pregnancy

The management of plural pregnancy is essentially the same as for singleton pregnancies. There is increased risk of hyperemesis gravidarum, polyhydramnios, macrocytic anaemia (folic acid deficiency), pregnancy-induced hypertension, malpresentation and preterm labour and unique risks of discordant fetal growth, twin to twin transfusion syndrome and specific twin delivery difficulties. The smaller fetus and the second twin at vaginal delivery are at greater risk of intrauterine and intrapartum hypoxia respectively so management decisions on timing and mode of delivery are made appropriately on assessment of the risk to the more vulnerable fetus. Plural pregnancies are routinely supplemented with iron and folic acid in order to maximize maternal oxygen transport in pregnancy and to prepare for postnatal demands and possible postpartum haemorrhage which is more common in twin pregnancies. Occasionally idiopathic polyhydramnios in one sac is found (unassociated with fetal malformation or poor metabolic control) which may be so severe as to restrict ambulation and necessitate prolonged inpatient additional nursing care.

Labour

Onset of Labour

The onset of spontaneous labour, despite its unpredictable timing, is ultimately most beneficial for the patient because it tends to result in a shorter labour, less need for analgesia and an increased chance of spontaneous delivery. The diabetologist or his deputy must be informed as soon as the patient is admitted so that the insulin and glucose requirements may be clearly documented for each patient. The on-call obstetric and midwifery staff should be left in no doubt as to the protocol of metabolic management. It is also mandatory to alert the neonatal intensive care medical and nursing staff of the impending delivery. Before induction and throughout labour micturition is encouraged in an effort to minimize the requirement for catheterization. Only in cases complicated either by severe pre-eclampsia under heavy sedation or hypovolaemia, e.g. following antepartum haemorrhage is an indwelling urethral catheter used.

Induction of Labour

If induction of labour is required our policy in Aberdeen is as follows. Prior cervical assessment is undertaken in the evening and a 3-mg prostaglandin E2 vaginal pessary inserted to ripen the cervix if the pelvic score (Bishop 1964) is less than 4. One hour after this a non-stress CTG is performed for at least 20 min. Forewater rupture (low amniotomy) is undertaken the following morning and intravenous syntocinon given according to the usual hospital regime (Table 27.1) along with the insulin and glucose requirements. If polyhydramnios is present, amniotomy is done with care and CTG immediately follows the procedure. Abnormal fetal lie or breech presentation indicates delivery by elective Caesarean section in women with diabetes in most circumstances.

Table 27.1. Aberdeen intravenous syntocinon regime. 30 units syntocinon injected into 500 ml normal saline which acts as reservoir for infusion pump (Injectomat 50)

Pump rate (ml/h)	Syntocinon dosage (mU/min)
1	1
2	2
4	4
8	8
16	16
32	32
64	64

Pump rate is doubled every 30 min until labour becomes established.

Duration of Labour

This should be no longer than 12 h irrespective of parity. Glycaemic control in women with IDDM may become more difficult after this time. The fetal heart rate must be monitored continuously and the patient should have a midwife in attendance throughout labour. The cervical dilatation and descent of the fetal head should progress in the normal way and the on-call obstetric team must be alert to secondary cervical arrest and the risk of cephalo-pelvic disproportion as a consequence of macrosomia. In order to achieve the best assessment of progress in labour, ideally each vaginal examination should be performed by the same person. The course of labour should be documented in the form of a partogram to facilitate review and alert the care team to the presence of dysfunction or delay (Fig. 27.2).

Analgesia in Labour

Requirements for pain relief naturally vary between individual patients and depend also on the progress of labour. If relief is required, then epidural analgesia is best for the diabetic patient because it reduces the tendency to ketosis and dehydration which results from hyperventilation and the muscular effort of labour; it reduces pain-induced catecholamine release which may adversely affect glucose metabolism; and it permits operative delivery, which is more often required in the diabetic parturient, and thus may avoid the need for general anaesthesia.

Fetal Monitoring in Labour

Following spontaneous rupture of the membranes or amniotomy a fetal scalp electrode should be attached to allow accurate CTG monitoring. In those with

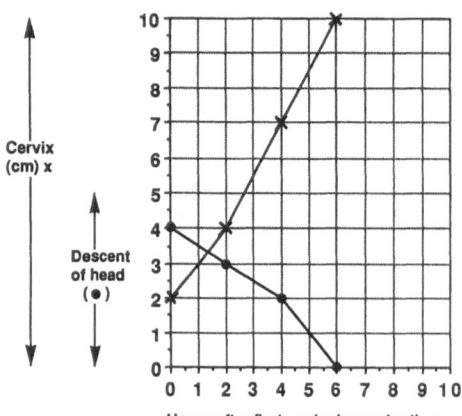

Fig. 27.2. Partogram showing normal progress of labour.

gross obesity or previous Caesarean section scar an intra-amniotic pressure transducer is preferred to the less accurate abdominal surface transducer. Scalp vein sampling to measure fetal blood pH is necessary when CTG tracings reflect fetal risk from hypoxia.

Mode of Delivery

Formerly in many centres 40% or more women with IDDM were delivered by Caesarean section (Kitzmiller et al. 1978) but the incidence in recent years has been falling due to better metabolic control and consequently fewer inductions of labour. The Caesarean section rate at Aberdeen Maternity Hospital 1984–1987 for women with IDDM was 38% (31/82) but critical retrospective review indicates that 42% (13) had less evidence of fetal distress (n=9) or less syntocinon stimulation (n=4) than would have applied to parturients without diabetes. It is expected that the Caesarean section rate will fall much further when a greater proportion of primigravidae with IDDM have vaginal deliveries at term.

Usually vaginal delivery should be anticipated from the outset but specific antenatal or intrapartum problems may alter this intention. In the second stage, maternal expulsive efforts (pushing) should be limited to 30 min and if delivery is not imminent, then assistance will be required.

If the fetus has an ultrasound-scan-predicted weight of more than 4000 g then the obstetrician should be present during the second stage. In anticipation of shoulder girdle dystocia, the patient should be placed in the lithotomy position and a generous episiotomy made. Thus, appropriate traction can be applied in the correct axis and, with maternal effort, delivery is usually achieved. Further measures to deal with shoulder girdle dystocia although rarely required, are as follows: check the cord is not tightly around the neck, if so, divide it; with the fetal shoulders ascertained to be in the antero-posterior diameter produced by the maternal expulsive effort, an assistant is required to apply suprapubic pressure while the obstetrician puts two fingers in the anterior axilla exerting traction downwards and backwards followed by "unscrewing" the shoulders by rotating them so that the anterior becomes the posterior and vice versa. This procedure produces the necessary disimpaction and allows descent and delivery of the body. On completion of this procedure, mucous extraction from the upper airways should be immediately done. The umbilical cord should be divided then (if not already vide supra) without the fetus being markedly raised or lowered (10 cm) from the level of the introitus.

Third Stage of Labour

Following delivery, it is important not only for the infant of the diabetic mother to be examined for malformation by a paediatric specialist but also that the placenta, cord and membranes are reviewed for abnormalities by the obstetrician and when present, notified to the paediatrician. Equally important are the proper supervision of the third stage of labour and the expert repair of perineal wounds in the woman with IDDM so that her recovery, ambulation and alimentation are not avoidably delayed.

The Puerperium

This time may be particularly stressful for the patient. She may have a new baby requiring much nursing and medical supervision (see Chap. 30) and her own metabolic requirements are returning to prepregnant levels. Ambulation and breast feeding should be encouraged. Insulin dosage will quickly return to pre-pregnant levels but insulin additional to this may be needed when breast feeding because the additional dietary intake, namely 2 kcal/kg/per d, for lactation may require this. Episodes of hypoglycaemia about 40 min following breast feeding may be troublesome. It is important to control maternal glycaemia by measurement of sugar in the blood and not by urinary non-specific testing because the misinterpretation of galactosuria may lead to iatrogenic hypoglycaemia. The insulin requirements may be increased further should any infection develop, e.g. mammary, respiratory or genital or urinary tract. Antibiotic treatment should be prescribed promptly.

Family planning advice should be given. The use of oral contraception is discussed in Chap. 28. When procreative desires are fulfilled, sterilization by tubal occlusion is advised particularly in women in White's classes D, F–R and T. In those with White's classes A, B and C diabetes the question of the husband having a vasectomy may be raised appropriately. If fallopian tubal occlusion is the method chosen, it is done as an interval procedure some 3 to 6 months following delivery in order to allow the patient to be sure of her decision and also to allow the baby to have a follow-up paediatric assessment.

References

Artal R, Platt LD, Sperling M et al. (1981) Exercise in pregnancy: maternal cardiovascular and metabolic responses in normal pregnancy. Am J Obstet Gynecol 140:123–127

Bishop EH (1964) Pelvic scoring for elective induction. Obstet Gynecol 24:266–268

Bracero L, Schulman H, Fleischer A et al. (1986) Umbilical artery velocimetry in diabetes and pregnancy. Obstet Gynecol 68:654–658

Diamond MP, Salyer SL, Vaughn WK, Cotton R, Boehm FH (1987) Reassessment of White's classification and Pedersen's prognostically bad signs of diabetic pregnancies in insulin dependent diabetic pregnancies. Am J Obstet Gynecol 156: 599–604

Drury MI (1986) Management of the pregnant diabetic patient – are the pundits right? Diabetologia 29:10–12

Elliot J, Garite T, Freeman R et al. (1982) Ultrasonic prediction of fetal macrosomia in diabetic patients. Obstet Gynecol 60:159–162

Farmer G, Russell G, Hamilton-Nicol DR et al. (1988) The influence of glucose metabolism on fetal growth, development and morbidity in 917 singleton pregnancies in non-diabetic women. Diabetologia 31:134–141

Kitzmiller JL, Cloherty JP, Younger MD et al. (1978) Diabetic pregnancy and perinatal morbidity. Am J Obstet Gynecol 131:560–580

Lavin JP, Lovelace DR, Miodovnik M, Knowles HC, Barden TP (1983) Clinical experience with 107 diabetic pregnancies. Am J Obstet Gynecol 147:742–752

Lufkin G, Nelson R, Hill L et al. (1984) An analysis of diabetic pregnancies at the Mayo Clinic 1950–1979. Diabetes Care 7:539–547

Mølsted-Pedersen L (1974) The transverse diameter of the pelvic inlet in diabetic women in relation to age at onset of diabetes. Acta Endocrinol (Suppl) 182:65–72

Mølsted-Pedersen L, Kuhl C (1986) Obstetrical management in diabetic pregnancy: the Copenhagen experience. Diabetologia 29:13–16

Pedersen J, Pedersen LM (1965) Prognosis of the outcome of pregnancies in diabetics: a new classification. Acta Endocrinol 50:70–78

Powrie JK, Pearson DWM, Ross IS, Sutherland HW (1987) Maternal serum alpha fetoprotein in diabetic pregnant women. Lancet II:856–857

Skyler JS, O'Sullivan MJ (1986) Diabetes and pregnancy. In: Kohler PO, Jordon RM (eds) Clinical endocrinology. Wiley, Chichester, New York, p 603–622

Sutherland HW (1986) Methods of fetal monitoring and assessment of placental function in diabetic pregnancy. Acta Endocrinol 112 (Suppl 277): 90–100

Traub AI, Harley JMG, Cooper TK, Maguiness S, Hadden DR (1986) Is centralized hospital care necessary for all insulin-dependent pregnant diabetics? Br J Obstet Gynaecol 94:957–962

Wald NJ, Cuckle HS, Boreham J, Stirrat G, Turnbull A (1979) Maternal serum alpha feto-protein in diabetes mellitus. Br J Obstet Gynaecol 86:101–105

White P (1949) Pregnancy complicating diabetes. Am J Med 7:609–616

Zabut T, Reed KL, Shenker L (1985) Incidence of premature labor in diabetic patients. Am J Perinatol 2:276–278

28. Management of Diabetes Mellitus in Pregnancy: Survey of Maternal–Fetal Medicine Subspecialists in the United States

S. G. Gabbe and M. B. Landon

Introduction

The management of pregnancies complicated by both insulin-dependent and gestational diabetes mellitus has changed dramatically in the United States during the past 15 years. Recommended programmes of care have been outlined in a Technical Bulletin published by the American College of Obstetricians and Gynecologists in 1986, as well as in the summary of the Second International Workshop Conference on Gestational Diabetes Mellitus in 1984 (Freinkel et al. 1985), at which the American College of Obstetricians and Gynecologists was also represented. However, even these documents do not agree, particularly in their approach to screening for gestational diabetes mellitus. This study was undertaken, therefore, to determine the state of the art in the care of pregnancies complicated by both gestational and insulin-dependent diabetes mellitus in the United States.

Materials and Methods

In September 1987, a questionnaire was mailed to all 356 full members of the Society of Perinatal Obstetricians. This Society, founded in 1977, requires that following residency training, its members complete a 2-year fellowship programme in maternal–fetal medicine which has been approved by the American Board of Obstetrics and Gynecology. They must then receive Board certification by passing both a written and an oral examination and writing a research thesis. At the time of this study, 80% of all those who had achieved this certification were members of the Society of Perinatal Obstetricians.

The questionnaire contained four questions characterizing the subspecialists' training and practice, 12 questions on the screening and management of gestational diabetes mellitus, 13 questions concerning the care of patients with insulin-dependent diabetes mellitus and two general questions regarding estimation of fetal weight and route of delivery in cases complicated by suspected macrosomia.

Results

Of the 356 questionnaires mailed to the membership, 273 were returned, a response rate of 77%. These 273 subspecialists represent 65% of all those who had received Board certification in maternal–fetal medicine at the time of the study. Almost 70% of the respondents reported that their clinical practice was university hospital-based, while 21% worked in community hospitals and 7% in private practice settings. The mean age of the respondents was 41 years with 54.8% having completed their residency training after 1975. Responses were received from a total of 44 states.

Gestational Diabetes Mellitus

Of the respondents, 89.7% (245/273) screen every pregnant patient for gestational diabetes mellitus. Of the 28 physicians who do not recommend universal screening, 79% test all pregnant patients over the age of 30. Ninety-three per cent of the respondents (254/272) utilize the 50-g oral glucose load followed by a glucose determination 1 h later to screen for gestational diabetes mellitus, while less than 6% employ glycosylated haemoglobin levels as a screening method. Almost one-third of the respondents (85/273) report that they screen patients for gestational diabetes mellitus at the initial prenatal visit. Screening is undertaken most commonly, however, between 24 and 28 weeks with 85.7% (234/273) of the respondents testing their patients at this time. The 50-g glucose screen is repeated after 28 weeks by 20.9% (57/216) of the perinatologists.

Once the diagnosis of gestational diabetes has been established, the subspecialists surveyed utilize a variety of methods to assess glucose control. The majority of respondents, 42.3% (115/272), evaluate weekly fasting and postprandial glucose levels or employ daily self-glucose monitoring (38.6%, 105/272). Only 10.3% of the subspecialists (28/272) rely solely on weekly fasting glucose measurements to assess diabetic control on the dietary regimen.

Insulin therapy is not widely employed in the care of patients with gestational diabetes mellitus (Table 28.1). Almost 40% of the subspecialists (107/269) reported that fewer than 10% of their patients with gestational diabetes mellitus require insulin therapy. Overall, nearly 90% of the respondents reported that 30% or less of their patients with gestational diabetes mellitus receive insulin therapy. Only four maternal–fetal subspecialists, or 1.5% of the respondents (4/269), stated that all women with gestational diabetes mellitus were offered prophylactic insulin treatment.

Table 28.1. Insulin therapy in GDM

Per cent treated	No.	Per cent
<10%	107	39.8
20%	83	30.9
30%	42	15.6
40%	19	7.1
>50%	14	5.2
All offered	4	1.5

The threshold at which insulin therapy is initiated in patients with gestational diabetes mellitus varied widely (Table 28.2). Half of the maternal–fetal subspecialists (102/204) would begin treatment with insulin if the fasting glucose level had reached 105 mg/dl. Of note, 9% would not recommend insulin therapy until the fasting glucose level had reached 120 mg/dl or higher. When questioned about the postprandial glucose level at which insulin therapy would be started, 23.7% (57/241) of the respondents reported that they would begin insulin if the 2-h postprandial value reached 120 mg/dl (Table 28.3). Over two-thirds of the respondents (68.9%, 166/241) would initiate treatment with insulin if the 2-h postprandial value reached 140 mg/dl. Yet, 10.8% of the membership (26/241) would not use insulin until the 2-h postprandial value reached or exceeded 160 mg/dl.

Table 28.2. Glucose threshold for insulin therapy in GDM (fasting)

Glucose (mg/dl)	No.	Per cent
90	5	1.8
95	9	3.3
100	9	28.6
101	3	1.1
105	102	37.4
106	3	1.1
110	44	16.1
115	1	0.4
120	16	5.9
140	1	0.4
150	1	0.4
No response	10	3.7

Table 28.3. Glucose threshold for insulin therapy in GDM (2-h postprandial)

Glucose (mg/dl)	No.	Per cent
120	57	23.7
121–130	28	11.6
131–140	81	33.6
141–150	49	20.3
≥160	26	10.8

Only 10% (27/273) of the responding maternal–fetal subspecialists electively deliver patients with gestational diabetes mellitus but no other complications prior to term. In such cases, approximately 50% (138/273) reported they would obtain pulmonary maturity studies prior to these elective deliveries. Of note, two-thirds of the subspecialists (180/273) would employ antepartum fetal testing routinely in patients with gestational diabetes mellitus prior to term.

Insulin-Dependent Diabetes Mellitus

The majority of the respondents (51.6%, 141/273) reported that each year they cared for at least 20 pregnancies complicated by insulin-dependent diabetes mellitus. However, a comparable figure (54.2%, 148/273) noted that they cared for no more than five patients annually whose diabetes was complicated by retinopathy and/or nephropathy. Only 17.8% (48/269) of the respondents stated that they consulted with an internist or diabetologist in the care of pregnancies complicated by insulin-dependent diabetes mellitus.

The results of the questionnaire indicate that few insulin-dependent diabetic women in the United States obtain preconceptional care. Almost 80% of the respondents noted that 20% or fewer of their patients seek preconceptional care and counselling (Table 28.4). Almost 90% of the respondents (88.1%, 238/270) reported that they routinely obtain a measurement of glycosylated haemoglobin in the first trimester to assist in counselling patients about the risk of fetal malformations. Of those who do obtain a glycosylated haemoglobin, 19.9% (47/236) stated that patients in their practice have elected to have a termination of pregnancy based on the results of the glycosylated haemoglobin level.

Table 28.4.   Women seeking preconceptional care

	No.	Per cent	Cumulative per cent
<10%	56	20.5	20.5
10%	104	38.1	58.6
20%	58	21.2	79.8
30%	24	8.8	88.6
40%	12	4.4	93.0
50%	5	1.8	94.8
Other	14	5.2	100.0

Self-glucose monitoring is a practice widely employed by maternal–fetal subspecialists in their care of the pregnancy complicated by insulin-dependent diabetes. Over 75% of the respondents (75.5%, 204/270) reported that all of their patients use self-glucose monitoring. However, only 37% (100/267) of the subspecialists noted that their patients uniformly utilize a reflectance meter as opposed to visual interpretation of the test strips. Almost 30% of the respondents (29.2%, 78/267) noted that no more than 50% of their patients rely on reflectance meters for self-glucose monitoring.

All of the subspecialists reported that they routinely perform antepartum fetal testing in patients with insulin-dependent diabetes mellitus. The preferred form of fetal assessment was the non-stress test which is utilized by 56.1% (137/244) of the subspecialists. The fetal biophysical profile was favoured by 27.9% (68/244) and the contraction stress test by 16.0% (39/244). Over three-quarters of the respondents reported that they usually initiate antepartum fetal testing by 32 weeks gestation (79.5%, 209/263), while another 18.6% (49/263) indicated that they waited until 34 weeks (Table 28.5). Only 2% (5/263) delayed the start of antepartum fetal testing until 36 weeks.

Table 28.5. Initiation of fetal testing, gestational age

Weeks	No.	Per cent	Cumulative per cent
<28	2	0.8	0.8
28	39	14.8	15.6
30	55	20.9	36.5
32	113	43.0	79.5
34	49	18.6	98.1
36	5	1.9	100.0

Elective delivery of the patient whose pregnancy is complicated by insulin-dependent diabetes remains a widespread practice. Half of the respondents (50%, 134/268) noted that 90% or more of their patients were delivered electively. This total includes 22% (59/268) who deliver all of their patients electively. Only 28.3% of the subspecialists (76/268) stated that 50% or fewer of their patients are delivered electively. Amniotic fluid tests for fetal pulmonary maturity are routinely performed by 84% (226/269) of subspecialists prior to undertaking the elective delivery of a woman with insulin-dependent diabetes mellitus.

Caesarean section is still a common route of delivery for patients with insulin-dependent diabetes mellitus. Over 70% of the respondents (70.9%, 190/268) reported that 50% or more of their patients are delivered by Caesarean section.

Estimation of Fetal Weight

Over 75% of the perinatologists (77.4%, 206/266) routinely perform an ultrasound at term to estimate fetal weight when a pregnancy is complicated by either gestational diabetes or insulin-dependent diabetes mellitus. Approximately one-third of the subspecialists (32.3%, 86/266) indicated they would perform an elective Caesarean section at a fetal weight of 4000 g. This figure increases to over 85% (227/266) if the fetal weight is estimated to be 4500 g. Only 13.6% (36/266) stated that there was no weight at which they would recommend a delivery by Caesarean section.

Discussion

The results of the present survey report for the first time the approach of maternal–fetal subspecialists in the United States in caring for patients whose pregnancy is complicated by diabetes mellitus. The 273 subspecialists who returned questionnaires, a 77% response rate, represent over two-thirds of all physicians with Board certification in maternal–fetal medicine at the time of this study. Therefore, the conclusions drawn from this database are likely to represent the true state of the art in the United States.

In 1985, Gabbe, addressing the Diabetic Pregnancy Study Group of the European Association for the Study of Diabetes, presented an overview of the American approach to the care of diabetes in pregnancy (Gabbe 1985). He proposed that the following trends characterized the management of patients in the United States whose pregnancies were complicated by diabetes mellitus:

1. Greater awareness of the association between maternal glycaemic control during embryogenesis and congenital malformations. Yet, few programmes for preconceptional treatment exist.
2. Increased application of uniform screening for gestational diabetes.
3. More intensive efforts to normalize maternal metabolism through home glucose monitoring and multiple insulin injections.
4. Increasing concern with both the perinatal impact of nephropathy and maternal outcome with retinopathy and coronary artery disease.
5. Wider application of outpatient care utilizing the non-stress test.
6. A significant reduction in the number of Caesarean sections for elective preterm delivery, and therefore less dependence on the L/S ratio and lung profile.
7. Increased concern with both immediate and long-term neonatal morbidity in infants of diabetic mothers.

The results of the present survey generally support the overview provided by Gabbe. Universal screening for gestational diabetes is recommended by almost 90% of maternal–fetal subspecialists. These results are in sharp contrast to a survey undertaken by Furman in Los Angeles (Furman and Steinberg 1987). In that study, Furman assessed the methods used for the detection of gestational diabetes mellitus by 180 respondents, 86% of whom were obstetricians. Furman found that only 41% screened all pregnant patients for diabetes. While 93% of the maternal–fetal subspecialists questioned in the present study utilized a 50-g glucose load followed by a glucose measurement 1 h later as a screening test, only 23% of the physicians surveyed by Furman followed this technique. In contrast, 24% employed a fasting blood glucose, 21% a 2-h postprandial glucose value, 13% the presence of glycosuria and 8% a random blood glucose as a screen for gestational diabetes. It should be pointed out that the most recent Technical Bulletin of the American College of Obstetricians and Gynecologists does not support universal screening. Rather, screening is recommended for women who are 30 years of age or older or who have historical or clinical clues suggesting the presence of gestational diabetes mellitus. The Technical Bulletin does advise the use of a 50-g oral glucose load and glucose determination 1 h later.

In our survey, over 85% of the subspecialists reported screening their patients for gestational diabetes mellitus between 24 and 28 weeks. In contrast, in Furman's report, only 33% of the physicians tested between 24 and 28 weeks. Overall, a comparison of our data with those reported by Furman suggests that there may be wide discrepancies between the practices employed by obstetrician–gynecologists in general practice and those who are maternal–fetal medicine subspecialists.

This study confirmed that relatively few American women with insulin-dependent diabetes mellitus are seeking preconceptional care. Only 2% of the respondents report that 50% of their patients are seen prior to pregnancy. Maternal–fetal medicine subspecialists are using a measurement of glycosylated haemoglobin in the first trimester to assess the patient's risk for a major fetal malformation. In several studies, a 20%–25% major malformation rate has been observed when the glycosylated haemoglobin level is significantly elevated (Ylinen et al. 1984; Hanson et al. 1985). These data can undoubtedly influence a patient's decision to elect termination of pregnancy when poor periconceptional control is documented by the glycosylated haemoglobin level. Almost one-fifth of the subspecialists reported that this had occurred in their practice.

More intensive efforts are being made to normalize maternal metabolism as assessed through self-glucose monitoring. Maternal–fetal medicine subspecialists are relying on their own expertise to control maternal diabetes mellitus with fewer than 20% asking for the assistance of an internist or diabetologist. Self-glucose monitoring not only plays an important role in the treatment of the patient with insulin-dependent diabetes mellitus, but was utilized by almost 40% of respondents in their surveillance of the patient with gestational diabetes mellitus. The number of patients with gestational diabetes mellitus being offered insulin therapy is relatively small, 71% of the respondents reporting that fewer than 20% of their patients receive insulin therapy. However, the thresholds at which insulin therapy should be initiated varied considerably. The fasting glucose level at which insulin therapy would be started ranged from a low of 90 mg/dl to as high as 150 mg/dl. Similarly, the 2-h postprandial level at which insulin therapy would be initiated ranged from a low of 120 mg/dl to as high as 200 mg/dl. The Second International Workshop Conference recommended that insulin therapy be started when the fasting plasma glucose level exceeded 105 mg/dl and the 2-h postprandial plasma glucose value exceeded 120 mg/dl.

While antepartum fetal testing is utilized to a limited extent in patients with gestational diabetes mellitus, it is being applied uniformly in pregnancies complicated by insulin-dependent diabetes mellitus. Despite such intensive antepartum fetal surveillance, intervention for suspected fetal distress now occurs in only 4% of these cases (Gabbe 1987). Most of the respondents utilize the non-stress test or the fetal biophysical profile.

In contrast to the trends suggested by Gabbe, elective delivery remains an important part of the management protocol for pregnancies complicated by insulin-dependent diabetes mellitus. Almost half of the respondents reported 90% or more of their patients with insulin-dependent diabetes are delivered electively and over 80% employ tests of fetal pulmonary maturity before such elective terminations of pregnancy. In contrast, only 10% of patients with gestational diabetes mellitus are delivered electively.

The overall Caesarean section rate for pregnancies complicated by insulin-dependent diabetes mellitus would appear to approach 50% or more in the majority of maternal–fetal medicine practices. Cousins reported a primary Caesarean section rate of 27.1% and a repeat Caesarean section rate of 14.3% in over 5000 pregnancies complicated by diabetes and reported between 1965 and 1985 (Cousins 1987). Olofsson calculated an average Caesarean section rate of 47.5% in his literature survey (Olofsson et al. 1984). He reported that at the University of Lund, Sweden, elective Caesarean sections were done in 20.9% of cases and that an amniocentesis to assess fetal lung maturity was performed before 70% of deliveries. Over three-quarters of the subspecialists utilize ultrasound to assess fetal weight and most would recommend an elective Caesarean section if the estimated fetal weight was 4000–4500 g. Acker has recently reported that 23% of infants of diabetic mothers weighing 4000–4499 g delivered vaginally suffer shoulder dystocia, a rate more than twice that of comparably sized neonates whose mothers did not have diabetes mellitus (Acker et al. 1985).

Conclusions

At the present time, the approach to the detection and management of patients with gestational diabetes mellitus utilized by maternal–fetal medicine subspecialists in the United States includes universal screening with a 50-g oral glucose load, followed by surveillance of maternal glucose levels with a variety of techniques once the diagnosis of gestational diabetes mellitus has been made. The criteria used to determine when insulin therapy is begun in these patients vary widely. Although antepartum fetal surveillance is commonly employed in pregnancies complicated by gestational diabetes mellitus, only 10% of these patients are delivered electively.

In managing pregnancies complicated by insulin-dependent diabetes mellitus, maternal–fetal medicine subspecialists consult with an internist or diabetologist infrequently. Few patients now seek preconceptional counselling, an area that must be addressed if pregnancy outcome in these high-risk women is to be improved. While self-glucose monitoring is widely employed in pregnant patients with insulin-dependent diabetes mellitus, reflectance meters are not being used uniformly. Despite the low incidence of intervention for suspected fetal distress reported in the literature, all subspecialists continue to utilize antepartum fetal surveillance in this patient population. Furthermore, most women with insulin-dependent diabetes mellitus will be delivered electively after the assessment of fetal pulmonary maturity by amniotic fluid analysis. Caesarean section is the route of delivery recommended by at least 50% of the perinatologists. Finally, most subspecialists routinely utilize ultrasound to assess fetal weight, preferring delivery by Caesarean section if the fetal weight is estimated to be 4500 g or more.

References

Acker DB, Sachs BP, Friedman EA (1985) Risk factors for shoulder dystocia. Obstet Gynecol 66:762–768
American College of Obstetricians and Gynecologists Technical Bulletin (1986) Management of diabetes in pregnancy. 92:1–5

Cousins L (1987) Pregnancy complications among diabetic women: review 1965–1985. Obstet Gynecol Surv 42:140–149

Freinkel N, Gabbe SG, Hadden DR et al. (1985) Summary and recommendations of the second international workshop – conference on gestational diabetes mellitus. Diabetes 34:123–126

Furman GI, Steinberg MC (1987) Diabetes screening during pregnancy. Diabetes 36:90

Gabbe SG (1985) The American approach to diabetes in pregnancy. In: Diabetic Pregnancy Study Group – XVI Annual meeting. The University of Malta, pp 4–5

Gabbe SG (1987) Antepartum fetal surveillance in the pregnancy complicated by diabetes mellitus. In: Infant of the diabetic mother. Ross Laboratories, Columbus, Ohio, pp 86–95

Hanson U, Persson B, Tunell S (1985) The relation between HbA$_{1c}$ in early diabetic pregnancy and occurrence of spontaneous abortion and congenital malformation in Sweden. In: Hanson U (ed) Diabetes and pregnancy – impact of blood glucose control and obstetrical management on fetal and neonatal outcome. SG Snabbtryck, Stockholm, pp I:1–I:13

Olofsson P, Liedholm H, Sartor G et al. (1984) Diabetes and pregnancy – a 21 year Swedish material. Acta Obstet Gynecol Scand [Suppl] 122

Ylinen K, Aula P, Stenman U-H et al. (1984) Risk of minor and major fetal malformations in diabetics with high haemoglobin A$_{1c}$ values in early pregnancy. Br Med J 289:345–346

29. Oral Contraceptives in Diabetic Women

S. O. Skouby

Introduction

In women predisposed to diabetes mellitus and in insulin-dependent diabetic women abnormalities of glucose metabolism following intake of oral contraceptives (OCs) obviously attract special attention. Previously there has been a negative attitude towards the use of OCs in these women due to the enhanced risk of unfavourable clinical events. As a consequence of the rapidly accumulating amount of scientific data available on the undesirable metabolic effects of contraceptive steroids it has become evident that the pharmacokinetic properties of the hormonal constituents and the amount, and type, of steroid are of fundamental significance for the observed effects. This chapter summarizes the influence on glucose metabolism of combined OCs with differences in the steroid content when administered to women with previous gestational diabetes mellitus (GDM) and to women with insulin-dependent diabetes mellitus (IDDM).

The Pharmacological Profile of Sex Steroids in Oral Contraceptives

In contraceptive compounds the oestrogens marketed today are either ethinyloestradiol or mestranol. Unconjugated ethinyloestradiol is the active substance in both compounds. Ethinyloestradiol undergoes enterohepatic recirculation and reabsorption. Approximately 30% of a given dose can be recovered in the faeces and the faecal/urine ratio is about 2:3. The half-life in plasma varies from 6 to 20 h (Orme et al. 1983).

Genuine or non-alkylated oestrogens, oestrone, 17-β-oestradiol and oestriol are not used in commercially available contraceptive compounds, whereas they have been used extensively for substitution therapy in climacteric women. Compared with artificial oestrogens higher doses of oestradiol must be used in oral compounds due to higher rates of metabolism in the gut wall and to first-pass effects in the liver. The use of microcrystalline forms, however, improves the absorption.

Most of the progestational components used in the combined contraceptive pills are 17-α-ethinyl derivatives of the reduced form of testosterone (19-nortestosterone). The 19-nortestosterone derivatives are classified in oestranes and gonanes. All progestogens of the oestrane type are converted to norethisterone after oral intake (Orme et al. 1983). The gonanes differ from other 19-nortestosterone products in having a beta-ethyl group at carbon 13 instead of the one-carbon chain unit present in the products, and thus, the pharmacokinetic properties are markedly different. The most widely used gonane is norgestrel or the active D-isomer, levonorgestrel. The bioavailability of oestranes is approximately 60% (Okerholm et al. 1978) whereas no first-pass effect seems to occur with the gonanes. The half-life of oestranes varies from 5 to 14 h compared with 10 to 24 h for the gonanes (Orme et al. 1983).

Oral Contraceptives and Glucose Metabolism in Women with Previous Gestational Diabetes Mellitus

It is well established that intake of OCs may decrease glucose tolerance and cause a rise in insulin levels in healthy non-diabetic women. Such changes have become evident in both intravenous and oral glucose tolerance tests (Kalkhoff 1975). The relative effects of oestrogens and progestogens on glucose metabolism have been debated from the very beginning of the OC period but today the consensus is that the progestogens are mainly responsible for the diabetogenic effect of the combined compounds (Spellacy et al. 1972) although the artificial oestrogens may modulate this effect. A possible decreased insulin sensitivity at cellular level in peripheral tissues has been suggested as the mechanism behind the altered glucose metabolism (De Pirro et al. 1978; Skouby et al. 1987).

Despite these adverse effects on glucose tolerance no risk of developing clinical diabetes has been found in epidemiological studies (Wingrave et al. 1979). However, in women with previous GDM an overall incidence of 44% of deterioration of glucose tolerance has been registered during intake of the traditional brands of OCs (Beck and Wells 1969; Szabo et al. 1970). Only a limited number of studies has been published on the effect of previously used low-dose OCs on glucose metabolism in pregnancy in women with previous GDM. We have previously reported the effects of a monophasic low-dose ethinyloestradiol/levonorgestrel preparation (Skouby et al. 1982). Before treatment the women with previous GDM displayed significantly elevated glucose values compared to non-diabetic controls. After hormonal intake for 6 months the insulin response to oral glucose increased significantly, but no deterioration of

Table 29.1. Insulin areas (min × nmol/l) (mean ± SEM) calculated from glucose tolerance tests performed in women with previous gestational diabetes ($n=10$) and in normal women ($n=10$) during intake of triphasic and monophasic low-dose oral contraceptives (ethinyloestradiol and levonorgestrel)

Months	Normal		Previous GDM	
	Monophasic	Triphasic	Monophasic	Triphasic
0	53 ± 5	63 ± 17	49 ± 9	53 ± 5
2	55 ± 8	58 ± 6	53 ± 6	62 ± 5
6	65 ± 6*	60 ± 9	69 ± 11*	63 ± 5

* 0 vs 6 months; $P<0.05$

glucose tolerance was observed. The glucagon response was similar in the women with previous GDM and in the controls. These findings are in accordance with the observations made in a small number of women with borderline abnormal glucose tolerance before intake of a monophasic low-dose ethinyloestradiol/ norethisterone preparation (Spellacy et al. 1979).

One of the strategies used for further reduction of the metabolic side-effects of OCs has been new administration regimens. The triphasic approach is a response to this view using the lowest possible dose of both hormones without a concomitant unacceptable uterine bleeding pattern (Upton 1983). When compared to the most widely used low-dose monophasic ethinyloestradiol/levonorgestrel combination the ethinyloestradiol ratio is 1.08 during one 3-week treatment period with the triphasic preparation whereas the levonorgestrel ratio is only 0.61. We have therefore examined the influence of such a triphasic compound on glucose tolerance in normal women and in women with previous GDM during a 6-month treatment period (Skouby et al. 1985a). In both the women with previous GDM and the normal women the triphasic preparation resulted in significantly lower insulin responses to oral glucose than the low-dose monophasic oestradiol/levonorgestrel preparation (Table 29.1).

Glycaemic Control and Clinical Effects of Oral Contraceptives in Women with Insulin-Dependent Diabetes Mellitus

In women with IDDM both the fertility rate and the length of the fertile period have risen significantly during the last decades due to improved metabolic control. However, a diabetic pregnancy still carries potential hazards to both the mother and the child and recent evidence suggests that optimal diabetes regulation around the time of conception plays an important role in normal fetal development. Consequently, the contraceptive method used before the first pregnancy and between each of the subsequent pregnancies should be as reliable as possible but also without any deleterious effects on the metabolic control.

Although a wide variety of metabolic changes, including the effects on glucose metabolism, has been demonstrated in users of different types of OCs much less is known about the effects on existing metabolic diseases, in particular diabetes mellitus. Osler and Wiese (1974) found increased difficulties in diabetes control during treatment with traditional combined compounds. Steel and Duncan (1980) found increased insulin requirements in 19% of diabetic women. Insulin requirements were not different using compounds containing 50 µg ethinyloestradiol versus low-dose compounds containing only 30 µg ethinyloestradiol and a reduced amount of progestogen. These authors also reported a high incidence of severe clinical side-effects during intake of the combined compounds (Steel and Duncan 1978). Rådberg et al. (1981) investigated the effects of 50 µg ethinyloestradiol plus 250 µg lynestrenol in women with IDDM. The insulin requirement increased by 7% without any change in body weight or blood glucose levels. The clinical events were comparable to those observed in non-diabetic women.

When combined compounds containing natural or genuine oestrogens are administered as hormonal replacement therapy to climacteric women less influence on glucose and lipid metabolism is seen compared with compounds containing artificial oestrogens (Larsson-Cohn and Wallentin 1977). We were therefore prompted to examine the clinical and biochemical effects on diabetes control of a monophasic oral contraceptive compound containing natural oestrogen (4 mg oestradiol plus 2 mg oestriol and 3 mg norethisterone) (Skouby et al. 1985b). Such a preparation has been reported previously to give efficient suppression of ovulation and fewer metabolic side-effects compared with a compound combining artificial oestrogen with identical progestational content (Lebech 1977; Samsioe et al. 1983). We observed no accidental pregnancies during the 12-month study period and the overall continuation rate of 60 compares well with the continuation rate normally found in non-diabetic women after administration of conventional type OCs. No difficulties were found with diabetes control and there were no significant changes in insulin requirement, 24-h urinary glucose excretion or concentration of glycated haemoglobin (HbA_{1c}). However, from a pharmacological point of view OCs with the least hormonal content appear the most attractive. In women with IDDM we have therefore compared the influence of the non-alkylated oestrogen/progestogen compound with the influence of (a) a low-dose monophasic ethinyloestradiol/norethisterone combination, (b) progestogen-only treatment with norethisterone and (c) a triphasic ethinyloestradiol/levonorgestrel combination.

Measurements were made on blood pressure, body weight, fasting plasma glucose, 24-h insulin requirements, HbA_{1c}, total plasma cortisol and plasma FFA levels before and during hormonal intake for 2 and 6 months (Skouby et al. 1986). The patients in each treatment group were matched with regard to age, weight, duration of diabetes and socioeconomic status. No significant changes in body weight or blood pressure were recorded between or within the groups during treatment and none of the participants experienced noticeable difficulties with their diabetes control. Fasting plasma glucose, 24-h insulin requirements (Fig. 29.1), HbA_{1c} levels (Fig. 29.2) and FFA concentrations (Fig. 29.3) were similar in all groups before and during treatment and no significant changes were observed within the groups during treatment. From this study it therefore appears that, in this group of patients, the glycaemic control was equally good during administration of the low-dose synthetic OCs as compared to the non-alkylated oestrogen/progestogen compound.

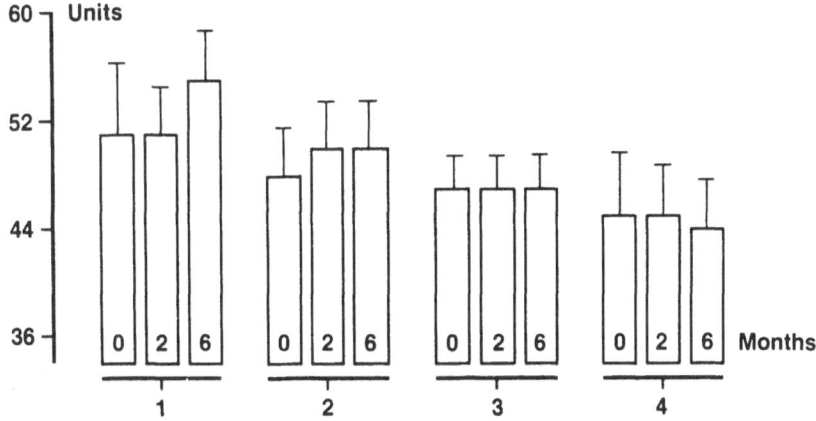

Insulin requirement/24-h Mean ± SEM

1.   4 mg 17-β E_2 + 2 mg E_3 + 3 mg NE   4. Triphasic EE + LNG.
2.   35 µg EE + 500 µg NE   (days 1-6 : 30 µg EE + 50 µg LNG,
3. 300 µg NE   days 7-12: 40 µg EE + 75 µg LNG,
                                                 days 13-21: 30 µg EE + 125 µg LNG)

Fig. 29.1.   24-h insulin requirements in insulin-dependent diabetic women during intake of four different OCs.

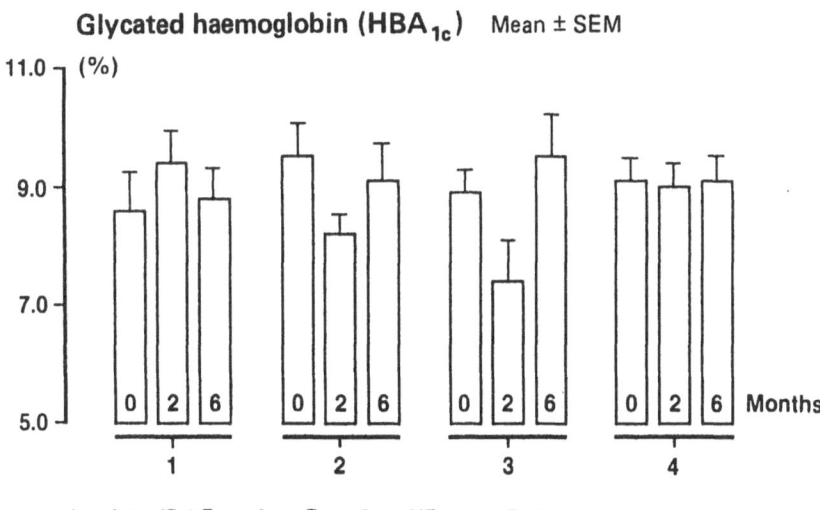

Glycated haemoglobin (HBA_{1c}) Mean ± SEM

1.   4 mg 17-β E_2 + 2 mg E_3 + 3 mg NE   4. Triphasic EE + LNG.
2.   35 µg EE + 500 µg NE   (days 1-6 : 30 µg EE + 50 µg LNG,
3. 300 µg NE   days 7-12: 40 µg EE + 75 µg LNG,
                                                 days 13-21: 30 µg EE + 125 µg LNG)

Fig. 29.2.   Fasting HbA_{1c} in insulin-dependent diabetic women during intake of four different OCs.

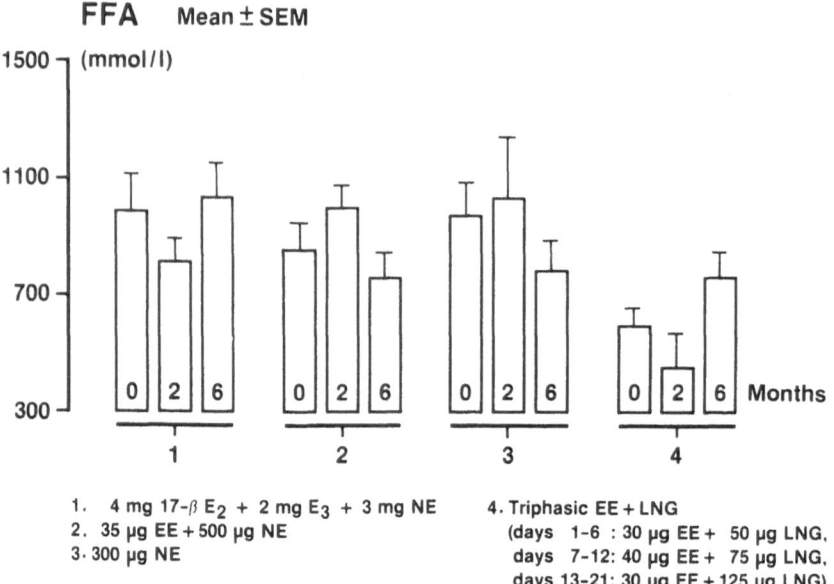

Fig. 29.3. Fasting FFA in insulin-dependent diabetic women during intake of four different OCs.

Conclusion

Low-dose oral contraceptive compounds may be administered to women of normal weight with previous GDM without running a risk of causing a deterioration of glucose tolerance, but the oestrogen/progestogen ratio significantly decreases the insulin response to oral glucose in both normal women and in women with previous GDM. Genuine oestrogens may be administered in combination with a progestogen as an efficient and acceptable mode of contraception in women with IDDM without any concomitant adverse effects on diabetic control. However, it also appears that administration of low-dose preparations of either triphasic ethinyloestradiol/levonorgestrel or monophasic ethinyloestradiol/norethisterone and progestogen only preparations with norethisterone is without any influence on glycaemic control in women with IDDM. These results appear promising for the more widespread use of low-dose oral contraceptive agents in preconception counselling and as an effective method for spacing pregnancies in women with IDDM and previous GDM.

References

Beck P, Wells SA (1969) Comparison of the mechanisms underlying carbohydrate intolerance in subclinical diabetic women during pregnancy and during post-partum oral contraceptive steroid treatment. J Clin Endocrinol Metab 29:807–810

De Pirro R, Fusco A, Bertoli A, Greco AV, Lauro R (1978) Insulin receptors during the menstrual cycle in normal women. J Clin Endocrinol Metab 47:1387–1389

Kalkhoff RK (1975) Effects of oral contraceptive agents on carbohydrate metabolism. J Steroid Biochem 6:949–952

Larsson-Cohn U, Wallentin L (1977) Metabolic and hormonal effect of post menopausal estrogen replacement treatment. Acta Endocrinol 86:583–596

Lebech PE (1977) Oral contraception with natural human oestrogen – differences between natural and artificial oestrogens. In: Haspels A (ed) Hormonal contraception. Excerpta Medica, Amsterdam, pp 33–38

Okerholm RA, Peterson FE, Keeley FJ, Smith TC, Glazko AJ (1978) Bioavailability of norethindrone in human subjects. Eur J Clin Pharmacol 13:35–39

Orme ML'E, Back DJ, Breckenridge AM (1983) Clinical pharmacokinetics of oral contraceptive steroids. Clin Pharmacokinet 8:95–136

Osler M, Wiese J (1974) Contraception in diabetic women. Acta Endocrinol [Suppl] (Copenh) 182:87–94

Rådberg T, Gustafson A, Skryten A, Karlsson, K (1981) Oral contraception in diabetic women. Diabetes control and high density lipoprotein lipids during low dosage progestogen, combined estrogen/progestogen and non-hormonal contraception. Acta Endocrinol (Copenh) 86:583–596

Samsioe G, Skryten A, Silverstolpe G (1983) Oral contraception with a nonalkylated estrogen component. Effect on lipid metabolism. Gynecol Obstet Invest 15:275–282

Skouby SO, Mølsted-Pedersen L, Kuhl C (1982) Low dosage oral contraception in women with previous gestational diabetes. Obstet Gynecol 59:325–328

Skouby SO, Kuhl C, Mølsted-Pedersen L, Petersen K, Christensen MS (1985a) Triphasic oral contraceptives: metabolic effects in normal women and those with previous gestational diabetes. Am J Obstet Gynecol 153:495–500

Skouby SO, Møller Jensen B, Kuhl C, Mølsted-Pedersen L, Svenstrup B (1985b) Hormonal contraception in diabetic women: acceptability, diabetes regulation and influence on ovarian function of a nonalkylated estrogen/progestogen compound. Contraception 32:23–31

Skouby SO, Mølsted-Pedersen L, Kuhl C, Bennett P (1986) Oral contraceptives in diabetic women: metabolic effects of four compounds with different estrogen/progestogen profiles. Fertil Steril 46:858–864

Skouby SO, Andersen O, Saurbrey N, Kuhl C (1987) Oral contraception and insulin sensitivity: in vivo assessment in normal women and in subjects with previous gestational diabetes. J Clin Endocrinol Metab 64:519–526

Spellacy WN, Buhi WC, Birk SA (1972) The effect of estrogens on carbohydrate metabolism: glucose, insulin and growth hormone studies on one hundred and seventy one women ingesting premarin, mestranol and ethinyl estradiol for six months. Am J Obstet Gynecol 114:378–384

Spellacy WN, Buhi WC, Birk SA (1979) Carbohydrate metabolism prospectively studied in women using a low-estrogen oral contraceptive for six months. Contraception 20:137–148

Steel JM, Duncan LJP (1978) Serious complications of oral contraception in insulin-dependent diabetics. Contraception 17:291–295

Steel JM, Duncan LJP (1980) Contraception for the insulin dependent diabetic woman: the view from one clinic. Diabetes Care 3:557–560

Szabo AJ, Cole HS, Grimaldi RD (1970) Glucose tolerance in gestational diabetic women during and after treatment with a combination-type oral contraceptive. New Engl J Med 282:646–650

Upton GV (1983) The phasic approach to oral contraception: the triphasic concept and its clinical application. Int J Fertil 28:121–140

Wingrave SJ, Kay CR, Vessy MP (1979) Oral contraceptives and diabetes mellitus. Br Med J I:23

30. The Infant of the Diabetic Mother: Recent Experience

P. Duffty and D. J. Lloyd

Introduction

At the time of the First International Colloquium on Carbohydrate Metabolism in Pregnancy and the Newborn held in Aberdeen in 1973, a Paediatric textbook (Mitchell 1974) quoted a perinatal mortality of 20% in infants of diabetic mothers.

Since then the management of the diabetic pregnant woman has been considerably improved by careful attention to her diabetic control throughout pregnancy and labour. Ultrasound scanning and electronic monitoring have allowed continuing assessment of fetal wellbeing and an accurate estimate of the gestational age so preventing iatrogenic prematurity and its associated complications.

In view of these developments the purpose of this chapter is to look at our recent experience with the infants of insulin-dependent diabetic mothers.

Patients

Forty-six infants of insulin-dependent diabetic mothers, all of whom had been on insulin prior to their pregnancy, were delivered in Aberdeen Maternity Hospital during the 2-year period January 1986 to December 1987. There were 26 male and 20 female infants with an average gestational age of 38.1 ± 1.8 weeks (± 1 SD). There were seven preterm infants: one of 31 weeks, four of 35 weeks and two of 36 weeks gestation. The mean birthweight was 3.43 ± 0.64 kg (± 1 SD) with a range of 1.79 to 4.75 kg.

Management

All the infants were admitted routinely to the neonatal unit.

Capillary blood glucose concentrations (BM-Test-Glycemie 20–800) were determined ½-hourly until either 3 h of age or the first feed. Provided there were no significant problems the first feed was given as early as possible followed by 3-hourly feeds of breast milk or proprietary formula for the first 36–48 h starting at a volume of 50 ml/kg per d and increasing by 25 ml/kg per d up to 150 ml/kg per d on the fourth day. The capillary blood glucose was checked before each feed for the first 15 h or until stable. A true plasma glucose concentration was obtained if the BM-stix reading was <2.2 mmol/l.

The haematocrit was determined at about 3 h of age on a free-flowing capillary sample and if >70% rechecked on a free-flowing venous sample. Serum calcium was measured daily for 2 d. Serum bilirubin and other investigations were done as clinically indicated.

Infants who had respiratory or other significant neonatal problems received an intravenous infusion of 10% dextrose and were managed by standard techniques. Neonatal jaundice was treated by phototherapy if the serum bilirubin was >275 μ mol/l.

The infants were discharged to the postnatal ward as soon as possible after they had established oral feeding and had a stable blood glucose.

Management of Hypoglycaemia

Hypoglycaemia was defined as a plasma glucose of <2.0 mmol/l during the first 48 h of life.

Early asymptomatic hypoglycaemia before the first feed was treated by feeding the infant and repeating the BM-stix 1.5 h later. If asymptomatic hypoglycaemia occurred after the first feed then the infant was changed to high-calorie formula feeds (SMA Low Birth Weight) with the volume of the feeds being increased by an extra 25 ml/kg per d. The frequency of the feeds was subsequently increased to 2-hourly if necessary. If this was unsuccessful then oral feeds were discontinued and replaced by an equivalent volume of 10% dextrose given as a continuous intravenous infusion after an initial bolus of 2 ml/kg. If the BM-stix 0.5 h later was still <2.0 mmol/l then the concentration of intravenous dextrose was increased to 12.5% (equivalent to 6.5 mg/kg per min of dextrose at 75 ml/kg per d).

Symptomatic hypoglycaemia at any age was treated similarly with an intravenous bolus of 2 ml/kg of 10% dextrose followed by a continuous infusion which was increased to 12.5% dextrose if necessary.

A continuous intravenous infusion of glucagon at 0.5 mg/d was started and increased as necessary in any infant who remained hypoglycaemic despite an intravenous infusion of 12.5% dextrose. If this was unsuccessful then hydrocortisone 10 mg/kg per d in four divided doses could be used either intravenously or intramuscularly.

Once the plasma glucose had become stable then milk feeds were gradually increased whilst the intravenous infusion of dextrose was decreased approximately. If a glucagon infusion had been necessary then this was slowly withdrawn over 24–36 h to prevent rebound hypoglycaemia.

Results

The method of delivery of the 46 infants is shown in Table 30.1. Only 15 (33%) were spontaneous vaginal deliveries with 21 (46%) being delivered by Caesarean section, 11 electively and 10 as emergencies.

Twelve infants (26%) were heavy for dates (Table 30.2), of whom all but one were above the 95th centile for their gestational age (Thomson et al. 1968).

Table 30.1. Mode of delivery

Method	No.	%
Spontaneous vaginal delivery	15	33
Forceps delivery	10	22
Caesarean section	21	46

Table 30.2. Birthweight centiles

Centile		No.	%
Heavy for dates	>90th	12	26
	>95th	11	24
Light for dates	<10th	4	9
	< 5th	3	7

Thirteen (28%) of the 46 infants had no neonatal problems whatsoever with a further 14 (30%) having only mild problems which would not normally have needed admission. Thirty-one (67%) of the infants were discharged to the postnatal wards within 48 h of birth. However, five infants (11%) required intensive care.

Hypoglycaemia was the most common neonatal problem affecting 18 (39%) of the 46 infants (Table 30.3) although none of them was symptomatic. In six of these 18 infants the hypoglycaemia occurred early and resolved with early feeding (Table 30.4). The other 12 hypoglycaemic infants were treated with an intravenous infusion of 10% dextrose although this had initially been started in six of these infants for reasons other than hypoglycaemia; respiratory problems in four, vomiting in one and mild asphyxia in one. In six infants an increase in the dextrose concentration to 12.5% was required whilst two of these infants also needed an intravenous infusion of glucagon to control their hypoglycaemia adequately (Table 30.4).

Hypocalcaemia (serum total calcium ≤1.75 mmol/l) occurred in four infants (Table 30.3), all of whom had other significant neonatal problems.

Table 30.3. Neonatal morbidity

Problem		No.
Hypoglycaemia	<2.0 mmol/l	18
	<1.5 mmol/l	9
	Symptomatic	0
Perinatal asphyxia – severe		3
– mild		9
Respiratory distress syndrome		2
Transient respiratory problems		8
Cardiomegaly – marked		2
Jaundice – phototherapy		4 (+1)[a]
Hypocalcaemia		4
Severe congenital anomalies		2
Died		1

[a] Prophylactic phototherapy was given to the 31-week gestation infant.

Table 30.4. Management of hypoglycaemia ($n=18$)

Management	No.
Early feeding	6
Intravenous 10% dextrose	12
Intravenous 12.5% dextrose	6
Intravenous glucagon infusion	2
Steroids	0

Phototherapy was used in four infants whose serum bilirubin rose to >270 μmol/l; one of these infants had an *E. coli* urinary tract infection. In addition prophylactic phototherapy was used for the 31-week gestation infant in view of her prematurity with her maximum serum bilirubin being 195 μmol/l.

Significant perinatal asphyxia was present in three infants with a further nine infants requiring bag and mask resuscitation at delivery.

Ten infants had neonatal respiratory problems (Table 30.3). In eight these problems were mild and transient but two infants developed respiratory distress syndrome and both infants required mechanical ventilation. One of these infants was the 31-week gestation 1.79 kg infant who also had several other problems related to her prematurity including a patent ductus arteriosus, recurrent apnoea and a possible *Klebsiella* pneumonia. However the other infant was a 37-week gestation 3.12 kg infant delivered by elective Casearean section for breech presentation and deteriorating maternal vision with Apgar scores of 9:9. This infant developed severe respiratory difficulties and required paralysis with pancuronium as well as mechanical ventilation in up to 100% oxygen.

Two further infants who presented with tachypnoea following mild perinatal asphyxia were shown to have marked cardiomegaly on chest X-ray. Echocardiograms showed both babies to have enlarged poorly functioning ventricles. In both cases the problems resolved within a few days although one infant required mechanical ventilation and the other supplementary oxygen. Both of these infants had persistent hypoglycaemia and they were the two infants who required intravenous infusions of glucagon (Table 30.4).

Two infants had significant congenital anomalies; one had multiple skeletal abnormalities whilst the other had a cleft palate and a grossly abnormal tongue. This caused upper airway problems necessitating intubation. It was subsequently found to be impossible to re-intubate him during an examination under anaesthesia. An emergency tracheostomy was performed but he later died from the consequences of severe asphyctic brain damage.

A comparison between the results of this study and our previous report (Lloyd and Duffty 1984) at the last Colloquium is shown in Table 30.5. There was an overall increase in the number of infants of diabetic mothers which was significantly more than could be explained by the increase in the birth rate between the two periods with 46 such infants being born during the 2-year period of this study compared with 41 during the 4-year period of the previous study. The only other significant change was a decrease in the incidence of hypoglycaemia from 68% of the infants in the previous study to 39% in this study ($P<0.01$).

Table 30.5. Comparison with previous experience (3)

Years	1986/1987	1979/1982
Total number	46	41*
Delivery – spontaneous vaginal	15	8
– forceps	10	15
– Caesarean section	21	18
Heavy for dates >90th centile	12	8
Light for dates <10th centile	4	3
Perinatal asphyxia	12	9
Respiratory problems	10	11
Hypoglycaemia <2.0 mmol/l	18	28*
<1.5 mmol/l	9	21*
Jaundice >275 μmol/l	4	3
Severe congenital abnormalities	2	0
Deaths	1	0
Discharged at <48 h of age	31	24

* $P<0.01$

Discussion

There has been an increase in the number of infants born to diabetic mothers in the Grampian region during the past few years. There were on average 10 such infants born per year during the 4-year period 1979–1982 of our previous report compared with an average of 23 per year during this study. This increase is most probably a reflection of the fact that the incidence of diabetes mellitus in Scottish girls aged 10–18 years doubled over the decade 1968–1978 with the present incidence of childhood diabetes in Grampian being one of the highest in the world at 26.3 per 100 000 (Patterson et al. 1988).

In retrospect 27 (59%) of the 46 infants did not require admission to the neonatal unit. On the other hand, 19 (41%) did with five of these infants requiring intensive care. It is not always possible to determine initially which infants will need special or intensive care so they all require careful monitoring especially during the first hours of life. Unfortunately we have neither the facilities nor sufficient nursing and medical staff to provide appropriate care for these infants outwith the neonatal unit.

The marked decrease in the incidence of hypoglycaemia between our two reports is gratifying. However as hypoglycaemia tends to occur early in these infants it is unlikely that this was related to our management, especially as that had not changed significantly during this time. It might however be indicative of better antenatal diabetic control of the mothers. If that were the reason then it is disappointing that no similar decrease occurred in any of the other neonatal problems. In particular the continuing high incidence of heavy-for-dates infants is puzzling and could indicate that fetal macrosomia is not directly related to the maternal diabetic control.

Of the five infants requiring intensive care, two had respiratory distress syndrome. Whilst this was not unexpected in the 31-week gestation baby, its occurrence in a relatively mature 37-week infant is a reminder that these infants remain at an increased risk for this condition (Robert et al. 1976). The reason for the severe cardiomegaly in the two affected infants remains unclear. Prolonged hypoglycaemia can cause cardiomegaly per se and both these infants had severe problems with hypoglycaemia necessitating an intravenous infusion of glucagon, but this seems unlikely to have been the cause as the cardiomegaly was present in both infants at the time of their first chest X-ray. Hypertrophic cardiomyopathy is well described in infants of diabetic mothers but in this condition the echocardiogram generally shows thickening of the intraventricular septum with normal or increased contractility (Naeye 1965) in contrast with the findings in our two infants. The fifth infant requiring intensive care was the child with upper airway anomalies who was our only death.

In conclusion infants of insulin-dependent diabetic mothers continue to have a higher than expected incidence of neonatal problems. Although most of these are mild the classical problems can still occur.

References

Lloyd DJ, Duffty P (1984) Management of the infant of the diabetic mother: recent experience. In: Sutherland HW, Stowers JM (eds) Carbohydrate metabolism in pregnancy and the newborn. Churchill Livingstone, Edinburgh, pp 144–149

Mitchell RG (1974) Disease in infancy and childhood. Churchill Livingstone, London

Naeye R (1965) Infants of diabetic mothers: a quantitative, morphologic study. Pediatrics 35:980–988

Patterson CC, Smith PG, Webb J, Heasman MA, Mann JI (1988) Geographical variation in the incidence of diabetes mellitus in Scottish children during the period 1977–1983. Diabetic Med 5:160–165

Robert M, Neff R, Hubbell J, Taeusch H, Avery M (1976) Association between maternal diabetes and the respiratory distress syndrome in the newborn. N Engl J Med 294:357–360

Thomson AM, Billewicz WZ, Hytten FE (1968) The assessment of fetal growth. J Obstet Gynaecol Br Commonw 75:903–916

31. The Future for Infants of Diabetic Mothers

R. Schwartz

The goals for reproduction in the diabetic are to abolish perinatal mortality and minimize neonatal morbidity. Additionally, normal growth, physical and psychological development and normal behavioural and psychosocial adjustment should be attained. Ultimately these aspirations will be fulfilled when sequencing of the human genome identifies the gene responsible for diabetes, so that techniques may be developed to eliminate this disorder. Since this is unlikely to occur in the next decade, we must strive to prevent the problems which exist currently.

Clues to solving future problems can be obtained from a retrospective view. Over 20 years ago, Gellis and Hsia (1959) analysed the Boston Lying-In experience with 934 pregnancies treated mainly by Priscilla White from 1 January 1940 to 30 June 1956.

They reported fetal mortality after 28 weeks gestation to be 23% for the decade 1940–1950, and 16.5% for the 6 years that followed (1950–1956). Pedersen and Brandstrup (1956) in a comparable large series from Copenhagen reported a 27% fetal mortality from 1946 to 1952, and a 15% mortality from 1953 to 1955.

In the 767 viable diabetic pregnancies, the Boston study reported a combined intrauterine and neonatal death rate of 19%. The most critical neonatal morbidity reported then was respiratory distress syndrome which was found in one-third of infants of diabetic mothers (IDMs). In their study, lethal congenital anomalies were found in only 1.8% of infants, a value about twice as large as that reported for the normal population from that institution at that time.

In a more extensive report, Pedersen (1977) noted a decline in perinatal mortality in Denmark from 22.1% to 7.4% by 1970–1972. In a remarkable series summarized from the recent literature (1983–1985), Gabbe (1987) noted four stillbirths in 777 pregnancies (0.5%) and no neonatal deaths, excluding anomalies and neglectors.

It is apparent that modern medical and obstetrical management has been associated with a striking improvement in perinatal mortality.

Similar positive results have occurred with several of the morbidities found in IDMs. The improvements may be attributed both to clinical care and to the application of scientific knowledge.

Respiratory Distress Syndrome

The understanding of the pathophysiological events associated with respiratory distress syndrome began with the electron microscopic observations of the terminal airspaces or alveoli at 26 to 28 weeks of gestation by Bertalanffy and LeBlond (1953) who identified type I and II alveolar cells. Subsequently, the lamellar bodies were identified. Clements (1957) and Mead et al. (1957) independently confirmed von Neergaards's very early observations from 1929 that lung fluid had unique surface-tension-reducing properties. Chemical analysis of lung fluids has been difficult; however, classes of substances consist mainly of phospholipids and proteins. Both classes are heterogeneous in composition. The biochemistry of the first clsss, i.e. of phospholipids, has been defined in detail. The specific enzymes necessary for synthesis and factors which modulate these have been characterized. The effects of corticoids, thyroxine and catecholamines have been described. As described below, these events have been critical to understanding the clinical role of phospholipids in surfactant production.

In 1972 King and Clements isolated several fractions, one of which turned out to be a surfactant-associated glycoprotein of molecular weight 30 000–40 000 which was specific for lung fluid. This apoprotein known as SAP 35 is synthesized from an $M_r = 26 000$ polypeptide precursor which is post-translationally modified by proteolytic cleavage of a leader sequence and the addition of complex carbohydrate (Weaver et al. 1986). Smaller molecular weight apoproteins of $M_r = 6000$, known as SAP 6, have recently been characterized by Whitsett et al. (1986). Both Glasser et al. (1988) and Hawgood et al. (1987) have identified cDNAs which encode specific apoproteins of lung surfactant. Reconstitution of small molecular weight surfactant proteins with synthetic phospholipids imparts virtually complete surfactant-like properties to the mixture, including rapid surface absorption and surface tension lowering during dynamic compression.

A variety of techniques were found to induce surfactant. The classical studies were made by Liggins (1969) in New Zealand. He astutely noted that fetal lambs delivered prematurely after glucocorticoid administration had more mature, partially aerated lungs. Controlled clinical trials (Liggins and Howie 1972) then verified that betamethasone administered preterm to the mother could prevent respiratory distress syndrome in premature infants. Notably, IDMs do not respond as well as those of non-diabetic mothers.

In the large series of 934 pregnancies from the Joslin Clinic, Boston, which were observed from 1 January 1940 to 30 June 1956 (16 years), Gellis and Hsia (1959) reported that 30.5% of viable infants had respiratory distress clinically. Of 104 IDMs who died, 95 were studied pathologically. Of these 71 (70%) had pulmonary hyaline membranes with or without atelectasis (Driscoll et al. 1960).

Subsequently in the decade from 1958 to 1968 at the Boston Hospital for Women (also referring mainly to the Joslin population), Robert et al. (1976) retrospectively compared 805 IDMs with 10 152 infants of non-diabetic mothers. She found respiratory distress syndrome (RDS) to be nearly 24 times as likely in an IDM than in an infant of a non-diabetic mother. When confounding factors of gestational age, route of delivery, maternal age, infant sex and birthweight were controlled, the relative risk of RDS in the diabetic group was 5.6 for infants delivered before 38 weeks.

A major advance in the diagnosis and management of respiratory distress syndrome was made by Gluck and Kulovich (1973) who recognized that lecithin/ sphingomyelin (L/S) ratios in amniotic fluid were predictive of lung maturation. They noted however, that diabetics from White's classes A, B and C (often associated with macrosomia and large placentas) had L/S ratios with delayed time of appearance of a mature ratio of 2.0 or greater. In contrast, classes D to F were associated with an accelerated mature ratio. An additional index for predictability of amniotic fluid phospholipids was provided by Hallman et al. (1977) who showed that phosphatidylglycerol provided another indicator of pulmonary maturation. The L/S ratio false mature value in diabetic pregnancies is minimized by analysis of phosphatidylglycerol. Studies in 88 diabetic pregnancies and 65 controls (Hallman and Teramo 1979) showed there were no differences in L/S ratios based on gestational ages. In diabetic pregnancies, phosphatidylglycerol may be absent or low even if the L/S ratio is >2. Respiratory distress syndrome coincided with an L/S ratio of between 2.0 and 3.0 only when phosphatidylglycerol was absent. They concluded that the fetus of the diabetic pregnancy can be safely delivered free of respiratory distress syndrome after phosphatidylglycerol appears, but in its absence RDS may complicate the neonatal course even if the L/S ratio is ≥2. Thus, phosphatidylglycerol may be another important biochemical marker of RDS.

Warburton (1983a) has studied the effects of chronic hyperglycaemia on the flux of surface active material in tracheal fluid of chronically catheterized fetal lambs at 112 to 145 d gestation. A mild elevation of serum glucose from 18 ± 2 mg/dl to 32 ± 2 mg/dl was associated with an increase in serum insulin from 12 ± 3 μU/ml to 38 ± 4 μU/ml. There were no perturbations of blood gases or haematocrit. Whereas surface active material began to appear in tracheal fluid by 123 d gestation and was present in all controls by 129 d, it did not appear at all in four hyperglycaemic fetuses carried to 145 d gestation, while two had only low levels at 142 d. In contrast to the controls, there was no rise in tracheal fluid phospholipid content, mixed lecithin content or disaturated phosphatidylcholine content. In a later series, he treated similar groups of hyperglycaemic and control fetal animals with infused cortisol (Warburton 1983b). This resulted in a 4.8-fold increase in surface active material in tracheal fluid from the controls, associated with a 7.7-fold increase in total phospholipid content, a 9.5-fold increase in mixed lecithin content, a 10.5-fold increase in disaturated phosphatidylcholine and a 5.6-fold increase in phosphatidylglycerol content. In the cortisol-treated, glucose-infused animals there was no change in surface active material flux, nor was there any increase in phospholipid fractions. These observations have obvious implications regarding management of the diabetic pregnancy and subsequent risk for respiratory distress syndrome.

The above technologies combined with improved obstetrical and neonatal management have resulted in an astounding decrease in the incidence of this once common and overwhelming problem. The occurrence of respiratory distress syndrome in the same institution (Boston Hospital for Women) from 1940 to 1977 decreased dramatically 10-fold from a 31% to a 3% incidence.

In the past decade, attention has turned to very early treatment of respiratory distress syndrome with surfactant-like materials. Those being studied at present include (a) human surfactant isolated from amniotic fluid, (b) calf lung washing isolates and (c) synthetic or semi-synthetic surfactant. While the lipid components are well characterized, the protein components remain to be finally defined.

From the above, it is evident that no single event has been responsible for the marked improvement in neonatal outcome relative to respiratory distress syndrome. Thus precise quantitative scientific discoveries have been combined with clinical judgement in altering modes of practice to produce the very good prognosis which exists currently.

Hypoxaemia

Hypoxaemia has been one of the vexing problems to those managing the diabetic pregnancy. Early evidence was inferential with recognition of high rates of unexplained stillbirths as noted above. In the 768 pregnancies over 28 weeks gestation reported by Gellis and Hsia (1959), there was a 7.6% stillbirth rate. In other series reported at that time, fetal mortality was as high as 25%,

Pedersen (1977) reported a similar experience among 1332 newborn IDMs. His perinatal mortality declined from 22.1% in 1946–1955 to 7.4% in 1970–1972. He stated: "In principle, the treatment of the Copenhagen series has remained unchanged since 1946 and has been supervised by a restricted number of doctors, midwifes and nurses. Naturally, the experience of the team has increased over the years. The time-related decrease in perinatal mortality over the thirty years cannot be precisely explained."

Another observation which may be related to hypoxia is the increase in extramedullary haematopoiesis noted over 40 years ago. Miller (1946) stated:

> The extramedullary erythropoiesis in infants born to diabetic mothers, which is most marked in the liver and spleen, is observed in almost all cases studied at postmortem. Since most of these infants are either stillborn or die within the first four days after birth, it is not known how long the extramedullary erythropoiesis persists. Studies of the peripheral blood and its normoblast content suggest that, as in erythroblastosis fetalis associated with Rh incompatibility, the extramedullary activity is short-lived. The differentiation between the extramedullary erythropoiesis associated with the blood incompatibilities of the mother and fetus and the extramedullary erythropoiesis seen in infants born to diabetic and prediabetic mothers has given some difficulty to clinicians and pathologists in the past. There are differences, however, which permit one to make the correct diagnosis in most instances. The infant born to a diabetic mother or prediabetic mother does not become anemic or develop marked jaundice. Macklin (1944) has pointed out that the amount of hemosiderin in the livers of infants born to diabetic mothers is small as contrasted to the large amount seen in infants with Rh incompatibilities in whom considerable hemolysis has occurred. Whenever excessive erythropoiesis is encountered in the newborn infant, red blood cell counts, tests for hemosiderin in the tissues, along with the appropriate tests for blood group incompatibility and tests for congenital syphilis are necessary.

Naeye (1965) examined autopsy material from 56 IDMs who were either stillborn or who died within the first 2 d of life. In 30 specimens with adequate material, he noted that overweight infants had liver weights which were 179% of control organs. Although in large measure this was due to an increase in hepatocyte cytoplasm, there was also a threefold increase in haematopoietic tissue compared with controls. Most of these haematopoietic cells were erythroid precursors. Figure 31.1 shows histology from livers of three IDMs of comparable gestational age. The one on the left is normal, while the one on the right shows a gross increase in extramedullary erythropoiesis. Singer (1986) has performed point counting of histological sections of liver of 40 controls and 16 IDMs. With this quantitative technique he showed a striking inverse relationship between the degree of hepatic erythropoiesis and gestational age from 22 to 40 weeks. Most of the IDMs were normal; however, three or four over 40 weeks gestation had clearly increased haematopoiesis.

A related problem may be neonatal polycythaemia. Mimouni et al. (1986) prospectively evaluated 34 pairs of IDMs and controls carefully matched for six variables, including site of sampling, time of sampling, time of cord clamping, gestational age, mode of delivery and Apgar scores. Polycythaemia was defined as a venous haematocrit greater than or equal to 65%. There was a significantly greater incidence of polycythaemia (29.4% vs 5.9%) in IDMs than the controls ($P<0.03$). They also found significantly high nucleated red blood cell counts in the IDMs. They noted no correlation with maternal haemoglobin-A_1 concentration or with increased infant weight percentile. There was a correlation with neonatal hypoglycaemia but no measurements of fetal insulin secretion were made.

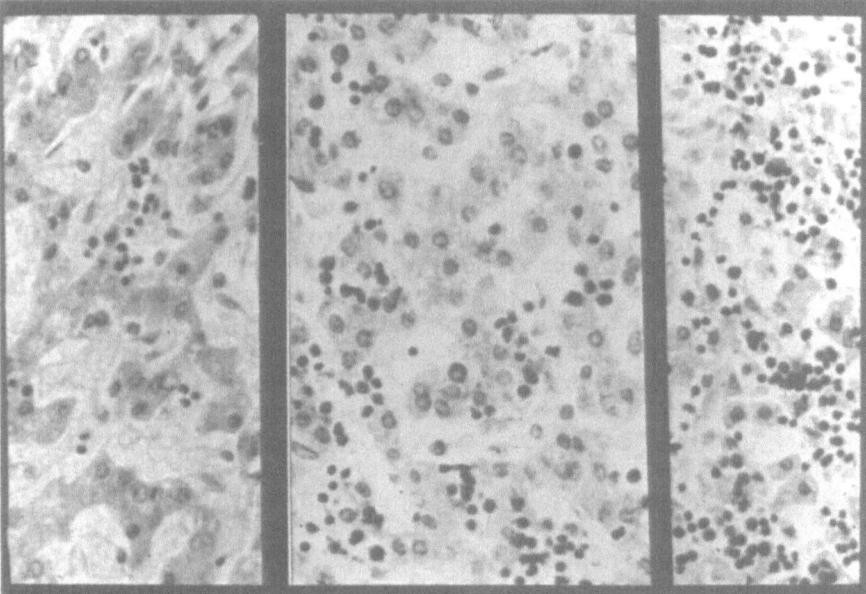

Fig. 31.1. Liver histology from three IDMs of the same gestational age. The *left* shows normal haematopoiesis, while the *right* shows grossly increased erythropoiesis. With permission of the Ross Laboratories, publishers of the 93rd Ross Conference, 1987.

The first definitive experimental studies of fetal hypoxaemia induced by chronic hyperinsulinaemia were made serendipidly by Carson et al. (1980). During studies to evaluate the metabolic effects of infusion of insulin to chronically catheterized fetal sheep, they compared not only the dose of insulin administered, but also the duration of infusion. An unexpected outcome was the development of fetal hypoxia in those animals infused for 2–4 d. The effects on oxygen content did not occur in the initial 4 h; however, by 24 h a highly significant decrease was observed. In contrast, plasma glucose decreased significantly within 4 h of the start of the insulin infusion, while the molar ratio of glucose to oxygen increased significantly. There was a significant relationship between the glucose to oxygen quotient and plasma insulin concentration (r = 0.68, $P<0.001$). There also was an inverse relationship between the oxygen content and plasma insulin concentration ($r = 0.60$, $P<0.001$). These events were reversible. Thus cessation of insulin infusion resulted in restoration to normal of plasma glucose concentration, the glucose to oxygen quotient and blood oxygen content. The mechanisms responsible for these changes were not clarified. Theoretically these could have been due to limitation of utero-placental-fetal oxygen transfer; alternatively there could have been enhanced fetal tissue oxygen uptake, or some combination. In addition, a redistribution of blood and oxygen delivery in the fetus could be a contributing event.

Milley et al. (1984) have confirmed these observations. They infused chronically catheterized fetal sheep with insulin at rates sufficient to produce hyperinsulinaemia, but at levels one to two magnitudes lower than reported by Carson. While they produced a definite decrease in oxygen content, no changes in plasma glucose concentration occurred. They speculated initially that this fetal arterial hypoxaemia could result from either of two mechanisms. First, oxygen delivery to the fetus by the placenta may be impaired; this could result if placental function deteriorated or umbilical blood flow decreased. The latter might decrease because fetal cardiac output either was decreased or was changed in its distribution. Alternatively, fetal oxygen consumption might increase without a corresponding increase in oxygen availability. Blood flow and cardiac output were analysed with the microsphere techniques. There was a decrease in umbilical blood flow as well as umbilical venous oxygen content associated with hyperinsulinaemia. The fall in umbilical blood flow was due to a change in the distribution of cardiac output so that placental perfusion decreased while blood flow to the fetal carcass increased. Fetal oxygen consumption increased. Since delivery of oxygen to the fetus did not increase, the increased use was associated with increased fetal extraction of available oxygen. The fetal arterial hypoxaemia is the result of this increased extraction of available oxygen.

In subsequent studies Milley et al. (1986) used the same model with well-fed sheep to evaluate the effects of chronic hyperinsulinaemia on substrate uptake. They observed an increased uptake of oxygen, glucose and alpha amino-nitrogen-containing substances (amino acids). The rise in oxygen uptake again occurred by increasing fetal oxygen extraction resulting in fetal arterial hypoxaemia. They also determined substrate-oxygen quotients for glucose and lactate. This molar ratio represents substrate uptake relative to oxygen corrected for the amount of oxygen required to oxidize a given substrate (i.e. 6 and 3 mol of oxygen per 1 mol of glucose and lactate respectively). This number represents the maximal fraction of oxidative metabolism that could be supported by the complete oxidation of that substrate. Under endogenous or basal condition the $G:O_2$ ratio was 0.61 ±

0.06 for well-fed animals. With insulin infusion, this ratio increased to 0.80. In contrast, the lactate:O_2 molar ratio remained unchanged at 0.23 ± 0.02. Total oxidative metabolism of these two substrates increased from 84% to 103%. Thus, no other substrates were necessary for metabolism. It was suggested that the increased uptake of amino acids could be used either for synthetic or oxidative purposes.

In a parallel series of studies, Philipps et al. (1982a, 1984) have evaluated the effects of continuous hyperglycaemia in chronically catheterized fetal sheep. Plasma glucose levels were elevated two fold above control values. Plasma insulin levels rose; however, responses in individual animals were variable. Whole blood oxygen content of the distal aorta was observed to have a consistent and striking fall by 33% of basal values. Thus, a rise in the venous–arterial oxygen difference was found. In several instances, pO_2 fell to life-threatening levels so that glucose infusion was terminated. Umbilical blood flow remained unchanged. Since fetal oxygen delivery remained constant, oxygen consumption rose from 34% during the control period to 51% after 3 d of hyperglycaemia. The increase in oxygen consumption was due to increased fetal oxygen extraction and not due to alterations in fetal blood oxygen affinity or in placental oxygen transport. Significant hyperpnoea and respiratory acidosis occurred; however, no metabolic acidosis was found. Philipps et al. (1985a,b) suggested that defined fetal glucose infusions induced stimulation of oxidative metabolism but had little effect upon placental oxygen consumption.

In parallel with and independently of these animal observations, our group has approached the problem of assessment of fetal hypoxaemia indirectly by measurement of fetal plasma erythropoietin concentration. In the adult this hormone is synthesized and released in response to hypoxaemia in the kidney. In contrast, the fetus produces the hormone in both liver and kidney. The only known significant stimulus is hypoxaemia. The hormone is not stored, so approximately 4–6 h of stimulation are necessary before elevation of the plasma level occurs. This release time has not been affected by using the highly specific and highly sensitive radioimmunoassay techniques for detection. The half-life of plasma erythropoietin is about 7–10 h. A small but significant fraction, 2%–9%, is excreted in urine in adult animals over 1–2 d.

In our original studies reported by Widness et al. (1981), we evaluated umbilical plasma erythropoietin concentrations at delivery in 28 controls and 61 diabetic pregnancies. We found one-third (22 of 61) of the infants of insulin-dependent mothers to have elevated umbilical plasma erythropoietin values, which exceeded the range of the controls. Strikingly, several infants had values several magnitudes above the controls (30 000 vs 30 mU/ml) at levels as high as any reported in man. In a subset of subjects, free-flowing umbilical blood was studied for blood elements as well as plasma glucose and insulin concentrations. A significant relationship was observed between umbilical plasma insulin and plasma erythropoietin, but not between umbilical plasma glucose and erythro-poietin. In the original human series, no relationships between plasma erythro-poietin and either red blood cell count, nucleated red blood cell counts or reticulocyte counts were found.

At that time we already had well developed a chronically hyperinsulinaemic rhesus fetus model. We found that hyperinsulinaemia in the absence of hypergly-caemia was associated with significant elevation of plasma erythropoietin. Furthermore, hepatic extramedullary haematopoiesis was minimally affected, but umbilical blood reticulocytes were significantly elevated ($P<0.007$). We inferred that chronic hyperinsulinaemia was associated with fetal hypoxaemia.

Further elaboration in the fetus of the relationships among the variables hyperglycaemia, hypoxaemia and erythropoietin was made by Philipps et al. (1982b) using the chronically catheterized fetal sheep. As noted above, glucose infusion raised plasma glucose concentration threefold from 18.8 ± 2.4 (mean $\pm$ SEM) mg/dl to 55.4 ± 3.7 mg/dl. Infusions were maintained for 3 to 11 d. Whole blood oxygen content fell by a third from 6.2 ± 1.2 ml/dl to 4.2 ± 1.0 ml/dl. Plasma erythropoietin was 13.2 ± 2.8 mU/ml during the control period and rose to 150.7 ± 35.9 mU/ml in those animals whose oxygen content fell to less than 60% of basal values. A reciprocal relationship was demonstrated between fetal arterial oxygen content and fetal plasma arterial Ep concentration ($P<0.001$) in the pooled data of infused fetuses. Although plasma insulin concentrations rose in the infused fetuses, the elevations were inconsistent and no relationship between fetal plasma insulin concentration and decrement in fetal oxygen content was evident. Similarly, no relationship was apparent between fetal arterial plasma insulin and erythropoietin concentrations. It was concluded that the glucose-induced hypoxaemia was responsible for the increase in plasma erythropoietin. The cellular mechanism(s) responsible for the glucose-induced fetal hypoxaemia remain to be defined.

The original human observations have been extended in collaboration with Teramo et al. (1987) in Helsinki. In a prospective study of 25 control subjects and 49 insulin-treated diabetic subjects, we have evaluated the relationship between amniotic fluid erythropoietin and umbilical plasma erythropoietin concentrations (Fig. 31.2). Amniotic fluid erythropoietin concentrations were consistently on average 38% lower than the plasma concentrations. The samples from the diabetic pregnancies were significantly elevated in both amniotic fluid and umbilical plasma compared to the controls. Furthermore, a very strong correlation was found between natural log transformed amniotic fluid erythropoietin and natural log transformed umbilical plasma erythropoietin concentrations ($r =$

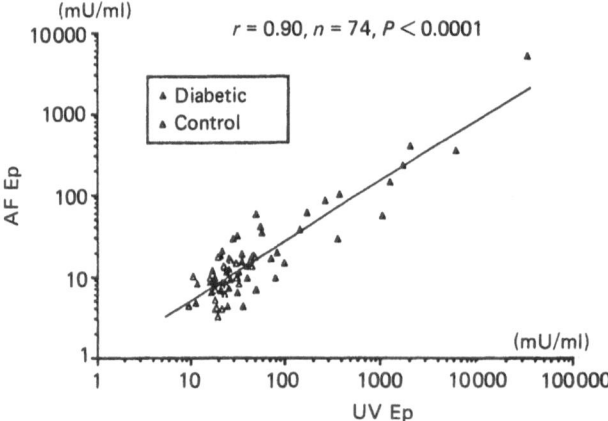

Fig. 31.2. Log-transformed amniotic fluid erythropoietin concentration relative to log-transformed umbilical plasma erythropoietin concentration in control infants and IDMs. (Modified from the observations of Teramo et al. 1987.)

0.90, $P<0.001$). Because Teramo evaluates haemoglobin A_{1c} bi-weekly in his pregnant diabetic subjects, we were able to analyse this measure of metabolic control. The mean values in individual subjects varied from 4.9% to 9.5% over the 5-month interval prior to delivery. Log transformed umbilical plasma erythropoietin and log transformed amniotic fluid erythropoietin each correlated with maternal HbA_{1c} determined during the final month of pregnancy ($r = 0.64$, $r = 0.58$, $P<0.0001$ respectively). Using forced stepwise multiple regression analysis, Widness et al. (1987) found maternal HbA_{1c} again to be highly correlated with fetal umbilical vein and amniotic fluid erythropoietin concentrations. Umbilical plasma glucose and insulin concentrations made significant contributions to the regressions, whereas umbilical plasma C-peptide did not. When amniotic fluid erythropoietin was utilized as the outcome variable, only amniotic fluid insulin contributed significantly to the relationship while glucose and C-peptide did not.

It is apparent from the foregoing review, that hypoxaemia is a significant risk for the fetus of a diabetic pregnancy. Since it is quite clear that either fetal hyperglycaemia or hyperinsulinaemia is associated with fetal hypoxaemia, rigid control of diabetes during pregnancy should abolish the morbidities due to this problem. The pathogenesis of the hypoxaemia is due to increased fetal oxygen consumption in the presence of constant fetal blood flow. The major substrate is glucose, although some increase in amino acid uptake has been reported.

Macrosomia

Macrosomia has been one of the hallmarks of diabetic fetopathy since its recognition over 150 years ago. It has served both as major evidence in understanding pathophysiological events as well as a marker for evaluating morbidity. Macrosomia has been found in as many as one-third of diabetic pregnancies. Studies from 1940 to 1960 (Farquhar 1962; Fee and Weil 1963), when rigid or tight control of diabetes was not common, indicate that approximately 25% of deliveries were macrosomic, when weight was corrected for gestational age using Babson et al's. (1970) 95th percentile of weight-for-gestational age for a sea-level population of mixed sexes as the reference. In more recent reports, although results have been highly variable, macrosomia continues to be a significant problem. Investigators in Cincinnati (S. Stys and R. C. Tsang 1987, personal communication) have had an ongoing study comparing diabetic pregnant women treated by standard care with a group under strict control. Their summary data indicate no difference in the frequency of macrosomia, which is still significant at 37%–38% in each group. Similar studies have been reported from Stockholm (Persson and Gentz 1984) and San Francisco (Shannon et al. 1986). Our own data from Helsinki (Schwartz and Teramo 1987) indicate a continuous 25% prevalence of macrosomia, defined as weight-for-gestation exceeding 2 SDs of body weight, derived from a large, recently surveyed Finnish reference population.

Early body composition studies of total body water or of body fat in infants or in fetuses of diabetic mothers indicated an altered composition with increased body fat. Later studies by King et al. (1971) indicated no difference in fatty acid composition of adipose tissue from IDMs and from normal infants. Naeye (1965) in a study of 21 macrosomic infants noted that body weight was increased 141% relative to controls. His measurements are summarized as follows: length 112%, heart 174%, liver 179%, lung and spleen 127% each, adrenal 158% and pancreas 110%. Notably, brain and kidneys were unaffected. From morphometric analyses, Naeye concluded that both hypertrophy and hyperplasia accounted for the organ enlargement, which is most consistent with increased protein synthesis.

Evidence has accumulated in the last 50 years to support the original Pedersen hypothesis (1977) that many of the pathophysiological events found in the IDM may be attributed to fetal hyperinsulinaemia secondary to inadequate maternal metabolic control. The clinical data currently available may be demonstrated by our recent experience in Helsinki. In this study designed to prospectively evaluate the relationship between amniotic fluid and umbilical plasma erythropoietin concentrations, patients were managed similarly, with tight control, but were segregated according to mode of delivery. Body weight at birth relative to gestational age and to the Helsinki normal population, which exceeded +2 SDs is considered macrosomic. Macrosomia, which was present in 25% of the total population, was distributed over all White's (1974) classes. This nomenclature was based primarily on age at onset, duration of the disorder and complications. Since haemoglobin A_{1c} in maternal blood reflects ambient glucose concentration over the previous 4 to 6 weeks, infant weight (SD units) was examined relative to

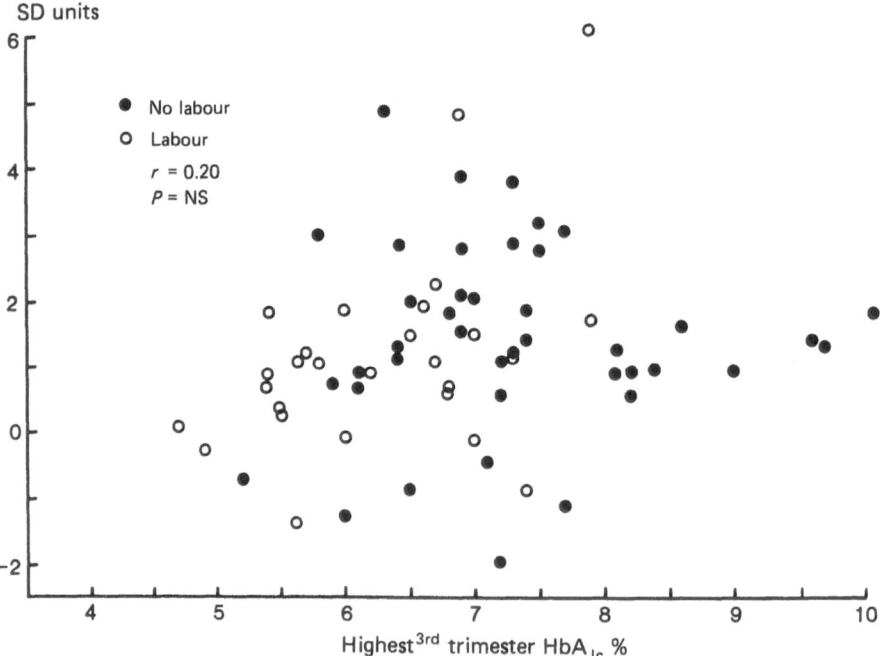

Fig. 31.3. Individual body weights of infants of diabetic mothers expressed as deviations from the mean of a normal population from Helsinki corrected for gestational age and sex. Body weight data expressed in SD units are shown relative to maternal third-trimester highest HbA_{1c}.

the highest haemoglobin A_{1c} found in the third trimester (Fig. 31.3). No relationship was found between these two variables. However, it is significant that of 17 infants whose highest maternal haemoglobin A_{1c} was within the normal range (<6%), only one was macrosomic. Similar analysis was found for mean haemoglobin A_{1c} determined every 2 weeks in the third trimester. Interestingly, a relationship was found between umbilical vein (UV) plasma C-peptide concentration (expressed as log number, LN) and highest maternal haemoglobin A_{1c} (%) in the third trimester ($r = 0.508$, $P<0.001$). When body weight in SD units was evaluated relative to LN UV C-peptide for both control infants and IDMs, a positive relationship ($r = 0.547$, $P<0.0001$) was found (Fig. 31.4). Similar clinical observations have been reported by others.

C-peptide is the product of post-translational proteolytic cleavage of dibasic amino acids at positions 31,32 and 64,65. It is released into the portal circulation in equimolar quantities with insulin. Since insulin is significantly removed by the liver, C-peptide which is physiologically inert has served as an indirect means of assessing insulin secretion. Studies of insulin in umbilical plasma from infants whose mothers have insulin antibodies have been confounded technically. Previous studies have assumed that C-peptide like insulin does not cross the placenta.

We (Gruppuso et al. 1987) have examined this question by administering ^{125}I-proinsulin or ^{125}I-tryosylated C-peptide by bolus and constant infusion to pregnant rhesus monkeys near term. In addition to sequential maternal blood samples, we analysed umbilical plasma at delivery to examine placental transfer

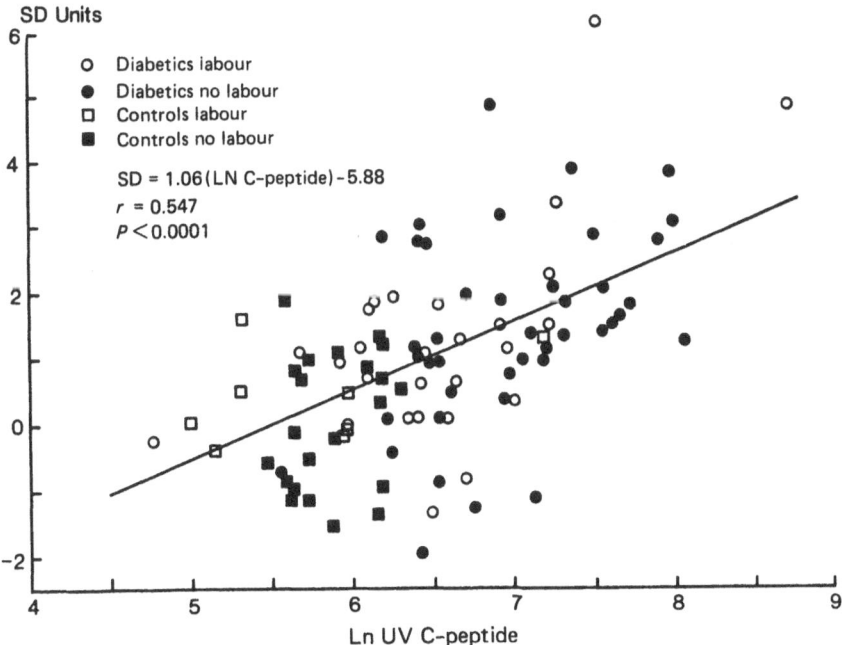

Fig. 31.4. Relationship of natural log-transformed umbilical plasma C-peptide and infant body weight expressed in SD units (see Fig. 31.3). With permission of the Ross Laboratories, publishers of the Report of the 93rd Ross Conference, 1987.

of these peptides. At the end of each infusion, fetuses were exsanguinated in situ via the umbilical vein. The bolus–constant infusion technique produced a steady state in maternal plasma of immunoprecipitable label, measured using excess insulin or C-peptide anti-serum. In animals infused with ^{125}I-proinsulin, analysis of umbilical venous plasma revealed no apparent transfer to the fetus of immunoprecipitable label. In contrast, in animals infused with ^{125}I-tyrosylated-C-peptide, 3%–13% of the umbilical venous plasma radioactivity was immunoprecipitable, representing 1.4%–5.8% of the immunoprecipitable radioactivity in maternal plasma at delivery. Gel filtration chromatography of umbilical venous plasma revealed that the immunoprecipitated moiety was not intact ^{125}I-tyrosylated-C-peptide, but a fragment of ^{125}I-tyrosylated-C-peptide (Fig. 31.5). Analysis of maternal plasma showed that the predominant peak of radioactivity represented intact C-peptide. However, a peak corresponding to the fetal immunoprecipitable peak (b) was also present. Analysis of simultaneously sampled maternal arterial and uterine vein plasma showed that degradation of ^{125}I-tyrosylated-C-peptide occurred across the uterus. Studies in one non-pregnant and three postpartum animals indicated that pregnancy increased the rate of metabolism of ^{125}I-tyrosylated-C-peptide. When ^{125}I-tyrosylated-C-peptide was incubated with trophoblastic cells in tissue culture, degradation to a

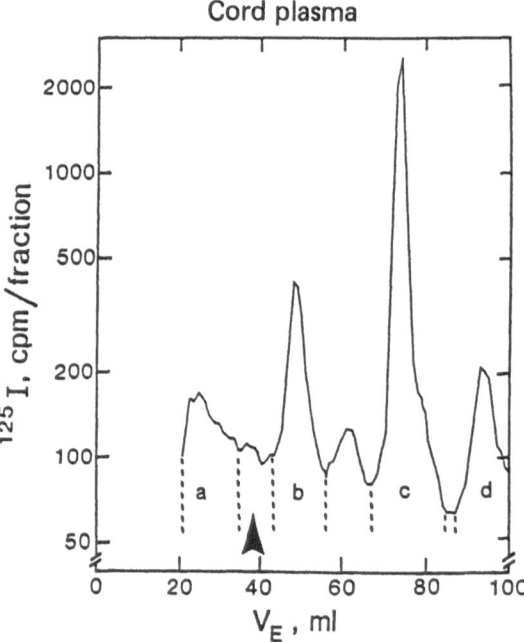

Fig. 31.5. Gel filtration chromatography of 1.0 ml umbilical venous plasma from an animal infused with ^{125}I-tyrosylated-C peptide for 2 h. Immunoprecipitation was carried out on four to six peak tubes from peaks a–d. The limits used to determine the percentage of total radioactivity per peak are shown by the *broken lines*. The *arrow* marks the position at which ^{125}I-tyrosylated-C-peptide should elute. Peak b, a smaller fragment, was immunoprecipitable, whereas peaks c and d were not. Reproduced from *The Journal of Clinical Investigation*, 1987, 80:1132–1137 by copyright permission of the American Society for Clinical Investigation.

species corresponding on gel filtration to the immunoprecipitable fetal metabolite was found. We conclude that proinsulin, like insulin, does not traverse the placenta. Immunoreactive fragments of C-peptide do cross, however, and pregnancy alters the metabolism of ^{125}I-tyrosylated-C-peptide, probably owing to placental degradation.

The metabolism of C-peptide by the placenta has implications for interpretation of plasma C-peptide concentrations. Since there is a difference between pregnant and non-pregnant animals in the percentage of administered ^{125}I-tyrosylated-C-peptide metabolized to non-immunoreactive forms, extrapolation from the non-pregnant to the pregnant state probably is not valid. Furthermore, the effect of the placenta would presumably be changing throughout gestation. Use of plasma C-peptide measurements to estimate the hepatic extraction of insulin and insulin secretion rate in pregnant subjects must take this into account. Application to estimates of fetal insulin secretion or fetal hepatic extraction must similarly be considered in light of the possible metabolism of fetal C-peptide by the placenta. The apparent ability of the placenta to extract and metabolize C-peptide must therefore be added to the list of variables that must be considered in the interpretation of peripheral plasma C-peptide concentrations (Polonsky and Rubenstein 1984).

One may conclude from these studies that macrosomia is related in large measure to fetal hyperinsulinism. Fetal hyperglycaemia may not be the sole aetiological stimulus for the endogenous fetal hyperinsulinaemia. In insulin-treated subjects, maternal antibody may transport insulin to the fetus as well. Furthermore the role of amino acids, especially those that are insulinogenic (Freinkel and Metzger 1979; Milner 1979), has not been firmly established in the fetus/infant of the diabetic mother.

Since insulin is the major anabolic hormone of the fetus, we have evaluated its role more directly. Our own studies with Susa over the last 10 years (Susa et al. 1979; Schwartz and Susa 1980) have clearly demonstrated the effects of primary fetal hyperinsulinaemia in the normal third-trimester rhesus monkey. We developed this model because (a) the primate placenta is impermeable to insulin, (b) the placenta is permeable to glucose and (c) the maternal glucose pool is large enough to sustain the fetal glucose requirement.

Rhesus fetuses from time-gestation normal mothers have been implanted with osmotic minipumps capable of continuous delivery of insulin subcutaneously for 28 d. After 3 weeks of continuous hyperinsulinaemia, fetuses have been found to have elevated plasma insulin but diminished endogenous plasma C-peptide and glucagon concentrations. Substrate changes include decreased umbilical arterial plasma glucose concentration and plasma total amino acid concentration, but unaltered plasma free fatty acids (FFA) and 3-hydroxybutyrate. Macrosomia has been a consistent observation at two insulin doses: mean plasma insulin concentration 340 uU/ml or 3625 uU/ml with fetal weights (mean ± SD) being 459 ± 53 g and 474 ± 48 g, as compared to 372 ± 54 g for age-matched controls (Schwartz and Teramo 1987) (Fig. 31.6). Although body composition studies were not performed, there was a gross increase in body fat on visual inspection. Interestingly, in contrast to human material, there were no measurable differences in body length. At the lower, physiological hyperinsulinaemia dose, among organ weights only cardiomegaly was significant. However, at the higher, supraphysiological dose, increased weight of liver and spleen was also noted. The brain was remarkably unaffected at any dose.

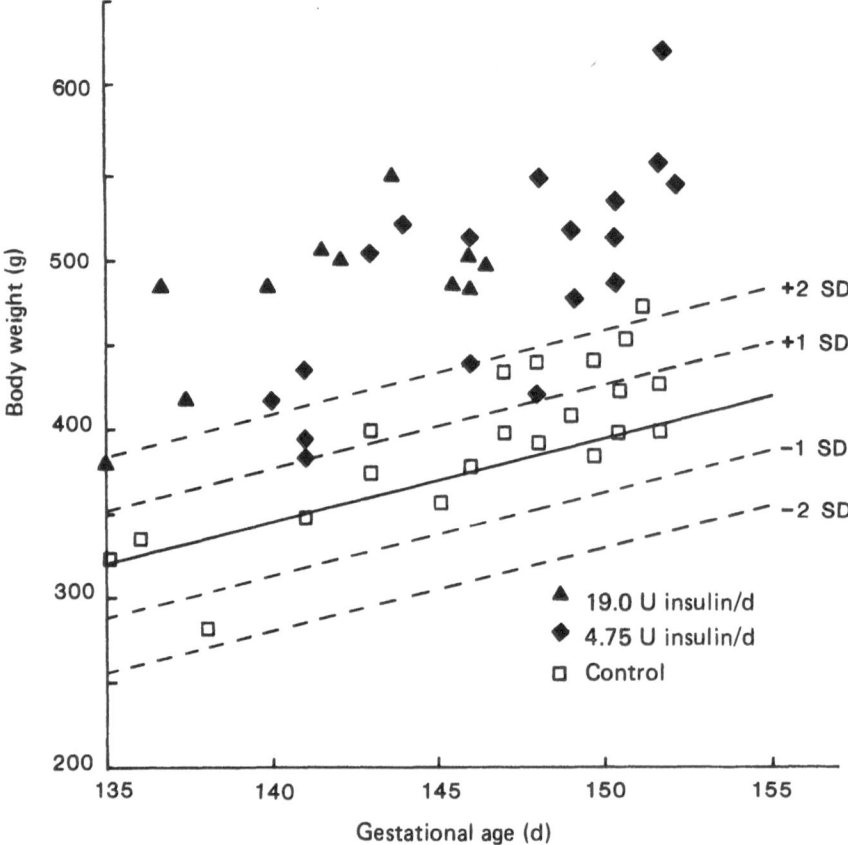

Fig. 31.6. Body weights of control and hyperinsulinaemic rhesus fetuses at delivery. The *lines* represent mean and per cent of a large control population. With permission of the Ross Laboratories, publishers of the Report of the 93rd Ross Conference, 1987.

A comparison of organ sizes at both insulin doses indicates that macrosomia and cardiomegaly are consistent findings, while enlarged liver, spleen and placenta only occur at supraphysiological insulin doses. A comparison of rhesus organ weights with human organ weights from IDMs from Naeye reveals a characteristic pattern of somatic and cardiac increase with normal brain and kidney mass.

In contrast to the morphometric findings of Naeye (1965), there was no difference in the ratio of protein to deoxyribonucleic acid in liver, skeletal muscle or heart. We conclude from these measurements that only cell hyperplasia, without hypertrophy, has occurred in these hyperinsulinaemic fetuses. Although we have no direct measurements of substrate flux, we believe that insulin has enhanced cellular uptake of all nutrients in these selected organs. Thus, insulin has been the stimulus for enhanced uptake in the absence of substrate excess, in contrast to the diabetic pregnancy.

The fetal rhesus studies and human observations reviewed here are consistent with macrosomia and selective organomegaly being attributed to fetal hyperinsulinaemia. In the human, glucose is only one of the substrates involved in stimulation of insulin production. Further studies of hormone–substrate–cell interaction are necessary to define the cell biology of the diabetic fetopathy.

Because of the structural homology between proinsulin and insulin-like growth factor I (also known as somatomedin-C, SM-C) and insulin-like growth factor II, recent attention has focused on the IGFs . Whether the insulin-like growth factors (IGFs) (e.g. IGF-I, IGF-II) are involved in the pathogenesis of macrosomia remains undefined. Inconsistent changes in umbilical plasma IGF-I or IGF-II have been found in IDMs (Susa et al. 1984). In our rhesus studies, plasma total somatomedin peptide content was similar in hyperinsulinaemic and control fetuses (Susa et al. 1984).

D'Ercole (1987) has recently summarized the data with reference to IGFs and macrosomia in offspring of diabetic mothers. He noted that SM-C/IGF-I concentrations in cord blood from normal infants correlate with birth size. However, SM/IGF concentrations are elevated in some but not all overgrown IDMs. He also reported that when diabetes was induced in pregnant rabbits with alloxan, fetal serum SM-C/IGF-I concentrations correlated with the degree of maternal glucose intolerance but not with the degree of fetal hyperinsulinaemia. In the previously described hyperinsulinaemic fetal monkeys (Susa et al. 1984), SM/IGF serum concentrations were elevated only when serum insulin levels were very high (>3000 uU/ml); however, there was great variability among animals. Hill and Milner (1980) reported an increase in bioassayable serum SM/IGF and cartilage metabolic activity (increased thymidine uptake) in fetal rabbits 48 h after the injection of a long-acting insulin preparation. Similarly, hyperinsulin-aemia produced in fetal pigs by implantation of osmotic minipumps caused an increase in bioassayable SM/IGF. D'Ercole concluded that in none of these studies was it possible to determine whether the insulin per se or the metabolic effect of insulin stimulated the increase in SM/IGF. Furthermore, fetal hyperin-sulinaemia induced by maternal glucose infusion or by maternal glibenclamide administration can also raise bioassayable SM/IGF in fetal rat serum (Heinze et al. 1982). In the fetal lamb, total pancreatectomy results in a modest decrease (28%) in circulating SM-C/IGF-I but an increase in IGF-II (Gluckman et al. 1987). The serum SM-C/IGF-I concentrations, however, may not reflect tissue levels, which presumably are the relevant physiological measure. Other explana-tions for such an apparent discrepancy are possible, including the actions of SM-C/IGF-I inhibitors. D'Ercole has concluded that it seems likely that the action of insulin on the synthesis of SM/IGFs is a consequence of the altered metabolic milieu and nutritional status, rather than a direct action. Although speculative, he considers it likely that SM/IGF-I plays some role in the overgrowth of the fetus of the diabetic pregnancy.

Since macrosomia does not appear to be solely due to hyperinsulinaemia, we considered the observations that elevated proinsulin in the fetus of the diabetic mother may act via insulin-like growth factor receptors I and II. Insulin-like growth factor-I (IGF-I) and proinsulin share similarities in both primary and tertiary structure. Proinsulin, endogenously secreted or exogenously adminis-tered, would therefore be expected to interact with IGF-I receptors. Gruppuso et al. (1988) in our group, determined the relative activities of IGF-I, insulin, proinsulin and the proinsulin conversion intermediates in IGF-I radioreceptor assays using term human placental membranes (Fig. 31.7). Insulin was approxi-mately 0.5% as potent as IGF-I and proinsulin was only 2% as potent as insulin.

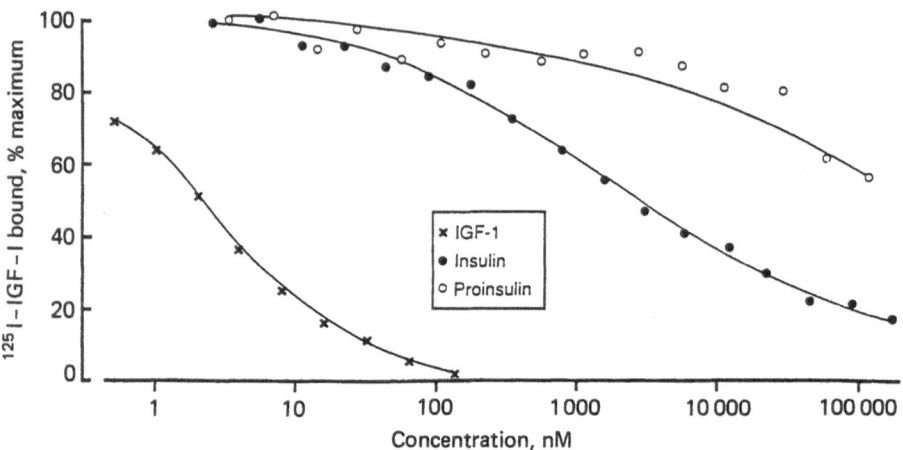

Fig. 31.7. Displacement of ^{125}I-IGF-I from four human placental membranes by IGF-I, insulin and proinsulin indicated that insulin had 0.5% of the activity of IGF-I in displacing bound ^{125}I-IGF. Proinsulin caused minimal displacement of ^{125}I-IGF-I. At the maximal concentrations studied (1 mg/ml, 111 μM), its potency in displacing labelled IGF-I from placental membranes was 2% that of insulin.

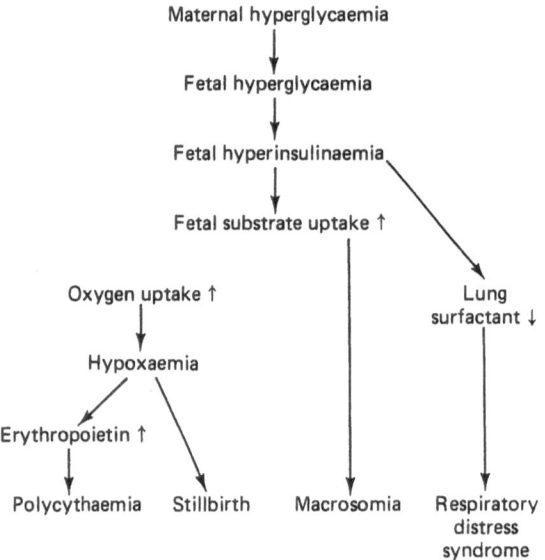

Fig. 31.8. Summary schema showing relationship of several fetal/neonatal morbidities to maternal hyperglycaemia and fetal hyperinsulinaemia.

The six major proinsulin conversion intermediates were studied; all had activities intermediate between insulin and proinsulin. We concluded that the binding of proinsulin and the proinsulin conversion intermediates to IGF-I receptors is not of physiological significance at the concentrations occurring endogenously or after exogenous administration of proinsulin.

The effects of maternal hyperglycaemia or substrate disequilibrium are summarized schematically in Fig. 31.8 which represents an expanded pathophysiological view of the Pedersen thesis. This is not all-inclusive, but rather represents those morbidities for which there is reasonable evidence.

Summary

Ultimately, our ability to abolish or minimize the problems of the fetus and newborn of the diabetic mother will depend on societal decisions as much as upon clinical science. Thus, further identification of the genetic factors associated with diabetes holds the prospect for ultimately eliminating these disorders. As noted earlier, allocation of resources for health care is essential for establishing screening and health maintenance during pregnancy; similarly, education of prospective parents is critical to the prevention of congenital anomalies and the increased morbidities associated with inadequate obstetrical care. While we have observed remarkable improvements in perinatal mortality and morbidities, especially in Western societies in the post-Second World War era, we have not yet solved all our problems.

References

Babson SG, Behrman RE, Lesel R (1970) Fetal growth: liveborn birth weights for gestational age of white, middle class infants. Pediatrics 45:937–944

Bertalanffy FD, LeBlond CP (1953) The continuous renewal of the two types of alveolar cells in the lung of the rat. Anat Rec 115:515–541

Carson BS, Philipps AF, Simmons MA, Battaglia FC, Meschia G (1980) Effects of a sustained insulin infusion upon glucose uptake and oxygenation of the ovine fetus. Pediatr Res 14:147–152

Clements JA (1957) Surface tension of lung extracts. Proc Soc Exp Biol Med 95:170–172

D'Ercole AJ (1987) Somatomedins/insulin-like growth factors: relationship to insulin and diabetes. In: Gabbe SG, Oh W (eds) Infant of the diabetic mother; report of the 93rd Ross Conference on Pediatric Research. Ross Laboratories, Columbus, Ohio, pp 50–60

Driscoll SG, Benirschke K, Curtis GW (1960) Neonatal deaths among infants of diabetic mothers. Am J Dis Child 100:818–835

Farquhar JW (1962) Birth weight and the survival of babies of diabetic women. Arch Dis Child 37:321–329

Fee BA, Weil WB Jr (1963) Body composition of infants of diabetic mothers by direct analysis. Ann NY Acad Sci 110:869–897

Freinkel N, Metzger BE (1979) Pregnancy as a tissue culture experience: the critical implications of maternal metabolism for fetal development. Ciba Found Symp 63:3–28

Gabbe SG (1987) Antepartum fetal surveillance in the pregnancy complicated by diabetes mellitus. In: Gabbe SG, Oh W (eds) Infant of the diabetic mother; report of the 93rd Ross Conference on Pediatric Research. Ross Laboratories, Columbus, Ohio, pp 86–95

Gellis SS, Hsia DYY (1959) The infant of the diabetic mother. Am J Dis Child 97:1–41

Glasser SW, Korfhagen TR, Weaver TE et al. (1988) cDNA, deduced polypeptide structure and chromosomal assignment of human pulmonary surfactant proteolipid, SPL (pVal). J Biol Chem 263:9–12

Gluck L, Kulovich MW (1973) Lecithin/sphingomyelin ratios in amniotic fluid in normal and abnormal pregnancy. Am J Obstet Gynecol 115:539–546

Gluckman PD, Butler JH, Comline R et al. (1987) The effects of pancreatectomy on plasma concentrations of insulin-like growth factors 1 and 2 in the sheep fetus. J Dev Physiol 9:79–88

Gruppuso PA, Susa JB, Sehgal P, Frank BN, Schwartz R (1987) Metabolism and placental transfer of ^{125}I-proinsulin and ^{125}I-tyrosylated c-peptide in the pregnant rhesus monkey. J Clin Invest 80:1132–1137

Gruppuso PA, Frank BH, Schwartz R (1988) Binding of proinsulin and proinsulin conversion intermediates to human placental IGF-1 receptors. J Clin Endocrinol Metab (in press)

Hallman M, Teramo K (1979) Amniotic fluid phospholipid profile as a predictor of fetal maturity in diabetic pregnancies. Obstet Gynecol 54:703–707

Hallman M, Teramo K (1981) Measurement of the lecithin/sphingomyelin ratio and phosphatidylglycerol in amniotic fluid: an accurate method for the assessment of fetal lung maturity. Br J Obstet Gynaecol 88:806–813

Hallman M, Feldman BH, Kirkpatrick E, Gluck L (1977) Absence of phosphatidylglycerol (PG) in respiratory distress syndrome in the newborn. Pediatr Res 11:714–720

Hawgood S, Benson BJ, Schilling J, Damm D, Clements JA, White RT (1987) Nucleotide and amino acid sequences of pulmonary surfactant protein SP 18 and evidence for cooperation between SP 18 and SP 28–36 in surfactant lipid adsorption. Proc Natl Acad Sci USA 84:66–70

Heinze E, Nguyen Thi C, Vetter U, Fussganger RD (1982) Interrelationship of insulin and somatomedin activity in fetal rats. Biol Neonate 41:240–245

Hill DJ, Milner RDG (1980) Increased somatomedin and cartilage metabolic activity in rabbit fetuses injected with insulin in utero. Diabetologia 19:143–147

King KC, Adam PAJ, Laskowski DE, Schwartz R (1971) Sources of fatty acids in the newborn. Pediatrics 47:192–198

King RJ, Clements JA (1972) Surface active materials from dog lung. II. Composition and physiological correlations. Am J Physiol 223:715–726

Liggins GC (1969) Premature delivery of foetal lambs infused with glucocorticoids. J Endocrinol 45:515–523

Liggins GC, Howie RN (1972) A controlled trial of antepartum glucocorticoid treatment for prevention of the respiratory distress syndrome in premature infants. Pediatrics 50:515–525

Macklin MT (1944) Diagnosis of Rh incompatibility, especially by microscopic appearances; its relation to syndrome formerly diagnosed as erythroblastosis. J Pediatr 25:533–554

Mead J, Whittenberger JL, Radford EP (1957) Surfact tension as a factor in pulmonary volume-pressure hysteresis. J Appl Physiol 10:191–196

Miller HC (1946) The effect of diabetic and prediabetic pregnancies on the fetus and newborn infant. J Pediatr 29:455–461

Milley JR, Rosenberg AA, Philipps AF, Morteni RA, Jones MD Jr, Simmons MA (1984) The effect of insulin on ovine fetal oxygen extraction. Am J Obstet Gynecol 149:673–678

Milley JR, Papacostas JS, Tabata BK (1986) Effect of insulin on uptake of metabolic substrates by the sheep fetus. Am J Physiol 251:E349–E356

Milner RDG (1979) Amino acids and beta cell growth in structure and function. In: Merkatz IR, Adam PAJ (eds) The diabetic pregnancy: a perinatal perspective. Grune and Stratton, New York, pp 145–153

Mimouni F, Miodovnik M, Siddiqi TA et al. (1986) Neonatal polycythemia in infants of insulin dependent diabetic mothers. Obstet Gynecol 68:370–372

Naeye RL (1965) Infants of diabetic mothers: a quantitative morphologic study. Pediatrics 35:980–988

Pederson J (1977) The pregnant diabetic and her newborn, 2nd edn. Williams and Wilkins, Baltimore

Pedersen J, Brandstrup E (1956) Foetal mortality in pregnant diabetics; strict control of diabetes with conservative obstetrical management. Lancet I:607–610

Persson B, Gentz J (1984) Follow-up of children of insulin-dependent and gestational diabetic mothers. Neuropsychological outcome. Acta Paediatr Scand 73:349–358

Phillips AF, Dubin JW, Matty PJ, Raye JR (1982a) Arterial hypoxemia and hyperinsulinemia in the chronically hyperglycemic fetal lamb. Pediatr Res 16:653–658

Philipps AF, Widness JA, Garcia JF, Raye JR, Schwartz R (1982b) Erythropoietin elevation in the chronically hyperglycemic fetal lamb. Proc Soc Exp Biol Med 170:42–47

Philipps AF, Porte PJ, Stabinsky S, Rosenkrantz TS, Raye JR (1984) Effects of chronic fetal hyperglycemia upon oxygen consumption in the ovine uterus and conceptus. J Clin Invest 74:279–286

Philipps AF, Rosenkrantz TS, Raye JR (1985a) Consequences of perturbations of fetal fuels in ovine pregnancy. Diabetes 34:32–35

Philipps AF, Rosenkrantz TS, Porte PJ, Raye JR (1985b) The effects of chronic fetal hyperglycemia on substrate uptake by the ovine fetus and conceptus. Pediatr Res 19:659–666

Polonsky KS, Rubenstein AH (1984) C-peptide as a measure of the secretion and hepatic extraction of insulin. Pitfalls and limitations. Diabetes 33:486–494

Robert MF, Neff RK, Hubbell JP, Taeusch HW, Avery ME (1976) Association between maternal diabetes and the respiratory distress syndrome in the newborn. N Engl J Med 294:357–360

Schwartz R, Susa JB (1980) Fetal macrosomia: animal models. Diabetes Care 3:430–432

Schwartz R, Teramo KA (1987) Primary hyperinsulinemia and macrosomia in infants of diabetic mothers. In: Gabbe SG, Oh W (eds) Infant of the diabetic mother, report of the 93rd Ross Conference on Pediatric Research. Ross Laboratories, Columbus, Ohio, pp 40–46

Shannon K, Davis LC, Kitzmiller JL et al. (1986) Erythropoiesis in infants of diabetic mothers. Pediatr Res 20:161–165

Singer DB (1986) Hepatic erythropoiesis in infants of diabetic mothers. Pediatr Pathol 5:471–479

Susa JB, McCormick KL, Widness JA et al. (1979) Chronic hyperinsulinemia in the fetal rhesus monkey. Effects on fetal growth and composition. Diabetes 28:1058–1063

Susa JB, Widness JA, Hintz R, Liu R, Sehgal P, Schwartz R (1984) Somatomedins and insulin in diabetic pregnancies: effects on fetal macrosomia in the human and rhesus monkey. J Clin Endocrinol Metab 58:1099–1105

Teramo KA, Widness JA, Clemons GK, Voutilainen P, McKinlay S, Schwartz R (1987) Amniotic fluid erythropoietin correlates with umbilical plasma erythropoietin in normal and abnormal pregnancy. Obstet Gynecol 69:710–716

Warburton D (1983a) Chronic hyperglycemia reduces surface active material flux in tracheal fluid of fetal lambs. J Clin Invest 71:550–555

Warburton D (1983b) Chronic hyperglycemia with secondary hyperinsulinemia inhibits the maturational response of fetal lamb lungs to cortisol. J Clin Invest 72:433–440

Weaver TE, Ross G, Daugherty C, Whitsett JA (1986) Synthesis of surfactant-associated protein, 35 000 daltons, in fetal lung. J Appl Physiol 61:694–700

White P (1974) Diabetes mellitus in pregnancy. Clin Perinatol 1:331–347

Whitsett JA, Hull WM, Ohning B, Ross G, Weaver JE (1986) Immunological identification of a pulmonary surfactant associated protein of molecular weight = 6000 daltons. Pediatr Res 20:744–749

Widness JA, Susa JB, Garcia JF et al. (1981) Increased erythropoiesis and elevated erythropoietin in infants born to diabetic mothers and in hyperinsulinemic rhesus fetuses. J Clin Invest 67:637–642

Widness JA, Teramo KA, Clemons GK, Voutilainen P, McKinlay SM, Schwartz R (1987) Direct association of maternal glycemic control (HbA$_{1c}$) with fetal erythropoietin (Ep) in diabetic pregnancy. Pediatr Res 21:349A

32. Status at 4–5 Years in 90 Children of Insulin-Dependent Diabetic Mothers

Minna Bloch Petersen

Introduction

This study of children of insulin-dependent diabetic mothers is part of an extensive follow-up study comprising two other groups: children born with low and very low birthweights, and a comparison group. The purpose of the study of the children of diabetic mothers was threefold, namely to continue monitoring the outcome of these children, to get a more detailed description of their psychomotor development and finally to compare their outcome with that of the children of non-diabetic mothers. In this chapter only some of these aspects will be presented.

Material and Methods

All the children were born between October 1980 and January 1983 at the Obstetrical Department, Rigshospitalet, Copenhagen. All 90 children born to insulin-dependent diabetic mothers entered the study. The children of the comparison group were randomly selected using the following criteria: (a) they were born after 37 completed weeks of gestation with birthweight above 2500 g; (b) their Apgar scores at 1 min were equal to or above 8 and at 5 min were above 8; and (c) there was no evidence of neonatal illness. The comparison group consisted of 115 children. The children in the low birthweight group were randomly selected also among newborn with birthweights between 1501 g and 2300 g, giving a study population of 166. All infants of diabetic mothers and all low birthweight infants were admitted to the neonatal intensive care unit.

When the children were 4–5 years old an invitation to attend for examination and a questionnaire (150 questions) were mailed to the families. All children were seen by one psychologist (RK) and one paediatrician (MBP). Data on children lost to follow-up were obtained from the general practitioner. A two-stage pilot study was carried out.

On the day of examination a number of investigations were made. The psychological test used was the McCarthy Scales of Children's Abilities (McCarthy 1972), a battery of 18 tests grouped for scoring into six ability scales. Three scales – Verbal, Perceptual–Performance and Quantitative – are combined in the General Cognitive Scale for determination of the General Cognitive Index, which is equivalent to IQ in other tests. The two remaining scales are Memory and Motor. A physical examination including anthropomorphic measures and blood pressure was performed. At the slightest doubt about vision (visual acuity assessed with Österberg's pictures) and hearing, the children were referred to an ophthalmologist and/or audiologist. Data were obtained on all children as to visual and hearing impairment. The neurological examination consisted of 36 items of which 23 were given a qualitative score from 1 to 3, 3 being given for a good and steady performance. The total score was registered as a Qualitative Motor Development Score. The items chosen were partly from a test developed by Stott et al. (1972) and partly from Touwen (1979). These tested coordination, fine and gross motor performance and balance. The Grooved Pegboard Test is one of four items in a Motor Steadiness Battery (Klöve and Matthews, personal communication). The total time in seconds the child spent on placing 10 pegs, one hand at a time, was registered. For consistent application, procedural details pertaining to each item of the neurological evaluation were defined in a manual. The 3½–4 h visit by the child was ended with a comprehensive semi-structured interview (about 45 min) of the parent(s). Both the psychologist and the paediatrician took part in the interview. The information so obtained, combined with the observations, gave an acceptable amount of insight to evaluate the child.

When the clinical study was completed the hospital records were studied to collect neonatal and maternal data.

Data Analysis. To compare incidences the Fisher exact test and chi-square corrected for continuity were used. The significance levels of difference between two means were determined by the *t*-test.

Results

Seventy-six children of diabetic mothers (84.4%), 92 children of non-diabetic mothers (80%) who constituted the comparison group and 139 low birthweight children of non-diabetic mothers (83.7%) were seen at mean ages of 54.9 months, 53.1 months and 52.6 months respectively. Some family and social background factors are presented in Table 32.1. More children in the diabetic group came from the lower social classes than did children in the comparison group ($P<0.025$), whereas the social class distribution of the diabetic group did not differ from that of the low birthweight group. In all three groups there were more families in the two upper social classes compared to the social class distribution of Danish families: 16% (I+II), 30% (III), 52% (IV+V) and 2% (unclassifiable) (Enevoldsen et al. 1980).

Table 32.1. Family and social background factors of children of diabetic and non-diabetic mothers. Results expressed as means (ranges) and percentages

	Diabetic study group	Non-diabetic study groups	
		Low birthweight	Normal birthweight
No. of families	76	139	92
Maternal age (years)	31.2 (24–41)	32.9 (22–47)	31.9 (23–44)
Education:			
Years of school			
mother	10.2 (7–13)	10.1 (7–13)	10.4 (7–13)
father	9.4	9.9	10.4
Years after school			
mother	2.2 (0–8)	3.3 (0–13)	3.4 (0–10)
father	3.1	4.0	4.8
Social class (%):			
I + II	25.0	29.5	39.1
III	23.7	23.0	28.3
IV + V	50.0	47.5	31.5
Unclassifiable	1.3		1.1
One-parent family (%)	11.8	11.4	15.7
Parents divorced (%)	21.1	19.3	21.7

Table 32.2. Status at 4–5 years of age in children of diabetic mothers and normal birthweight children of non-diabetic mothers

	Children of diabetic mothers	Children of non-diabetic mothers
No. of children	76	92
Mean age in months (range)	54.9 (44–70)	53.1 (48–60)
Gestational age ± SD, mean completed weeks (range)	35.9 ± 2.2 (27–39)	39.7 ± 1.2 (37–42)
Birthweight in g ± SD (range)	3089 ± 825 (1205–4600)	3585 ± 450 (2720–4700)
Normal physical examination, no. (%)	61 (80.3)	83 (90.2)
Congenital malformations, no. (%)[a]	5 (5.6)	1 (0.9)
Normal ophthalmological examination, no. (%)	60 (78.9)	83 (90.2)
Squint, no. (%)	8 (10.5)	3 (3.3)
Blind, no.	1	0
Normal neurological evaluation, no. (%)	35 (46.1)[b]	59 (64.1)
Cerebral palsy, no.	2	0
Hearing loss, severe, no.	1	0
Major handicap, no. (%)[a]	5 (5.6)	1 (0.9)
Intellectually subnormal, no. (%)	11 (14.5)[c]	3 (3.3)
Deviant behaviour and few emotional resources, no. (%)	5 (6.6)	11 (11.9)

[a] Including information obtained.
[b] $P<0.05$.
[c] $P<0.025$.

Table 32.2 shows status in the children of diabetic mothers and in the children of the comparison group at follow-up. The mean gestational age and mean birthweight of the 139 low birthweight children was 34.2 completed weeks (±2.9, range 29–42) and 1955 g (±236, range 1515–2300 g), respectively. More low birthweight children had normal physical (84.2%) and ophthalmological (88.5%) examinations than did the children of diabetic mothers. The three groups, however, did not differ significantly. None of the children of diabetic mothers had developed diabetes.

The children described as being neurologically normal had no impairment of vision or hearing, had a normal neurological examination including no soft neurological signs and the Qualitative Motor Development Score was equal to or above −1 SD of the scoring mean of the comparison group. The diabetic group did not differ significantly from the low birthweight group (50.8% normal).

Subnormal intellect was defined here as General Cognitive Index being equal to or below −2 SD of the scoring mean of the comparison group. The children of diabetic mothers did not differ significantly from the low birthweight children, 13 (9.4%) of whom were intellectually subnormal. The following congenital malformations were found in the diabetic group: two had had anorectal atresia – one had perineal fistula and the other had hypospadias; another was operated on for cleft palate; ventricular septal defect was found in one child; and hypertrophy of the right leg and foot was found in another. Only one of these children had had a low birthweight (light for gestational age) and two were born prematurely (35 weeks). In 5.4% of the low birthweight children congenital malformations were found.

The major handicaps found in five children of diabetic mothers included blindness from retrolental fibroplasia in a girl. A hearing aid was used by one mature born boy; severe perinatal asphyxia was the most likely cause of the sensorineural hearing loss. Spastic diplegia and epilepsy were seen in one girl and mild to moderate spastic tetraplegia was seen in another. Both girls were born prematurely (29 and 32 weeks) and the latter was intellectually subnormal. Paralysis of the right arm was reported in one girl. She had sustained a severe lesion of the right brachial plexus during a very complicated birth. In the low birthweight group 4.2% had major handicaps.

Table 32.3 gives the results of the McCarthy Scales of Children's Abilities, the Qualitative Motor Developmental Score and the Grooved Pegboard Test. Transforming the resuts into z-scores of the scoring *mean* of the children in the comparison group thereby indicating deviations from a norm, the following were the results of the children of diabetic mothers with the numbers in parentheses giving the z-scores of the low birthweight children: General Cognitive Index −0.45 (−0.54), Verbal −0.10 (−0.32), Perceptual–Performance −0.52 (−0.46), Quantitative −0.59 (−0.32), Memory −0.07 (−0.33), Motor −0.61 (−0.51), Qualitative Motor Development Score −0.70 (−0.70) and Pegboard −0.27 (−0.51). The percentage of children of diabetic mothers performing well was equal to that of the children of the comparison group, whereas the percentage of poorly performing children was very similar to that of the low birthweight children (Table 32.4).

In all, 22 (29%) of the examined children of the diabetic mothers had problems which later may give difficulties in school. Eleven were intellectually subnormal, i.e. they may need some remedial instruction at some time during their schooling. Ten of the 11 children, including the girl with spastic tetraplegia, also scored

Table 32.3. Results of McCarthy Scales of Children's Abilities, Qualitative Motor Development Score (QDS) and Pegboard (expressed in seconds) at 4–5 years of age in 76 children of diabetic mothers and 92 children of non-diabetic mothers. Results expressed as mean ± SD and (range)

	Children of diabetic mothers	Children of non-diabetic mothers[a]
General Cognitive Index[b]	109.8 ± 13.7 (78–137)	115.5 ± 12.7 (84–150)
Verbal	54.2 ± 8.1 (40–76)	55.2 ± 9.9 (31–78)
Perceptual–Performance	58.5 ± 10.2 (22–75)	62.7 ± 8.1 (44–78)
Quantitative[c]	52.3 ± 7.4 (34–69)	56.5 ± 7.1 (40–75)
Memory	47.9 ± 7.3 (35–70)	48.6 ± 9.4 (31–78)
Motor[c]	45.0 ± 9.1 (22–61)	50.3 ± 8.7 (33–73)
QDS[c]	52.5 ± 7.8 (25–65)	56.2 ± 5.3 (41–66)
Pegboard	126.0 (61–395)	112.0 (69–213)

[a] Normal birthweight children.
[b] $P<0.01$.
[c] $P<0.001$.

Table 32.4. Children with scores at or above the scoring median of children born mature with normal birthweight to non-diabetic mothers.[a] Scoring was within three fields: General Cognitive, Qualitative Motor Development and Pegboard. Results expressed as numbers (percentages) of children

	Children of diabetic mothers	Children of non-diabetic mothers	
		Low birthweight[b]	Normal birthweight
Below in all three fields	20 (27.4)	43 (31.6)	16 (17.4)
At or above in one field	25 (34.2)	38 (27.9)	23 (25.0)
At or above in two fields	10 (13.7)	33 (24.3)	29 (31.5)
At or above in all three fields	15 (20.5)	15 (11.0)	17 (18.5)

[a] Children with definite handicap excluded.
[b] Low birthweight: 1501–2300 g.

poorly in Qualitative Motor Development. Nine other children scored poorly in Qualitative Motor Development, five of whom, including the boy with a hearing aid, had other problems such as excessive mirror movements, subnormal vision, squint or poor articulation. One child had excessive mirror movements and poor articulation and finally the girl with spastic diplegia scored poorly in Qualitative Motor Development.

In the children of non-diabetic mothers, 44 (31.7%) of the low birthweight children and 11 (12%) of the normal birthweight children i.e. the comparison group, had problems which later may give difficulties in school. The diabetic group differed significantly from the comparison group ($0.01<P<0.025$).

In evaluating the results of the children of diabetic mothers, those doing well and those doing poorly, we found no association with maternal White's class and metabolic compensation in pregnancy; nor did we find any association with the presence of pre-, peri- or neonatal asphyxia. Birthweight below 2400 g and gestational age below 37 completed weeks were significantly correlated with a poor performance ($P<0.05$ and $P<0.01$, respectively). Five (22.7%) of the children of diabetic mothers having problems had been mechanically ventilated compared to three (5.6%) of the children without problems, i.e. in all, 10.5% of the children of diabetic mothers compared with 18% of the low birthweight children had been treated in a respirator.

Three of the children in the diabetic group were classified as intellectually subnormal, with few resources and no neonatal problems. Their parents had only 8 years of school and no further education and belonged to social class V.

We have the following information on children lost to follow-up. One diabetic mother gave birth to a normal stillborn baby in the 32nd week of pregnancy. Three of the remaining 13 children of diabetic mothers had major problems: one boy had recurrent pneumonia with atelectasis secondary to bronchiectasis, retarded language development and short attention span; one boy had a behaviour disorder and delayed development; and the girl with paralysis of the right arm, mentioned above, had no major development problems. Another two girls had delayed speech and language development. Five children were normal. Of these children only two were of low birthweight (2025 g and 2100 g), two were born after 34 completed weeks and two had been mechanically ventilated. Two of 27 low birthweight children had major problems and two had minor problems. Fifteen low birthweight children were reported to be normal. From the comparison group one of 23 children had delayed psychomotor development and 17 were reported normal.

We have insufficient information on three children of diabetic mothers, on eight low birthweight children and on five from the comparison group. All children were alive and had no major problems at age 9 months – 2 years.

Discussion

At our hospital the obstetrical management in diabetic pregnancy as described by Mølsted-Pedersen and Kühl (1986) has resulted in a substantial decrease in perinatal mortality from 12%–13% in the late 1960s to a total of 2% in the period January 1981 to June 1985 and in this study 1.1%. In Denmark the perinatal mortality of newborns weighing 1000 g or more was 0.77% in 1981 and 0.74% in 1982 (Knudsen and Frimodt-Møller 1987). The incidence of congenital malformations has also declined, although less markedly. In this study the incidence was 5.6%, still two to four times the incidence in Danish children as a whole, but equal to the incidence in the low birthweight children in this study.

Whether or not the obstetrical efforts also have had a positive effect on the long-term prognosis for children of diabetic mothers is not an easy question to answer. In 1980 Freinkel discussed the subject of fuel-mediated teratogenesis and suggested that the concept of "behavioural teratology" (Werboff and Gottlieb 1963) be extended to include potential effects upon the brain via quantitatively or qualitatively altered fuel mixtures during the critical periods of fetal brain development (Dobbing and Sands 1979). Freinkel (1980) asked the question if "lesions" arise, do they persist into childhood or even later?

In a recent study we have shown that children who were smaller than normal in very early diabetic pregnancy performed worse at 4 years of age in developmental evaluation than children who had had normal early fetal growth in diabetic pregnancy (Petersen et al. 1988). The growth-retarded fetuses also had an increased risk of malformations (Pedersen and Mølsted-Pedersen 1981). These results agree with Freinkel's suggestion of considering fuel-mediated teratogenesis in broader terms than only organ teratology.

In the present study the overall impression is that concerning general health (with the exception of the five children with major handicaps), behaviour and emotional resources, the children of diabetic mothers do not differ from normal birthweight children of non-diabetic mothers, whereas children of diabetic mothers functionally resemble the low birthweight children who form a heterogeneous group considered to be at risk for their development.

Unlikely to be influenced by social conditions, the three non-cognitive factors, namely the Grooved Pegboard Test, the McCarthy Scales and the Qualitative Motor Development Score, may indicate some type of neurological immaturity or sequelae after some adverse influence on the development of the fetal brain, as both the diabetic and the low birthweight group scored poorly or very poorly ($P<0.001$) in these items compared to the normal birthweight children. In a prospective follow-up study of very low birthweight children Michelsson and Noronen (1983) found a significant correlation between the neurodevelopmental score at 5 and at 9 years of age. When comparing the children at 9 years of age with matched controls Michelsson et al. (1984) also found a significant correlation between the Test of Motor Impairment (Stott et al. 1972), school achievement and IQ. She suggested that an organic lesion which causes motor disturbances also is responsible for the dysfunction in learning and behaviour. If this statement holds we can expect the children of the diabetic mothers, who scored poorly in the three non-cognitive areas mentioned, to have school difficulties later.

In our study the mean General Cognitive Index (IQ) of the children of diabetic mothers differed significantly ($P<0.01$) from the mean of the normal birthweight children of non-diabetic mothers (comparison group). Part of, but not the entire difference may be explained by the difference in social class distribution. The mean IQ of all three groups of children as well as the one found in the two-stage pilot study was above the mean of the test. The same unexpectedly high mean IQ was found by Persson and Gentz (1984) and they concluded that children of diabetic mothers are intellectually normal. They did not have a comparison group which could explain the disagreement between their conclusion and ours. We found 14.5% of the children of diabetic mothers to be intellectually subnormal, and excluding three children from poor social backgrounds the percentage was 10.5%. This result is in line with those found by Stehbens et al. (1977) and Yssing (1975). Yssing also found 10% to have reading difficulties. Churchill et al. (1969) also reported that children of diabetic mothers have significantly lower IQs than matched controls at 4 years of age. The high mean IQ in the present study may be explained by either or both of the following factors: (a) the family social class distribution was skewed towards the upper social classes compared with the general family social class distribution (Persson and Gentz did not report on social class in their study); (b) the mean IQ seems to increase in the Scandinavian preschool and school children as mentioned by Persson and Gentz. Cummins and Norrish (1980) found a normal distribution of full-scale IQs, which seemed consistent with the distribution of parental social class which was similar to that in the general population. They found only two (4.2%) children to be intellectually subnormal (IQ less than 75). It would have been interesting if they had had a comparison group. All works referred to have included children of gestational diabetic mothers.

In all, we found 29% of the examined children of diabetic mothers and 30.8% of the children lost to follow-up to have problems indicating cerebral dysfunction which are findings similar to those of Yssing (1975) who found 36% of the children of diabetic mothers had signs of cerebral dysfunction (major and minor). Our battery of tests and items for examination/evaluation were, however, more extensive than those of Yssing. The difference between our results and those of Yssing may, therefore, be greater than the percentages indicate, i.e. more children seen by Yssing might have had signs of cerebral dysfunction.

Neither we, Persson, nor Cummins found any obvious relationship between IQ of the children and maternal White's class and metabolic compensation. Like Yssing (1975) and Stehbens et al. (1977) we found low birthweight to be related to poor performance and the latter also to be related to low gestational age. Mechanical ventilation as an indicator of neonatal illness seemed related to adverse outcome.

Our observations indicate that children of insulin-dependent diabetic mothers should still be considered as a group of children who risk psychomotor developmental problems. Similar to the low birthweight children, the children of diabetic mothers represent a heterogeneous group. The poor performance within the three non-cognitive fields (the Grooved Pegboard Test, the McCarthy Motor and the Qualitative Motor Development Score) suggests a neurological immaturity or sequelae to some adverse influence on the development of the fetal brain. The children born prematurely and/or with low birthweight are at greatest risk. Although the obstetrical efforts have resulted in a substantial decline in perinatal mortality and congenital malformations, the efforts have not, to the same degree, improved the long-term prognosis.

Acknowledgements. I wish to thank Professor B. Friis-Hansen, Department of Neonatology, Rigshospitalet, for encouraging me to initiate and accomplish the extensive follow-up study and I thank also Dr. L. Mølsted-Pedersen, Department of Obstetrics and Gynaecology, Rigshospitalet, for support and assistance in the study of children of diabetic mothers. Special thanks to psychologist Rosi Kovacs for seeing all the children, to senior research fellow psychologist Hanna Munck, The Institute of Clinical Psychology, and research associate Gorm Greisen, MD, Department of Neonatology, Rigshospitalet, for their contributions in the planning of this project. The study of children of diabetic mothers was supported by grants from market gardener Ove Villiam Buhl Olesen and his wife Edith Buhl Olesen's Commemorative Fund (J No. 3555), the Danish Diabetes Association (November 1985), Queen Louise's Children's Hospital Fund (J No. 15/85) and Mrs. Karen Cathrine Pedersen's Fund (J No. 228–5/79 II). The study of children of non-diabetic mothers was supported by grants from Dagmar Marshall's Foundation and Gerda and Aage Haensch's Foundation.

The study was approved by The scientific-ethical Committee for the Municipalities of Copenhagen and Frederiksberg.

References

Churchill JA, Berendes HW, Nemore J (1969) Neuropsychological deficits in children of diabetic mothers. Am J Obstet Gynecol 105:257–268

Cummins M, Norrish M (1980) Follow-up of children of diabetic mothers. Arch Dis Child 55:259–264

Dobbing J, Sands J (1979) Comparative aspects of the brain growth spurt. Early Hum Dev 3:79–83

Enevoldsen B, Michelsen N, Friis-Hasché E, Kamper-Jørgensen F (1980) Social classification (in Danish). Ugeskr Laeger 142:544–550

Freinkel N (1980) Of pregnancy and progeny (Banting Lecture 1980). Diabetes 29:1023–1035

Knudsen LB, Frimodt-Møller B (1987) Scandinavian birth statistics (in Danish). Ugeskr Laeger 149:3291–3292

McCarthy D (1972) McCarthy scales of children's abilities. The Psychological Corporation, New York

Michelsson K, Lindahl E, Parre M, Helenius M (1984) Nine-year follow-up of infants weighing 1500 g or less at birth. Acta Paediatr Scand 73:835–841

Michelsson K, Noronen M (1983) Neurological, psychological and articulatory impairment in five-year-old children with birthweight of 2000 g or less. Eur J Pediatr 141:96–100

Mølsted-Pedersen L, Kühl C (1986) Obstetrical management in diabetic pregnancy: the Copenhagen experience. Diabetologia 29:13–16

Pedersen JF, Mølsted-Pedersen L (1981) Early fetal growth delay detected by ultrasound marks increased risk of congenital malformation in diabetic pregnancy. Br Med J 283:269–271

Persson B, Gentz J (1984) Follow-up of children of insulin-dependent and gestational diabetic mothers. Acta Paediatr Scand 73:349–358

Petersen MB, Pedersen SA, Greisen G, Pedersen JF, Mølsted-Pedersen L (1988) Early growth delay in diabetic pregnancy: relation to psychomotor development at age 4. Br Med J 296:598–600

Stehbens JA, Baker GL, Kitchell M (1977) Outcome at ages 1, 3 and 5 years of children born to diabetic women. Am J Obstet Gynecol 127:408–413

Stott DH, Moyes FA, Henderson SA (1972) A test of motor impairment. Brook Educational Publishing, Guelph, Ontario

Touwen BCL (1979) Examination of the child with minor neurological dysfunctions, 2nd edn. Spastics International Medical Publications, William Heinemann Medical Books, London (Clinics in Developmental Medicine No 71)

Werboff J, Gottlieb JS (1963) Drugs in pregnancy: behavioral teratology. Obstet Gynecol Surv 18:420–423

Yssing M (1975) Long-term prognosis of children born to mothers diabetic when pregnant. In: Camerini-Davalos RA, Cole HS (eds) Early diabetes in early life. Academic Press, New York, pp 575–586

33. Diabetes and Pregnancy: Consensus and Controversy

J. S. Skyler

On the occasion of the Third Aberdeen International Colloquium on Carbohydrate Metabolism in Pregnancy and the Newborn in 1983, I was assigned the task of summarizing the meeting and projecting future directions in this important area of scientific inquiry and medical practice. My meagre efforts at crystal ball gazing appeared in the proceedings of that notable meeting (Skyler 1984). For the Fourth Aberdeen International Colloquium on Carbohydrate Metabolism in Pregnancy and the Newborn in 1988, my assignment was to identify those areas of consensus in management strategy, and those areas in which controversy remains. The task was made somewhat easier by the appearance in the month before the Colloquium of the first full report of the US Diabetes in Early Pregnancy Study in the *New England Journal of Medicine* (Mills et al. 1988). It is not that the participants necessarily needed this trigger to engender controversy. This was a vocal enough group in its own right. Nonetheless, this controversial report focused the debate rather sharply on at least the issue of congenital malformations.

In the time between the last two Aberdeen Colloquia, the Second Chicago Conference on Gestational Diabetes was held and was reported in a supplement to *Diabetes* (Freinkel 1985). Although it might have been projected that this Conference would have yielded consensus on several key issues, particularly screening approaches and diagnostic criteria, it was clear from the 1988 Aberdeen Colloquium that a number of areas of controversy yet remain, with some clear differences being demarcated by the Atlantic Ocean. In spite of extensive international participation in the Chicago meeting, the meeting "consensus" appears to have gained widespread acceptance principally in the North American continent. Thus, the issues of screening, diagnostic criteria and classification of gestational diabetes continue to linger as areas of controversy, in addition to well-known controversies concerning diet and insulin therapies.

In this commentary, I will divide my remarks into two main sections, one dealing with issues relating to pregestational diabetes, the other dealing with issues relating to gestational diabetes. I will pay particular attention to those areas which engendered the most discussion at the Aberdeen Colloquium, and will cite data presented there.

Pregestational Diabetes

Therapeutic Strategies

Over the past decade, there has been a dramatic change in the management approach to diabetes during pregnancy and to the management of such pregnancies as well. The introduction of patient self-monitoring of blood glucose (SMBG) launched the current era of meticulous glycaemic control during pregnancy without prolonged hospitalization. The attainment of excellent glycaemic control has facilitated permitting diabetic women to continue their gestation to term and have spontaneous vaginal deliveries. The previously common problem of intrauterine demise during late gestation has nearly vanished. Overall perinatal survival rates are approaching those of healthy women. The classical cherubic IDM baby today is a rarity in the nurseries of major centres. Neonatal complications are dwindling markedly. Optimism prevails, and the young woman with diabetes no longer needs to fear pregnancy.

One aspect of treatment that remains controversial is the use of continuous subcutaneous insulin infusion (CSII) during pregnancy. In reviewing the Copenhagen experience in which 43 women were randomly allocated either to CSII or to multiple daily insulin injections (MDII) prior to conception, Kuhl (Chap. 15) noted that pregnancy outcome was identical in both groups. The only differences seen were that in the CSII group free insulin levels were higher and beta-hydroxybutyrate levels were lower. In an earlier randomized series comparing CSII and MDII during 22 pregnancies, both glycaemic control and pregnancy outcome also were the same (Coustan et al. 1986). Similar findings were also reported in a prospective but non-randomized Israeli series of 52 pregnancies (Dicker et al. 1987). Thus, it would seem that to date no unique advantages have been demonstrated with CSII during pregnancy. On the other hand, the use of CSII during pregnancy carries a unique risk not shared with MDII, that of potential catheter occlusion or pump failure, with consequent interruption of insulin delivery. Because there is no subcutaneous depot of insulin during CSII, interruption of insulin delivery imposes the risk of diabetic ketoacidosis. During pregnancy, a state of "accelerated starvation", there is the possibility of rapid development of ketoacidosis, and its potentially disastrous consquences. For this reason, it would seem to me that CSII should be used during pregnancy only in conjunction with very frequent blood glucose monitoring (no more than 4–6 h between measurements) and careful attention paid to avoid interruption of insulin delivery. At the current time, in my opinion, the usual course during pregnancy should be the more prudent approach of MDII.

Congenital Malformations

Does preconceptional or early gestational glycaemic control lessen the risk of congenital malformations in infants of diabetic mothers? Apparent earlier consensus has been converted to renewed controversy on this issue, due to the publication of a report of the findings of the US Diabetes in Early Pregnancy Study (DIEPS) (Mills et al. 1988). Based on the elegant work of the Upsalla group in their rat model (reviewed by Erikkson in this volume) and the early human reports of Fuhrmann et al. (1983, 1984), Miller et al. (1981) and Steel (1985), most authorities had come to accept the tenets: (a) that hyperglycaemia early in gestation is a critical determinant of risk of congenital malformations, and (b) that meticulous glycaemic control early in gestation, or better still preconception, lessens that risk. Yet the DIEPS report was titled "Lack of Relation of Increased Malformation Rates in Infants of Diabetic Mothers to Glycemic Control during Organogenesis" (Mills et al. 1988). That report, appearing just a few weeks before the Aberdeen Colloquium, provoked lively debate at the Colloquium, triggered a flurry of letters to the editor and was rebuffed by a *Lancet* editorial as having a misleading title and being a statistical aberration (*Lancet* 1988). The DIEPS report found a malformation rate of 4.9% amongst 347 diabetic women enrolled with 21 d of conception, in contrast to a rate of 9.0% amongst 279 diabetic women enrolled beyond that time frame, a highly significant difference which supports the concept of early enrolment. On the other hand, the malformation rate in the early enrolment group was nonetheless significantly greater than the 2.1% rate for 389 non-diabetic control women. This led the DIEPS investigators to perform some post hoc analyses amongst diabetic women in the early enrolment group, comparing glycaemic control in those women having babies with malformations to that in those women having babies without malformations. This analysis failed to detect differences in glycaemic control and led to the unfortunate title of the paper. Yet, such a conclusion is unwarranted. First, the analyses were post hoc and not the primary aim of the study, which was to compare malformation rates between the three groups. Second, the appearance of malformations is a low-frequency event. In spite of exposure to potential teratogens, only a small minority of exposed women will deliver infants who manifest malformations. Thus, the group without malformations would be expected to include the vast majority of women who were exposed to any potential risk factor. This makes such subgroup analysis impossible. Third, no specific attempt was made to implement meticulous glycaemic control per se, or to manage glycaemia in a uniform manner. As a consequence, excellent glycaemic control was not achieved. The 50th percentile for mean plasma glucose was approximately 200 mg/dl (11.1 mmol/l) in the early-entry subjects while at least 193 of the 347 women (56%) in that group had glycosylated haemoglobin levels at least 2 SD above the mean for non-diabetic women. This could clearly account for the difference in malformation rates between early-entry diabetic women and control subjects. Thus, as noted in the *Lancet* editorial, "the findings are in complete accord with expectations", i.e. that one would expect that if glycaemia contributes to malformations, there would be a higher malformation rate in late-entry than early-entry diabetic women, and that the malformation rate in both groups would be higher than in non-diabetic control women.

The DIEPS Study represents the first prospective controlled trial of malformations that includes a non-diabetic control group, followed concomitantly and with malformations ascertained in an identical manner. Yet, it would seem worthwhile to mention a number of other studies that have examined malformation rates in diabetic women, particularly in relation to time of enrolment. In this regard, several series were reported or discussed at the Aberdeen meeting. Kuhl et al. (Chap 15) reported a malformation rate of 2.8% in 547 pregnancies in diabetic women seen in Copenhagen between 1979 and 1983 compared with good data of the Danish general population with a malformation rate of 1.7%. Thus, the rate in diabetic pregnancies is not dramatically different from that in non-diabetic pregnancies in Denmark. This is similar to Aberdeen data (this volume) that found a malformation rate of 2.9% amongst 103 pregnancies in diabetic women who were delivered between 1979 and 1986, in the setting of a background malformation rate of 2.0%. Fuhrmann's data from East Germany comprise 658 pregnancies in diabetic women who delivered between 1977 and 1983 (Fuhrmann et al. 1983, 1984). Amongst the 185 pregnancies in diabetic women enrolled prior to conception, the malformation rate was 1.1%, in comparison with a rate of 6.6% in the 473 pregnancies in women enrolled after conception, and a putative rate in the background population of 1.4%. The Edinburgh series of Steel et al. (Chap. 13), now up to 200 patients, had a malformation rate of 1.8% in 114 pregnancies in diabetic women enrolled prior to conception, compared with a rate of 10.5% in 86 pregnancies in diabetic women enrolled after conception. A similar study from Israel, reported by Goldman et al. (1986), found a malformation rate of 9.6% amongst 31 pregnancies in diabetic women enrolled late, compared with no malformations in 44 pregnancies in women enrolled prior to conception [and still no malformations in the next eight such pregnancies (Dicker et al. 1987)]. Tamas et al. (1985), from Hungary, found a malformation rate of 3.3% in 92 pregnancies in diabetic women enrolled prior to conception, and a rate of 7.1% in 479 pregnancies in diabetic women enrolled postconception. Further evidence of the importance of early control is gleaned from the UK Confidential Enquiry Study, reported by Lowy et al. (1983), in which the malformation rate was 5.0% amongst 460 diabetic women who had first-trimester blood glucose determinations, versus a rate of 10.2% amongst 313 diabetic women who did not have first-trimester blood glucose values recorded. Moreover, a number of studies have found a relationship between increased rates of malformation and higher levels of glycohaemoglobin in the first trimester (Miller et al. 1981; Ylinen et al. 1984; Hare et al. 1988). In Table 33.1, I have tabulated the data from the five series that have compared early and late enrolment. Inspection of the data clearly supports the desirability of planned pregnancies and early enrolment prior to conception. By inference, meticulous control would seem desirable. Is there a controversy? Should there be? I think not.

Table 33.1. Congenital malformation rates in offspring of diabetic women in five series comparing "early" (often preconceptional) and "late" enrolment

Study	"Early" enrolment		"Late" enrolment	
	No. of malformations	%	No. of malformations	%
DIEPS	17/347	4.9	25/279	9.0
Fuhrmann	2/185	1.1	31/473	6.6
Steel	2/114	1.8	9/86	10.5
Goldman	0/52	0	3/31	9.6
Tamas	3/92	3.3	34/479	7.1
Total	24/790	3.0	102/1348	7.6

Glycaemic Control: Targets

A related question is what degree of glycaemic control will minimize the risk of malformations. The available data give little information on this issue. In

Furhmann's series (1983, 1984), 88.3% of women in the prepregnancy group had first-trimester blood glucose profiles with mean values of 70–110 mg/dl (3.9–6.1 mmol/l). In contrast, only 20.7% of diabetic women first seen at 8–14 weeks gestation had values in that range. In that series the 50th percentile mean blood glucose was approximately 90 mg/dl (5.0 mmol/l) in the prepregnancy group, compared to 130 mg/dl (7.2 mmol/l) in the 8–14 week group. In Goldman's series (1986), first-trimester mean blood glucose was 110 ± 6.9 (SD) mg/dl (6.1 ± 0.4 mmol/l) in the preconception group, and 163 ± 10.2 mg/dl (9.0 ± 0.6 mmol/l) in the late entry group. These two series had the lower malformation rates of the five series summarized in Table 33.1. These data would suggest that malformations might be minimized if the mean blood glucose profile was 110 mg/dl (6.1 mmol/l) or less. Interestingly, Landon et al. (1987) found that when they examined neonatal morbidity in infants of diabetic mothers, there was an overall frequency of infant morbidity of 33% in 43 women with a mean blood glucose of less than 110 mg/dl (6.1 mmol/l), and an overall frequency of infant morbidity of 53% in 32 women with a mean blood glucose of greater than 110 mg/dl (6.1 mmol/l). Significant differences were observed for the frequency of neonatal hypoglycaemia, macrosomia and respiratory distress syndrome. The figure of 110 mg/dl (6.1 mmol/l) as an upper limit for mean maternal blood glucose seems to keep recurring.

Yet, concern has been raised that maternal hypoglycaemia may have an adverse influence on fetal outcome. Although there are no direct data on this issue in human beings, Freinkel's group has found that maternal hypoglycaemia has embryotoxic effects in the rat, at least during a critical window of exposure (Buchanan et al. 1986). That window corresponds to days 16 to 26 of human gestation, which includes a period prior to the time of the first missed period and diagnosis of pregnancy. This calls into question the practice of "maximal tolerated insulin" therapy advocated by Roversi et al. (1980). Indeed, employing this approach, Steel et al. (Chap. 13) found that 43% of pregnant women had severe hypoglycaemia requiring intervention by another person. Others have advocated very low blood glucose targets without apparent concern about hypoglycaemia (Jovanovic and Peterson 1982). Given the information available to date, to me it would seem that we cannot be cavalier about hypoglycaemia, nor should we crusade against it in such a way as to jeopardize the message that meticulous glycaemic control indeed is quite important. A compromise position might be to aim for glucose targets similar to those in Table 33.2, while diligently striving to avert hypoglycaemia. These targets, if attained, should yield a mean blood glucose of less than 110 mg/dl (6.1 mmol/l).

Table 33.2. Blood glucose targets for use during pregnancy

	mg/dl	mmol/l
Fasting	60–90	3.3–5.0
Preprandial	60–105	3.3–5.8
1-h postprandial	70–140	3.9–7.8
2-h postprandial	60–120	3.3–6.7
Overnight (2 a.m.–4 a.m.)	60–120	3.3–6.7

Gestational Diabetes

Diagnosis

One area of continuing controversy is the criteria to be used to establish a diagnosis of gestational diabetes. The American view, supported by the National Diabetes Data Group (1979) and the American Diabetes Association (1986), is based on the criteria of O'Sullivan and Mahan (1964). Those criteria utilize a 100-g oral glucose load, and require for definitive diagnosis that two or more of the venous plasma glucose determinations meet or exceed the following: fasting, 105 mg/dl (5.8 mmol/l); 1 h, 190 mg/dl (10.6 mmol/l); 2-h, 165 mg/dl (9.2 mmol/l); 3-h, 145 mg/dl (8.1 mmol/l). [It should be noted that Carpenter and Coustan (1982) have argued that these numbers do not consider that there has been a change in methodology for glucose determination, and that the criteria should be adjusted to: fasting, 95 mg/dl (5.3 mmol/l); 1 h, 180 mg/dl (10.0 mmol/l); 2 h, 155 mg/dl (8.6 mmol/l); 3 h, 140 mg/dl (7.8 mmol/l)]. The European view is based on World Health Organization (WHO) recommendations (1980; 1985). Those criteria establish a definitive diagnosis either with a fasting plasma glucose equal to or in excess of 140 mg/dl (7.8 mmol/l) or with a venous plasma glucose determination 2 h after a 75-g oral glucose load which meets or exceeds 200 mg/dl (11.1 mmol/l). However, the WHO (1980, 1985) has recommended that impaired glucose tolerance (IGT) during pregnancy be treated the same as gestational diabetes. This effectively reduces the 2-h postglucose value from 200 mg/dl (11.1 mmol/l) to 140 mg/dl (7.8 mmol/l).

It should be obvious that some women diagnosed as having gestational diabetes by the O'Sullivan and Mahan criteria would not meet the WHO criteria, and vice versa (if we include IGT). The unique feature of the O'Sullivan criteria is that the women on whom they are based have now been followed for 22 to 28 years, as reviewed by O'Sullivan (Chap 26). The criteria not only predict pregnancy outcome, but also predict future health of the mother, particularly in regard to development of diabetes and cardiovascular disease. The issue is one of public health practice. Even if one argued that pregnancy outcome was indistinguishable whether one used O'Sullivan or WHO criteria, there may be a difference in long-term maternal health. Unfortunately, no answer can be forthcoming to this question.

There are pragmatic issues to consider. The 75-g glucose load is much more easily tolerated than the 100-g glucose load. The WHO test spans but 2 h, the O'Sullivan test takes 3 h. Even simpler is the meal test championed by the Aberdeen group and discussed in detail elsewhere in this volume. The meal test is even more palatable and better tolerated than either size glucose load and appears to be more reproducible. The test meal, consisting of 453 kcal, divided as 61% carbohydrate, 18% fat and 16% protein, is clearly more physiological than a glucose load, and thus perhaps more relevant to glucose control during pregnancy. More work is needed to establish its utility as a potential replacement for an oral glucose load.

Yet, it must be appreciated that any diagnostic criteria are somewhat arbitrary. What proportion of a given population is likely to develop gestational diabetes? This cannot be statistically defined and limited to a particular frequency of the population. Rather, it should be outcome defined, based on what level of glycaemia confers added risk to mother or fetus. For example, it should be noted that some authors have found increased risk with mild hyperglycaemia not fulfilling the O'Sullivan criteria (Skyler et al. 1980; Tallarigo et al. 1986; Langer et al. 1987). In the long run, this requires that we have more sensitive outcome measures than we generally use today. It requires that we consider confounding variables, such as ethnic background, maternal obesity and nutrition. It also implies that we have interventions that can be applied to influence outcome.

Screening

Supposedly, there is a consensus view on screening (Freinkel 1985; American Diabetes Association 1986). That consensus would hold that: (a) all pregnant women should be screened for glucose intolerance; (b) those not identified prior to the 24th week of gestation should have a 50-g oral glucose screening test between weeks 24 and 28, given without regard to time of last meal or time of day; (c) a venous plasma glucose of 140 mg/dl (7.8 mmol/l) or more, taken 1 h after such a load, signifies need for a full diagnostic glucose tolerance test. In Aberdeen, Gabbe (Chap. 28) reported that approximately 90% of perinatal obstetrical specialists in the United States are actually following the consensus view in their practices. He noted, however, that in a survey in the Los Angeles area, only a minority of general obstetricians had implemented universal screening, and only a small minority were using the 50-g oral glucose screening test. Thus, in the United States, there seems to be a wide discrepancy between specialists and generalists concerning screening practices.

From the discussions in Aberdeen, it would appear that outside the United States, even the experts have not yet formed a consensus. Thus, in Copenhagen, rather than universal screening, the approach is to base further testing on the fasting plasma glucose and the presence of potential features of diabetes. Others use potential features of diabetes alone, glycosylated serum protein determinations, random plasma glucose levels or a short oral glucose tolerance test. Some have proposed that a meal tolerance test could be used at once for both screening and diagnosis. No doubt it would be nice to be able to screen on the basis of a single venous sample without any kind of loading. The hope was that glycosylated serum protein or fructosamine might qualify as being simple, convenient, inexpensive and with both sufficiently high sensitivity and specificity as to be able to serve as the optimal screening test. To date, however, these assessments have met with mixed reviews, and generally lacked the high sensitivity and specificity which has been found with the 50-g oral glucose load. Thus, this must remain as the standard until sufficient data emerge to warrant a different consensus.

Classification

Over the past several years, many authors have finally abandoned trying to apply the White classification of diabetes during pregnancy to gestational diabetes. Initially, White (1949) had not included gestational diabetes in her classification, which looked at the influence on pregnancy outcome of duration of diabetes and presence of diabetic complications. Unfortunately, in later papers White sometimes did include women with gestational diabetes in her classification. This was not logical, since such women obviously had no known prepregnancy diabetes duration nor had they diabetic complications. Thus, the determining variables of interest were not present. Later, White recognized this and together with Hare reaffirmed that gestational diabetes should not be included in the alphabetic portion of her classification (Hare and White 1980). But, it was too late. Too many authorities and too many textbooks had applied the White letters to gestational diabetes. Practices had become ingrained, and thus would be slow to change, in spite of protestations by several authors (Schwartz and Brenner 1982; Leveno and Whalley 1982).

Yet, gestational diabetes does not lend itself to the definitions in the White classes. Hare and White (1980) emphasized that the early classes should be as follows:

Gestational diabetes mellitus
Class A – Pregestational diabetes treated with diet (and/or sulphonylureas)
Class B – Pregestational diabetes (of short duration) treated with insulin.

Yet, some authors persist in including gestational diabetes within class A, such that class A would include two major groups, gestational diabetes and pregestational diabetes treated without insulin. Others have used class A to denote gestational diabetes treated without insulin, class B1 to denote gestational diabetes treated with insulin and class B2 to denote pregestational diabetes of short duration. Another scheme has used class A to denote gestational diabetes treated without insulin, and variously either class AB, class B, "Gestational class B" or class Bg to denote gestational diabetes treated with insulin. Yet others have used class A1 for gestational diabetes with fasting plasma glucose less than 105 mg/dl (5.8 mmol/l), class A2 for gestational diabetes with fasting plasma glucose 105–130 mg/dl (5.8–7.2 mmol/l) and class B1 for gestational diabetes with fasting plasma glucose greater than 130 mg/dl (7.2 mmol/l). The array of classification schemes is bewildering, but does not pose much of a problem provided the definitions are stated explicitly in any given paper, and provided that in any tabulation one does not lump together women with gestational diabetes and women with pregestational diabetes. Such mixing distorts interpretation. Nevertheless, it would seem wise if we did not include gestational diabetes in the White classification, and rather divided gestational diabetes into subgroups based on either treatment used for fasting plasma glucose, if subclassification is used at all.

Interventions

Intervention in gestational diabetes remains an area without consensus. The area of diet and weight control is one. It is not clear whether pregnancy is a time where weight reduction or weight maintenance should be permitted, or whether all pregnant women, regardless of prepregnancy weight, should have some predetermined desired weight gain. Most authorities would not use oral hypoglycaemic agents during pregnancy, yet these have been used in a few centres without apparent adverse effects. When to initiate insulin therapy is an area of considerable controversy. The extremes range from prophylactic insulin therapy in all women with gestational diabetes, on the one hand, to withholding of insulin therapy unless the fasting plasma glucose exceeds 140 mg/dl (7.8 mmol/l), on the other hand. More work is needed to define more carefully the appropriate dietary recommendations for gestational diabetes, the glucose targets that should be sought in these women and the criteria for instituting insulin therapy.

Concluding Comments

The Aberdeen Colloquia have become seminal points for critical review and reassessment of investigations on carbohydrate metabolism in pregnancy and the newborn. The volumes that have chronicled these four colloquia stand as classical treatises on the state of the art each half decade. The Colloquia also have served as an important forum for investigators in this field to form friendships and interact in a close and meaningful way. To a great extent, the social atmosphere engendered in Aberdeen, and the hospitality that Colloquia participants have come to cherish, have been an important component of the success of these meetings. The credit for this goes to the organizers, who have continually put forth extra special effort to make everyone feel at home in Aberdeen. In particular, Hamish and Frances Sutherland have become the symbols of Scottish hospitality to those of us who attend these meetings. Of that, there is surely not consensus, but unanimity. Thus, we who have come to know them are immensely saddened by the tragic death of their 21-year-old son Stuart, who was working on the oil rig off the coast of Aberdeen at the time of its explosion just a few weeks after the Aberdeen Colloquium. Surely, such tragedies, about which we often read, touch the lives of many families throughout the world. Occasionally, as in this instance, they touch someone we know and love. The Sutherlands' loss reminds us yet again of the frailty of human life and of how dear life is. Such a loss reminds us too that in the healing professions, our mission is to save lives and improve life for all who seek our help.

To those of us who care for pregnant women with diabetes and their offspring, may this serve to cause us to rededicate our efforts. To Hamish and Frances Sutherland, goes our deepest sympathy. To the memory of Stuart Sutherland, this treatise is dedicated.

References

American Diabetes Association (1986) Gestational diabetes mellitus. Ann Intern Med 105:461

Buchanan TA, Schemmer JK, Freinkel N (1986) Embryotoxic effects of brief maternal insulin-hypoglycemia during organogenesis in the rat. J Clin Invest 78:643–649

Carpenter MW, Coustan DR (1982) Criteria for screening tests for gestational diabetes. Am J Obstet Gynecol 144:768–771

Coustan DR, Reece EA, Sherwin RS et al. (1986) A randomized clinical trial of the insulin pump vs intensive conventional therapy in diabetic pregnancies. J Am Med Ass 255:631–636

Dicker D, Feldberg D, Karp M et al. (1987) Preconceptional diabetes control in insulin-dependent diabetes mellitus patients with continuous subcutaneous insulin infusion therapy. J Perinat Med 15:161–167

Freinkel N (ed) (1985) Proceedings of the Second International Workshop-Conference on Gestational Diabetes Mellitus. Diabetes 34 (Suppl 2):1–130

Fuhrmann K, Reiher H, Semonier K et al. (1983) Prevention of congenital malformations in infants of insulin-dependent diabetic mothers. Diabetes Care 6:219–223

Fuhrmann K, Reiher H, Semmler K et al. (1984) The effect of intensified conventional insulin therapy before and during pregnancy on the malformation rate in offspring of diabetic mothers. Exp Clin Endocrinol 83:173–177

Goldman JA, Dicker D, Feldberg D et al. (1986) Pregnancy outcome in patients with insulin-dependent diabetes mellitus with preconceptional diabetic control: a comparative study. Am J Obstet Gynecol 155:293–297

Hare JW, White P (1980) Gestational diabetes and the White classification. Diabetes Care 3:394

Hare JW, Green MF, Cloherty JP et al. (1988) First trimester glycemic risk for major malformations and spontaneous abortions. Aberdeen Colloquium, Poster Abstracts, p 7

Jovanovic L, Peterson CM (1982) Optimal insulin delivery for the pregnant diabetic patient. Diabetes Care 5 (Suppl 1):24–37

Lancet (1988) Congenital abnormalities in infants of diabetic mothers. Lancet I:1313–1315

Landon MB, Gabbe SG, Piana R et al. (1987) Neonatal morbidity in pregnancy complicated by diabetes mellitus: predictive value of maternal glycemic profiles. Am J Obstet Gynecol 156:1089–1095

Langer O, Brustman L, Anyaegbunam A et al. (1987) The significance of one abnormal glucose tolerance test value on adverse outcome in pregnancy. Am J Obstet Gynecol 157:758–763

Leveno K, Whalley P (1982) Dilemmas in the management of pregnancy complicated by diabetes. Med Clin North Am 66:1325–1346

Lowy C, Beard RW, Goldschmidt JU (1983) The confidential United Kingdom enquiry into the outcome of babies of diabetic mothers (1979–1980). Diabetologia 25:177

Miller E, Hare JW, Cloherty et al. (1981) Elevated maternal hemoglobin A_{1c} in early pregnancy and major congenital anomalies in infants of diabetic mothers. N Engl J Med 304:1331–1334

Mills JL, Knopp RH, Simpson JL et al. (1988) Lack of relation of increased malformation rates in infants of diabetic mothers to glycemic control during organogenesis. N Engl J Med 318:671–676

National Diabetes Data Group (1979) Classification and diagnosis of diabetes mellitus and other categories of glucose intolerance. Diabetes 28:1039–1057

O'Sullivan JB, Mahan CM (1964) Criteria for the oral glucose tolerance test in pregnancy. Diabetes 13:278–285

Roversi GD, Gargiulo M, Nicolini U et al. (1980) Maximal tolerated insulin therapy in gestational diabetes. Diabetes Care 3:489–494

Schwartz M, Brenner W (1982) The need for adequate and consistent diagnostic classification for diabetes mellitus diagnosed during pregnancy. Am J Obstet Gynecol 143:119–124

Skyler JS (1984) Diabetes and pregnancy – the 1980s and beyond. In: Sutherland HW, Stowers JM (eds) Carbohydrate metabolism in pregnancy and the newborn. Churchill Livingstone, Edinburgh, pp 226–234

Skyler JS, O'Sullivan MJ, Holsinger KK (1980) The relationship between maternal glycemia and macrosomia. Diabetes Care 3:433–434

Steel JM (1985) Prepregnancy counselling and contraception in the insulin-dependent diabetic patient. Clin Obstet Gynecol 28:553–566

Tallarigo L, Giampietro O, Penno G et al. (1986) Relation of glucose tolerance to complications of pregnancy in non-diabetic women. N Engl J Med 315:989–992

Tamas G, Demeter J, Baranyi E et al. (1985) Use of NovoPen in pregnant diabetic women: first clinical experiences. Presented at the Third International Hvidore Symposium, May 28–29, Copenhagen, Denmark

White P (1949) Pregnancy complicating diabetes. Am J Med 7:609–616

World Health Organization (WHO) Expert Committee (1980) Diabetes mellitus technical report series 646. World Health Organization, Geneva.

World Health Organization (WHO) Study Group (1985) Diabetes mellitus technical report series 727. World Health Organization, Geneva

Ylinen K, Aula P, Stenman U-H et al. (1984) Risk of minor and major fetal malformations in diabetics with high haemoglobin A_{1c} values in early pregnancy. Br Med J 289:345–346

Subject Index